Perioperative Inflammation as Triggering Origin of Metastasis Development

Michael W. Retsky • Romano Demicheli
Editors

Perioperative Inflammation as Triggering Origin of Metastasis Development

Springer

Editors
Michael W. Retsky
Harvard TH Chan School of Public Health
Boston, MA, USA

University College London
London, UK

Romano Demicheli
Istituto Nazionale Tumori di Milano
Fondazione IRCCS
Milan, Italy

ISBN 978-3-319-57942-9 ISBN 978-3-319-57943-6 (eBook)
DOI 10.1007/978-3-319-57943-6

Library of Congress Control Number: 2017943514

Printed on acid-free paper

This Springer imprint is published by Springer Nature
The registered company is Springer International Publishing AG
The registered company address is: Gewerbestrasse 11, 6330 Cham, Switzerland

Foreword

The trajectory of modern cancer research has changed dramatically over the past four decades. The beginning of this time period can be demarcated with some precision—the publication by Varmus, Bishop and colleagues in 1976 that demonstrated that normal genes residing within our genome, proto-oncogenes, have the potential to be corrupted and become genetic agents that actively drive neoplastic cell growth, the oncogenes. This discovery led to a massive effort to document these genes during the following decades. By now, we are aware of more than 50 commonly occurring genes that can be documented, when in altered form, to function as oncogenes as well as an even larger cohort of genes that work in the opposite direction, the so-called tumour suppressor genes. Oncogenes become hyperactive in the genomes of cancer cells, whereas the growth-constraining actions of tumour suppressor genes are lost during tumour pathogenesis.

These discoveries led to a simple and powerful paradigm, specifically that the behaviour of cancer cells and the tumours that they form can be understood in terms of the mutant genes that they carry in their genomes. During the 1990s, however, diverse lines of research led to the realization that this paradigm represented a gross oversimplification, simply because cancer cells do not exist in a biological vacuum. Instead, as pathologists knew for a century, cancer cells reside in the complex tissues termed tumours, which, in addition to neoplastic cells, carry a variety of recruited host cells that together constitute the tumour-associated stroma. Indeed, the complex heterotypic signalling interactions between cancer cells and stromal cells led increasingly to the conclusion that the tumour stroma also represents a key determinant of tumour behaviour. Moreover, the variety of inflammatory cells recruited to the tumour stroma led to the simple conclusion that 'tumours are wounds that do not heal' and that the cellular and tissue programmes that enable the complex reconstruction of wounded tissues are co-opted by cancer cells—notably carcinoma cells—in order to progress to high-grade malignancies. As was learned in the first decade of the new century, signals released by recruited stromal cells can profoundly perturb the biological phenotypes of the cancer cells that previously recruited them.

Even this model soon required refinement, in that the perturbations of the systemic physiology of the host also required attention. Notably, cancer cells release systemic signals that enable them to perturb various components of the bone marrow, which in turn results in the mobilization into the circulation and subsequent recruitment of a variety of stromal cells that populate the 'reactive stroma' of an advanced tumour; such cells perturb the signalling environment of the nearby cancer cells that had previously recruited them into the tumour-associated stroma.

Even this depiction falls short of encompassing the full spectrum of complexity because of an additional facet of tumour/host interactions. Over the past decades, cancer biologists have repeatedly ignored the actions of the adaptive immune system in controlling tumour outgrowth. Many were persuaded that the immune system was tolerant to the presence of tumour-associated antigens and thereby ignored or overlooked tumour outgrowth. As we now realize, the absence of readily observable immune attack is often the result of multiple layers of defence that tumours mount to neutralize immune attack.

This immunological control of tumour outgrowth now begins to converge directly on the process that is the central theme of the current volume: how do disseminated tumour cells enter into dormancy, and how do the processes involved in treating primary tumours awaken them, resulting in life-threatening metastases? Why do disseminated tumour cells (DTCs) remain unapparent for days and months and then, either spontaneously or in response to certain perturbations, spawn rapidly growing metastases?

In the context of breast cancer pathogenesis, these questions are particularly acute. Perhaps one-third of breast cancer patients presenting in the oncology clinic carry myriad micrometastatic deposits of carcinoma cells in their marrow, and one-half of these women will eventually develop metastatic disease. Most interesting is the question of why the other half of women fail to do so. To be sure, the carcinoma cells in many micrometastatic deposits remain dormant and thus clinically inapparent because these cells, having arrived in the marrow (and in numerous other sites throughout the body), are poorly adapted to thrive in a tissue microenvironment that is foreign to them. After all, why should a mammary epithelial cell upon arrival in the marrow possess the traits that enable it to proliferate in such an unfamiliar and potentially inhospitable tissue microenvironment?

Yet another mechanism may explain the inability of the vast majority of DTCs to proliferate in sites of dissemination: the immune system may hold them in check. Such immune-imposed control may represent a centrally important mechanism that can be derailed by systemic perturbations, including those wrought by the wounding at distant sites associated with primary tumour resection and, perhaps more importantly, the postsurgical wound-healing response. Whilst the innate and adaptive arms of the immune system possess multiple mechanisms for recognizing and controlling the outgrowth of DTCs, their actions might be disrupted by countervailing mechanisms, specifically immunosuppressive mechanisms such as those exerted by regulatory T-cells (Tregs) and myeloid-derived suppressor cells (MDSCs).

When depicted this way, the outgrowth of DTCs may be the result of a finely tuned balance between immunological attack and the immunosuppressive actions that normally serve to hold immune attack in check. This balance may well be disrupted by the significant changes in bone marrow physiology that occur, usually transiently, in response to localized wound healing at various sites throughout the body. If demonstrated definitively, this leads to a notion that is likely to be accepted only reluctantly by many in the clinical oncology community: primary tumour resection does not provide an undiluted benefit to the breast cancer patient in terms of long-term survival, simply because postsurgical wound healing may upset the finely tuned physiologic balances that keep DTCs in check. Indeed, more extensive wounding and subsequent wound healing may result in an even greater likelihood of subsequent eruption of previously inapparent micrometastatic deposits. Various aspects of these fascinating interactions are described in this volume, which is likely to profoundly influence future surgical oncology and postsurgical treatment protocols.

Robert A. Weinberg
MIT Ludwig Center for Molecular Oncology
Whitehead Institute for Biomedical Research
Cambridge, MA, USA

Preface

The authors of the chapters in this book are from the UK, USA, Italy, Nigeria, Australia, USA by way of Russia and Israel, UK by way of India, Denmark, Germany, Greece, and Belgium. One would think our intention was to have a geographically diverse representation of authors so as to get a worldwide perspective similar to the United Nations. But that was purely an accident. We did want a diverse group of authors and perspectives, but the topic for diversity was scientific investigation not geographic location.

Let us explain. Our research has been by discovery rather than hypothesis. We were trying to understand the implications of anomalous clinical breast cancer data. We did not know where it was taking us, but we just followed our scientific instincts. With the aid of knowledge from various medical specialties, mathematical tools and other resources, we have gradually come to the conclusion that something dramatic happens at or about the time of primary surgery that precipitates most relapses in breast, lung and other cancers.

It also seems that this effect was known 2000 years ago but somehow got overlooked. Regardless of that, this topic must be considered a new field. Hopefully, this book will stimulate new thinking and the generation of new data.

We looked around. Who else is doing some work that may be related to what we have found about the perioperative window? It turned out that there are some. What scientific tools are used? All available tools! Actually, the diversity of tools and approaches attracted us since we promoted to the publisher that this book would be a jumping-off point for continued research as well as a reference for clinicians and scientists. We wanted to be inclusive with minimal overlap of research or clinical specialties. We have already crossed several medical boundaries so that is no longer a barrier.

There are a number of possible mechanisms that could account for this effect, but we do not know which are most involved or even if we know them all. We do know that systemic inflammation plays a key role and that this lasts for about 1 week after surgery. We think the metastatic initiation process is amplified by approximately 100-fold during the week post-surgery. Based on a retrospective study, a perioperative anti-inflammatory intervention properly timed to the surgery would probably prevent early relapses and that these would not come back later. We strongly recommend that this needs to be verified, and if it works as we think, it could reduce the world's breast cancer problem by 25–50% at almost no cost or toxicity. Some egos will be bruised, and pocketbooks will be lighter, but that should not prevent this investigation from being pursued.

Sub-Saharan Africa would be an ideal place to conduct a clinical trial because of the high incidence of triple negative breast cancer (TNBC) since that category should respond best to a perioperative NSAID. Breast and lung cancers have been the most investigated, and there are a number of other malignancies for which this should also work, but evidence has not as yet been fully examined. This type of therapy would be ideal for developing countries where there is 70% of the cancer burden but only 5% of the resources.

It needs to be stated that even if this project works as well as possible, it will not solve the cancer problem. It will dramatically and inexpensively reduce the number of patients who relapse, but there will still be a need for treatments to prevent death from metastatic disease. We are not in competition with the excellent work underway to use immunotherapy to curtail tumour growth after relapse.

Boston, MA, USA Michael W. Retsky
London, UK
Milan, Italy Romano Demicheli

Contents

Contributors

Yakubu Abdulrahaman Faculty of Medical Laboratory Science, Department of Haematology and Blood Transfusion Science, Usmanu Danfodiyo University, Sokoto, Nigeria

Department of Human Physiology, University of Benin, Benin, Nigeria

Department of Medical Laboratory Science, University of Benin, Benin, Nigeria

Emokpae Abiodun Department of Medical Laboratory Science, University of Benin, Benin, Nigeria

Teddy Charles Adias Department of Microbiology, Federal University Otuoke, Otuoke, Bayelsa State, Nigeria

Olutayo Ifedayo Ajayi Department of Human Physiology, University of Benin, Benin, Nigeria

Michael Baum University College London, London, UK

Marie Louise Bønnelykke-Behrndtz, M.D., Ph.D. Department of Plastic and Breast Surgery, Aarhus University Hospital, Aarhus, Denmark

Evangelos Briasoulis, M.D., Ph.D. Department of Haematology, University of Ioannina Medical School, Ioannina, Greece

Amos Dangana Department of Haematology, University of Abuja Teaching Hospital, Abuja, Nigeria

Marc De Kock, M.D., Ph.D. Anesthesiology, Centre Hospitalier de Wallonie Picarde (CHWAPI), Tournai, Belgium

Romano Demicheli Istituto Nazionale Tumori di Milano, Fondazione IRCCS, Milan, Italy

Bibiana Nonye Egenti Department of Community Medicine, College of Health Sciences, University of Abuja, Abuja, Nigeria

Osaro Erhabor Faculty of Medical Laboratory Science, Department of Haematology and Blood Transfusion Science, Usmanu Danfodiyo University, Sokoto, Nigeria

Department of Human Physiology, University of Benin, Benin, Nigeria

Department of Medical Laboratory Science, University of Benin, Benin, Nigeria

Tosan Erhabor Medical Laboratory Science Council of Nigeria, Abuja, Nigeria

Yi Feng MRC Centre for Inflammation Research, University of Edinburgh, Edinburgh, UK

Patrice Forget, M.D., Ph.D. Anesthesiology and Perioperative Medicine, Vrije Universiteit Brussel (VUB), Universitair Ziekenhuis Brussel (UZ Brussel), Brussels, Belgium

Christy Fredrick Department of Pathology, College of Health Sciences, University of Abuja, Abuja, Nigeria

Ekaterina I. Galanzha Winthrop P. Rockefeller Cancer Institute, Arkansas Nanomedicine Center, University of Arkansas for Medical Sciences (UAMS), Little Rock, AR, USA

Georgios K. Georgiou, M.D., M.Sc., Ph.D. Department of Surgery, University of Ioannina Medical School, Ioannina, Greece

Leonid Hanin Department of Mathematics and Statistics, Idaho State University, Pocatello, ID, USA

Jonathan Hiller, MBBS (Hons.), GCEpi, FANZCA Department of Anaesthesia, Perioperative and Pain Medicine, Peter MacCallum Cancer Centre, Melbourne, VIC, Australia

University of Melbourne, Parkville, VIC, Australia

Monash University, Clayton, VIC, Australia

Momodu Imoru Faculty of Medical Laboratory Science, Department of Haematology and Blood Transfusion Science, Usmanu Danfodiyo University, Sokoto, Nigeria

Department of Human Physiology, University of Benin, Benin, Nigeria

Department of Medical Laboratory Science, University of Benin, Benin, Nigeria

Ikechukwu Iwueke Department of Pathology, Federal Neuro Psychiatric Hospital Kware, Kware, Sokoto, Nigeria

Lori J. Department of Chemistry, Bingham University, Karu, Nigeria

Mazen A. Juratli Department of General and Visceral Surgery, Goethe-University Hospital of Frankfurt, Frankfurt am Main, Germany

Winthrop P. Rockefeller Cancer Institute, Arkansas Nanomedicine Center, University of Arkansas for Medical Sciences (UAMS), Little Rock, AR, USA

Paul Martin School of Biochemistry, University of Bristol, Bristol, UK

School of Physiology and Pharmacology, University of Bristol, Bristol, UK

School of Medicine, University of Cardiff, Cardiff, UK

Dmitry A. Nedosekin Winthrop P. Rockefeller Cancer Institute, Arkansas Nanomedicine Center, University of Arkansas for Medical Sciences (UAMS), Little Rock, AR, USA

Godswill Chikwendu Okara Dr. Hassan's Hospital and Diagnostic Centre, Abuja, Nigeria

Michael W. Retsky, PhD Harvard TH Chan School of Public Health, Boston, MA, USA

University College London, London, UK

Bernhard Riedel, MBChB, FCA, FANZCA, PhD Department of Anaesthesia, Perioperative and Pain Medicine, Peter MacCallum Cancer Centre, Melbourne, VIC, Australia

University of Melbourne, Parkville, VIC, Australia

Mustafa Sarimollaoglu Winthrop P. Rockefeller Cancer Institute, Arkansas Nanomedicine Center, University of Arkansas for Medical Sciences (UAMS), Little Rock, AR, USA

Robert Schier, M.D., Ph.D. Department of Anaesthesiology and Intensive Care Medicine, University Hospital of Cologne, Cologne, Germany

Henrik Schmidt, M.D., Dr.Med. Department of Oncology, Aarhus University Hospital, Aarhus, Denmark

Department of Clinical Medicine, Aarhus University, Aarhus, Denmark

Eric R. Siegel Winthrop P. Rockefeller Cancer Institute, Arkansas Nanomedicine Center, University of Arkansas for Medical Sciences (UAMS), Little Rock, AR, USA

Frank Udomah Faculty of Medical Laboratory Science, Department of Haematology and Blood Transfusion Science, Usmanu Danfodiyo University, Sokoto, Nigeria

Department of Human Physiology, University of Benin, Benin, Nigeria

Department of Medical Laboratory Science, University of Benin, Benin, Nigeria

Jayant S. Vaidya, MBBS, MS, DNB, FRCS, PhD Professor of Surgery and Oncology, Division of Surgery and Interventional Science, University College London, London, UK

Consultant Surgeon, Whittington Health, Royal Free Hospital and University College London Hospital, London, UK

Isaac Zama Faculty of Medical Laboratory Science, Department of Haematology and Blood Transfusion Science, Usmanu Danfodiyo University, Sokoto, Nigeria

Department of Human Physiology, University of Benin, Benin, Nigeria

Department of Medical Laboratory Science, University of Benin, Benin, Nigeria

Vladimir P. Zharov Winthrop P. Rockefeller Cancer Institute, Arkansas Nanomedicine Center, University of Arkansas for Medical Sciences (UAMS), Little Rock, AR, USA

Introduction

Chapter 1. We have been collaborating on a cancer research project that will be discussed in this book that can trace its origin to an event in 1993. Retsky was attending a cancer conference in Europe and happened to notice a poster in the hallway outside the lecture hall presented by Demicheli. The poster showed a bimodal relapse hazard for patients treated at Demicheli's institution in Milan. The patients (N = 1073) were treated with mastectomy after diagnosis of breast cancer and followed up for over 15 years. These data were intriguing in that there was apparently a wave of relapses in the first 3 years after surgery, then there was a period at 4 years with few relapses, and that was followed by a second wave of relapses that had a shallow peak at about 5–6 years after surgery and continued for 15 and more years.

Retsky had been doing research in breast cancer for about 10 years prior to this time, and Demicheli was on the staff of Milan National Cancer Institute as a clinical researcher for longer than that. Retsky had never seen data such as Demicheli was showing.

It is not incidental, but as we discovered later, both Retsky and Demicheli have PhDs in physics (Demicheli also has an MD). Among many other descriptions, physics is a way of thinking, and pursuing the implication of anomalous data plays a central role. To illustrate, the most important discoveries by the most highly regarded physicists in history can be traced to understanding the meaning of anomalous data.

For one example of the importance of anomalous data in scientific discovery, in the 1600s, Tycho Brache spent a number of years recording the position of the planets visible to him relative to the sun. Brache never got enough credit for what happened next, but Johannes Kepler obtained Brache's data and analysed it and to his surprise found the trajectories have distinct similarities that he reported as what are now known as Kepler's Laws. As one of these laws, Kepler found the planets orbited in an elliptical path with the sun as one of the two focal points. As another law, Kepler reported that the area swept by the planet's orbit per unit of time was constant. The third law was that the square of the period of the orbit was proportional to the cube of the semi-major axis of the ellipse. Isaac Newton considered these laws of Kepler based on the data from Brache and after inventing calculus derived the famous result that gravity holds the planets in their orbits with an inverse square dependence on separation and is proportional to the product of the masses of the sun and the specific planet.

As another example, in 1887, Michelson and Morley were measuring the velocity of light from different stars and found to some amazement that the velocity of light did not depend on the velocity of the star relative to the Earth. Albert Einstein considered that and ultimately derived the dramatic law of Special Relativity in 1905.

Not to place ourselves in the same category as Newton and Einstein, this serves to show the historic importance of pursuing anomalous data in the field of physics. Getting back to Demicheli's poster showing a bimodal relapse pattern, this was important anomalous data in breast cancer. Retsky and Demicheli spent the next two decades trying to interpret what the bimodal relapse data were telling us.

This bimodal pattern of hazard of relapse among early-stage breast cancer patients has now been identified in multiple databases from the USA, Europe and Asia. We are studying these data to determine if this can lead to new ideas on how to prevent relapse in breast cancer. Using computer simulation of this very high-quality database from Milan for patients treated with mastectomy only, we proposed that relapses within 3 years of surgery are stimulated somehow by the surgical procedure. Most relapses in breast cancer are in this early category. Retrospective data from a Brussels anaesthesiology group suggested a plausible mechanism. The use of ketorolac, a fairly common NSAID analgesic sometimes used before and after surgery, was associated with far superior disease-free survival in the first 5 years after surgery. The expected prominent early relapse events in months 9–18 are reduced fivefold in the Brussels data. Transient systemic inflammation accompanying surgery (identified by IL-6 in serum) could facilitate angiogenesis of dormant micrometastases, proliferation of dormant single cells and seeding of circulating cancer stem cells (perhaps in part released from the bone marrow) resulting in early relapse and could have been effectively blocked by the perioperative anti-inflammatory agent. If this observation holds up to further scrutiny, it could mean that the simple use of this safe, inexpensive and effective anti-inflammatory agent at surgery might eliminate early relapses. We suggest this would be most effective for triple negative breast cancer and would be especially valuable in low- and middle-income countries. Similar bimodal patterns have been identified in other cancers suggesting a general effect.

This will be discussed in detail in the following chapters, but the point we wish to make here is who best could we ask to discuss this? We have already invited Robert Weinberg who is perhaps the world's most renowned thought leader in cancer biology to write a foreword for this book. Who do we know in the clinical realm with the proper background to think in the manner needed to put this in perspective? The answer of course is our cancer researcher, medical historian, philosopher and breast surgeon colleague Michael Baum who has written extensively on this subject.

In Chap. 1, we present excerpts from Michael Baum's publications that have been strung together to provide a chronological narrative that relates to the topic that is the central theme to be discussed in this book. Some of the texts in this chapter are taken verbatim, and other texts are modified from references 43 and 48–50 in the chapter by Baum. In addition, at the end of his chapter, Baum has added some fresh insights that challenge the received wisdom of the somatic gene mutations as the driving force of oncogenesis and how indirectly it provides some insights into the nature of the anomalous observations that have provoked us to produce this book.

Chapter 2 is written by editor Retsky and coeditor Demicheli that we hope will adequately sum up our knowledge base on this subject.

Chapter 3 is written by Georgios K. Georgiou and Evangelos Briasoulis. We predicted that primary surgery would initiate angiogenesis so we were much interested in a study that dealt with this. Georgiou and Briasoulis looked ideal to write a chapter describing their project. They measured circulating angioactive factors in blood before and after surgery in women with breast cancer and in other women with non-malignant fibroadenoma. It is a small study, but they find intriguing results. We hope that this study motivates others to conduct larger studies since there is much to learn. We note with regret that the initiator of this project, Prof. Briasoulis, died recently from cancer of unknown primary.

Chapter 4 is by Jonathan Hiller, Robert Schier and Bernhard Riedel. The chapter by Hiller et al. discusses the perioperative window from the perspective of clinical anaesthesiology. This would be a good place to start reading on a major clinical component of this book. The authors present the science and practice of anaesthesiology in cancer surgery with emphasis on the teleological aspect. This fascinating viewpoint describes our ancestral hard-wired response to trauma, injury and infection and how this impacts the oncologic effect of surgical removal of malignancy. Note in particular the section on NET (neutrophil extracellular traps) that trap bacteria and parasites but quite interestingly circulating cancer cells. This seems to be one of several processes involving neutrophils reported in this book that could explain surgery-induced metastatic activity. We were quite taken by a comment in Hiller et al. (2013) in *Best Practices* that 'The perioperative period can be considered a 'perfect storm' of immunosuppression and inflammation in the presence of residual or circulating tumour cells'.

Chapter 5 is written by Mazen A. Juratli, Dmitry A. Nedosekin, Mustafa Sarimollaoglu, Eric R. Siegel, Ekaterina I. Galanzha and Vladimir P. Zharov. When we started this project, the original computer simulation used a time increment of 5 days. That is, the simulation updated tumour size and other malignant processes every 5 days. We thought that was reasonable given that breast cancer takes at least 10 years to run its course. But now, we think just after surgery things happen very rapidly. Thus, one of our criterions for these chapters was to include some research activity dealing with cancer development involving perhaps circulating tumour cells or initiation of capillary leakage with time scale of fractions of 1 day. The chapter by Juratli et al. fits that description. They describe some interesting technology that can measure circulating tumour-cell activity within minutes of a biopsy or surgical intervention. Their experiments are on mice, but we are told as of this writing that the authors are obtaining data from cancer patients. We look forward to their publications.

Their animal data show evidence of tumour cells injected into circulation from biopsy but do not show cells injected into circulation from tumour surgery. This is consistent with data from delayed reconstruction compared to reconstruction performed currently with mastectomy as reported by Dillekas and Demicheli et al. in a Norwegian study. The paper by Dillekas and Demicheli et al. is discussed in both the chapter by Retsky-Demicheli and the chapter by Vaidya. It is good to see a correlation between animal models and clinical data.

Chapter 6 Osaro Erhabor et al. This chapter is a dramatic and sobering document that should be required reading for any researcher who is planning or even thinking about conducting a clinical trial in Nigeria or sub-Saharan Africa. Retsky has been in Nigeria twice in the past few years and will be there again soon. Several things need to be discussed.

There is considerable redundancy in this chapter. For example, 'triple' appears 16 times. It was apparent to Retsky in editing that 4–6 individuals each wrote portions of this chapter that were more or less patched together to make the document. This is an advantage to us in that we get a number of independent scientific/medical viewpoints on breast cancer from clinicians and other professionals from various sections of western Nigeria. There are different opinions on what needs to be done, but every one of the authors reports triple negative breast cancer is the dominant type in their community and is a major therapeutic challenge. Presentation with locally advanced cancer is common, and it seems that women fear mastectomy and choose to avoid it for a variety of reasons.

They are requesting help from the West in solving the poor outcome for many women in Nigeria. That is extremely well justified in our opinion, and we would add that this could be an *opportunity* for the West to learn how to better treat TNBC. If we could learn how to treat TNBC in Nigeria, it would be a major help to treating all types of breast cancer in all countries in the world whether resources are limited or not. Based on Retsky's participation in cancer patient web-based groups, he does not want to mention names, but there are places in the world including the USA that are not too dissimilar to Nigeria.

In Nigeria, Retsky would frequently walk around alone and can personally verify that, as indicated in the chapter, there are shanty towns where street names and addresses are absent. As noted in the chapter, it will be difficult to follow up patients if you cannot locate their residence. Thus, some patients will be lost to follow up, and that needs to be considered in trial design. However, Nigeria has a diverse socio-economic population, and there are other areas where communities look identical to those in upper-scale USA.

Chapter 7 Hanin. This paper includes some mathematical equations and will scare away many readers. Hanin is originally from Russia, and as a general statement many Russians seem to love mathematics. Retsky has seen many older papers with extensive mathematical equations published by Russian authors that mention cancer in the title and in the first and last paragraph but nowhere else. The paper by Hanin uses mathematics, but the author actually uses it to analyze clinical data. He raises an interesting clinically relevant question. The reader may not need to understand details of the mathematics but should know enough to capture the author's intent and may cause him or her to think about this issue.

That leads to another reason why we include a mathematically oriented document here. Mathematics is considered the Queen of Sciences, but it seems to us that it too rarely appears in biological science papers. That is changing, and we hope this chapter will add more interest in the use of mathematics in clinical cancer research.

Chapter 8 Marie L. Bønnelykke-Behrndtz, Henrik Schmidt, Yi Feng, and Paul Martin. We wanted to include several chapters that deal with animal models and cancer. The chapter by Bønnelykke-Behrndtz et al. intrigued us since it used zebrafish models that are translucent and it also reported a new mechanism that might explain surgery-induced metastatic activity in a melanoma model. This mechanism involves neutrophils that are discussed again in the chapters by Forget and De Kock and by Hiller et al.

The mechanism seen in zebrafish is that preneoplastic cells attract neutrophils resulting from systemic inflammation. The preneoplastic cells then start dividing. This is an intriguing effect. This was one of the chapters we submitted to Prof Bob Weinberg to provoke his thoughts in writing the foreword. Bob Weinberg has been very helpful over the past years in this research. It has been extremely valuable to bounce these counterintuitive ideas off a world-renowned cancer biologist.

It is only at the talking stage, but there is interest in a possible paired clinical trial of perioperative NSAID for breast cancer in Denmark and in Nigeria. Both countries would have the same or nearly same protocol, and the trialists would meet occasionally. Denmark has the highest incidence of breast cancer in the world, and health care is provided by the government so it is easy to understand their particularly high interest in reducing the morbidity and mortality from that disease.

Chapter 9. Patrice Forget and Marc De Kock. That something happened at or around the time of surgery to provoke early relapses was strongly indicated, but up until 2010, we had only vague notions of mechanisms and much less in the way of ideas on how to prevent these from occurring. A paper by Patrice Forget and Mark De Kock in 2010 produced a revolutionary change in our thinking. This is described in the chapter by Retsky-Demicheli.

To present an interesting descriptive event, Patrice Forget came to Boston with his family during the summer of 2012 or 2013 for a month. Retsky arranged meetings and seminars with some Harvard and MIT groups. One meeting in particular occurred at MIT where Retsky and Forget each gave 20-min presentations on the breast cancer project to a small group of postdocs and students at the Broad Institute. The moderator of the meeting was postdoc Jordan Krall of Weinberg's lab who is now doing some experimental work in this field. Retsky gave his talk and Forget did likewise. Questions were then invited. One person sitting in the back row said, 'Breast cancer is a disease that runs its course in over 10 years. Are you telling us that most of the events leading to relapse years later occur in the first week after surgery?' That short comment captured the essence of our research! We never did get this person's name, but we have used that comment in one form or another in our papers since then. After the meeting, Retsky reported that episode by e-mail to his colleagues in distant cities and countries. Mike Baum wrote back that this was an example of 'the butterfly effect'. In case you do not know what that means, it refers to the comment that a butterfly might flap its wings in Mexico and cause a thunderstorm in Canada. It may indeed turn out to be scientifically possible, but on the surface, it is a preposterous connection. This book was almost titled 'Breast Cancer and the Butterfly Effect'.

It is a pleasure to introduce this chapter by Forget and De Kock. What are they working on now? They discuss the neutrophil to lymphocyte ratio (NLR) that shows relevance as a preoperative biomarker of systemic inflammation for breast, renal and lung cancers. They also report on short-term morbidity (septic and cardiovascular) and long-term mortality from cardiovascular disease (after lung cancer surgery and after hip fracture). Forget and De Kock suggest there is a need for new biomarkers and a need for a paradigm shift, and they have been right in the past.

Forget and De Kock also discuss postoperative peripheral neuropathy as a possible result of systemic inflammation. Permit Retsky to provide a patient's perspective on postoperative peripheral neuropathy. He is a long-term survivor of stage IIIc colon cancer and is a founder and director of the Colon Cancer Alliance. For several years, he participated in web-based discussion groups for colon and breast cancer patients. Among fellow cancer patients, they would candidly discuss intimate details of their disease and treatment. (Retsky recommends that lab-based cancer researchers join a patient website—as a lurker—with permission of the site 'owner'. They will learn much about clinical cancer.)

Richard Farrell was also a patient and founder of the Colon Cancer Alliance. Richard who ultimately died from metastatic colon cancer was very open with his cancer experience especially after he relapsed with hepatic metastases. The situation is better now, but 20 years ago, hepatic relapse was almost always fatal. He lived in Pennsylvania and since retirement was a very active fisherman. He would catch and release—not wanting to kill fish for sport. Richard knew where his disease was heading, and to aid fellow patients, he would frequently discuss his situation openly so they could benefit from his experience. He would ominously begin his reports with 'The journey continues…'. At one point, he was operated upon by a well-regarded hepatic surgeon at Memorial Sloan Kettering Cancer Center. The patients would often discuss both good and bad skills of surgeons and staff in detail. So we all knew Richard was getting extremely competent treatment. (The point of this story will become apparent later.)

Richard's surgery was considered successful, and he lived another year before eventually dying from metastatic colon cancer. He reported on the patient website that treatment at MSKCC was first class, but he also noted that after recovery he had peripheral neuropathy. Retsky remembers speaking to Richard about that. They happened to meet on a train station waiting for a train to a meeting somewhere and had a chance to talk. Retsky was curious about the peripheral neuropathy. Richard was operated upon whilst lying flat on his back with arms spread out. The operation was 6 or 8 h long. The explanation given to him afterwards was that someone must have been leaning over the operating table and inadvertently cut off circulation to his hands for extended periods of time, and that caused the permanent nerve damage in his hands.

We need to emphasize that this was not a life and death situation. It was only a quality of life side effect. Richard could not button a shirt, tie his shoes or much less go fishing for the year he lived after the hepatic surgery. Retsky had never heard about peripheral neuropathy before, and this stuck in his mind. Why did this happen in both hands he wondered. He asked Richard if he could tell this story to others. Not surprisingly, Richard emphatically gave Retsky permission to do so.

In 2010, Retsky happened to see a paper from a group at Mayo Clinic on postoperative peripheral neuropathy (Staff et al., 2010) describing it as mainly inflammation driven. He wondered if this could explain what happened to Richard Farrell. He asked the question and passed the paper to Patrice Forget. Forget replied probably so but such an effect is quite variable from one case to another. This paper is discussed in the chapter by Forget and De Kock. During Retsky's review of the chapter by Vaidya, he also sent the paper by Staff et al. to him.

Retsky does not want to go into details here but suspects there is a connection among the chapters by Forget and De Kock, by Vaidya and Richard Farrell's perioperative neuropathy. The medical issue involved is mortality from cardiac disease soon or even years after surgery as the result of inflammation-driven postoperative neuropathy.

Chapter 10. As coeditor and equal partner in the breast cancer project, Demicheli dives deep into the cancer biology literature and reports that cancer in the undisturbed state shows some similarity to normal tissue and organs. It may be closer to normal than usually thought at least in that undisturbed state.

Chapter 11. Vaidya. The chapter by Jayant Vaidya starts far removed from the subject of this book. It considers two separate subjects: first, there is consideration of breast reconstruction after mastectomy, and second, there is consideration of intraoperative radiation instead of external beam radiation to prevent local relapses after lumpectomy. How each of these diverse subjects arrives at useful information regarding intervention-induced inflammation and early relapse is a remarkable story. As someone who considers himself quite skilled in extracting all the useful information possible from data, Retsky is impressed with the project described in this chapter.

In addition, as soon as it gets to be public knowledge, it will be an important clinical issue. Imagine that each year for the past few decades, it is possible that over a thousand people have died from previously unknown side effects of breast cancer treatment. Furthermore, this may be connected to the Richard Farrell peripheral neuropathy and likewise be simply testable and resolvable. Clinical trials in most cancers including breast do not include all-cause mortality, only breast cancer-specific mortality. From the lessons of this chapter, that may need to be reconsidered.

There is no need to say anymore. Read the chapter by Vaidya and experience scientific discovery and excitement at a very high level.

Chapter 1
The Natural History of Breast Cancer

Michael Baum

Abstract To study the "natural history" of breast cancer implies observing a large number of patients over a long period without any medical intervention. Clearly this has been considered unethical in the modern era yet without knowing the natural history of the untreated disease it becomes impossible to judge the impact of treatment. The modern era can be considered to start in the early 19th century with the innovations in anaesthesia and antisepsis that within a few decades allowed for the introduction of the Halsted radical mastectomy. Since then we have had to deduce the natural history of disease in retrospect. Along the way a better understanding of the nature and biology of cancer has emerged that contributed to the replacement of radical surgery with ultraconservative techniques together with the elaboration of adjuvant systemic therapies. This chapter charts the paradigm shifts in our conceptual understanding of breast cancer with their therapeutic consequences and concludes that the time is ripe for another paradigm shift and a new era of treatment that relies on chaos theory rather than an obsolete notion of linear dynamics to explain the "unpredictability" of the disease.

Keywords Breast cancer • Historical background • Natural history • Conceptual models • Influence of surgery • Biological revolution • Adjuvant systemic therapy • Wrong mathematics • A new model

1.1 Introduction

The expression "Natural History" has two meanings. Historically it has come to mean the systematic study of all natural objects, hence the famous collection of dinosaur skeletons, trilobite fossils and Darwin's specimens from the Galapagos Islands in the Natural History Museum in London.

Another meaning to this expression used as a medical term, is the behaviour of a disease in the absence of treatment or in other words *left to nature.*

M. Baum (✉)
University College London, London, UK
e-mail: baum.michael3@gmail.com

M.W. Retsky, R. Demicheli (eds.), *Perioperative Inflammation as Triggering Origin of Metastasis Development*, DOI 10.1007/978-3-319-57943-6_1

In the modern world we accept the concept that many minor ailments are self limiting but with more serious conditions that are life threatening or could lead to chronic dysfunction we treat in order to influence this natural history in a favourable direction and rely on the history books to tell us what would have happened in the absence of treatment but with careful observation alone. Unfortunately in the days before active treatment of serious disease, careful and systematic observation were also exceptional. And this applies in particular to carcinoma of the breast.

Another relevant issue here is that we don't always see in a dispassionate way the objective reality of that which we observe but more likely a distortion, refracted through the prism of our personal prejudices. Observations that reinforce our prejudices are embraced and those that challenge our beliefs are ignored or rationalized away.

But why should we have a prior set of beliefs so powerful as to impair our observation of something so fundamental as the natural history of a life threatening disease? The simple answer to that is "human nature".

Part of our success in evolution from the lower primates is the capacity to make order out of the myriad daily observations of our busy lives. We constantly but subconsciously create hypotheses or models of objective reality- some are silly, most have a survival advantage and some in the fullness of time are found to have misled us all along.

However in this chapter I wish to concentrate on the natural history of breast cancer and the evolution of "conceptual models" to explain its behaviour. I propose that all this is fundamental to improving the lot of our suffering patients for the simple reason that our treatments are the therapeutic consequence of our belief in the underlying mechanisms of disease. In other words belief systems and treatment modalities are two sides of the same coin.

1.2 The Nature of Models and Models of Nature

A model car we understand but a model of nature, what can that mean? Let me explain. Models are not just mechanical miniatures of the real thing; they can be anything else which helps to capture the very essence of the subject of our scrutiny. They can be metaphysical, mechanistic or mathematical and you can also include biological models of organic objects for good measure. The rose bush I see from my study window and in particular one rose of an enchanting hue like the blush on the cheeks of Raphael's Madonna. *"What's in a name? That which we call a rose by any other name would smell as sweet"*, is a Shakespearian metaphysical model of this organic object. Easier to handle is the mechanistic model in a children's primary school botany book. Here the rose is built up of petals, sepals, stamens, filament, anther and carpel all connected to a stalk with leaves, thorns and roots. It loses its poetry when broken down this way. Even more so when the reductionists do their worst and the rose is described as a molecular model. Curiously enough much of the beauty and mystery of the rose reappears in its mathematical model. The new mathematics of Fibonacci numbers, fractals and

Lindenmayer systems allow us to generate beautiful floribunda on our computer screens thus linking the mathematical model of the rose to the greater symmetries and complex patterns of all of God's creation [1]. I will return to this conceptual model towards the end of this chapter.

1.2.1 The Natural History of a Rose

The rose has a complex natural history. Left to nature it will enjoy an annual cycle of renewal, flowering every summer, resting every winter and springing into bud each spring. In addition, left to nature it grows into angry knots; it develops suckers with seven leaves instead of five on each stem, which grow to prodigious lengths. Then holes appear in the leaves, brown patches of rust add to their disfigurement and green flies infest and destroy the buds. In the bad old days you could accuse your neighbour of witchcraft for blighting your bushes (a metaphysical model of disease) but in this modern era I know that the "rust" is a fungus (*Puccinia basdiomycetes*) and the holes are thanks to the caterpillars. I can influence this natural history with the aid of scientific horticulture, by pruning in February, putting phosphates down in March and spraying with inorganic chemicals all summer. This way their expectation of life can be 40–50 years with blooms as big as cabbages.

1.2.2 Breast Cancer

After that long preamble, the relevance of which will become immediately clear, I wish to return to the natural history of breast cancer. If left untreated what would happen and of equal importance, why?

In the Louvre, Paris hangs a large and beguiling masterpiece by Rembrandt, "Bathsheba at her toilet" (Fig. 1.1). Completed in 1655, the painting shows a naked Bathsheba looking wistfully into the middle distance left, whilst holding a letter in her right hand. Her attendant bathes her feet in a pool and the background is dark and ambiguous. Perhaps she has just learnt of her husband's death in battle as a result of King David's treachery, leaving her free to join the long list of the royal concubines. The model for Bathsheba in this painting shows the classical stigmata of cancer in the upper outer quadrant of her left breast. A description of this observation first appeared in print in 1983 [2] since when Bathsheba has become an icon of the breast cancer movement. In short the model was Hendrejke Stoffles who doubled up as mistress and housekeeper for Rembrandt. She was in her thirties when the picture was completed and died 8 years later. Her mode of dying was characteristic of breast cancer with secondaries to the liver. There is no record of her being treated, but in any case treatment in those days was a futile hocus-pocus based on the metaphysical doctrines of Aristotle and Galen, yet she lived 8 years after the clinically obvious disease, unknowingly portrayed in the painting, became apparent.

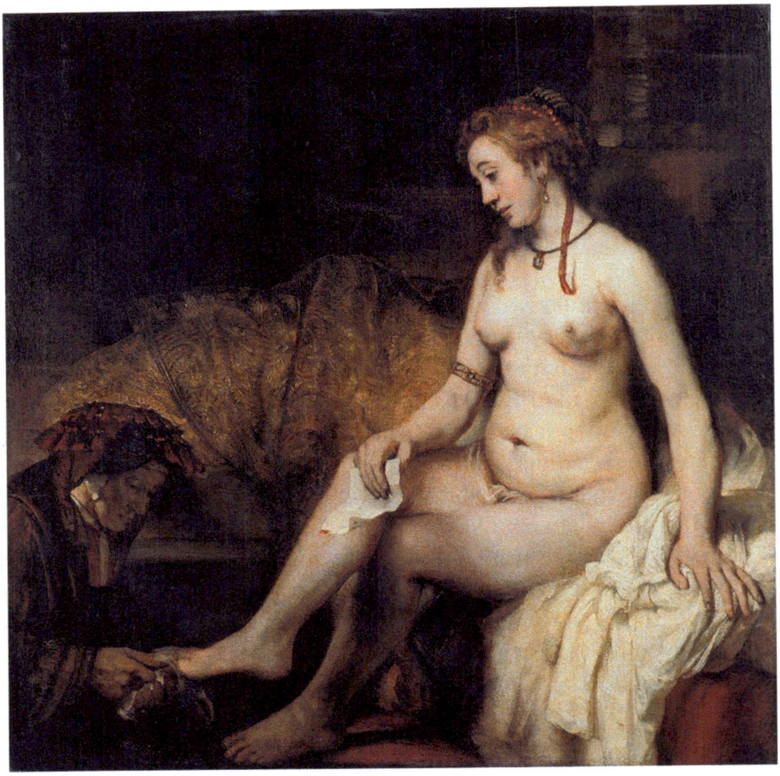

Fig. 1.1 "Bathsheba at her toilet", Rembrandt van Rijn, 1654

1.2.3 Breast Cancer in the Nineteenth Century and Early Twentieth Century

In 1970 whilst working with Dr. Bernard Fisher in Pittsburgh, I visited the library of the NIH in Bethesda with the object of completing an historical review for my thesis. Whilst searching for one reference a more important one literally fell in my lap. This happened to be a treatise on breast cancer by Dr. Gross of Philadelphia published in 1880 (Fig. 1.2) [3]. Gross' treatise provides a clear insight into the status of the disease in the era immediately before the developments in anaesthesia and antisepsis which allowed surgeons to attempt a radical cure of breast cancer. He describes a series of 616 cases, 70% of who had skin infiltration on presentation that had ulcerated through in 25% of the patients. 64% had extensive involvement of axillary nodes and 27% had obvious supra-clavicular nodal involvement. Accepting that the meagre benefits of surgery seldom outweighed the risks in those days, he judged it ethical to follow the natural course of 97 cases that received nothing other than" constitutional support".

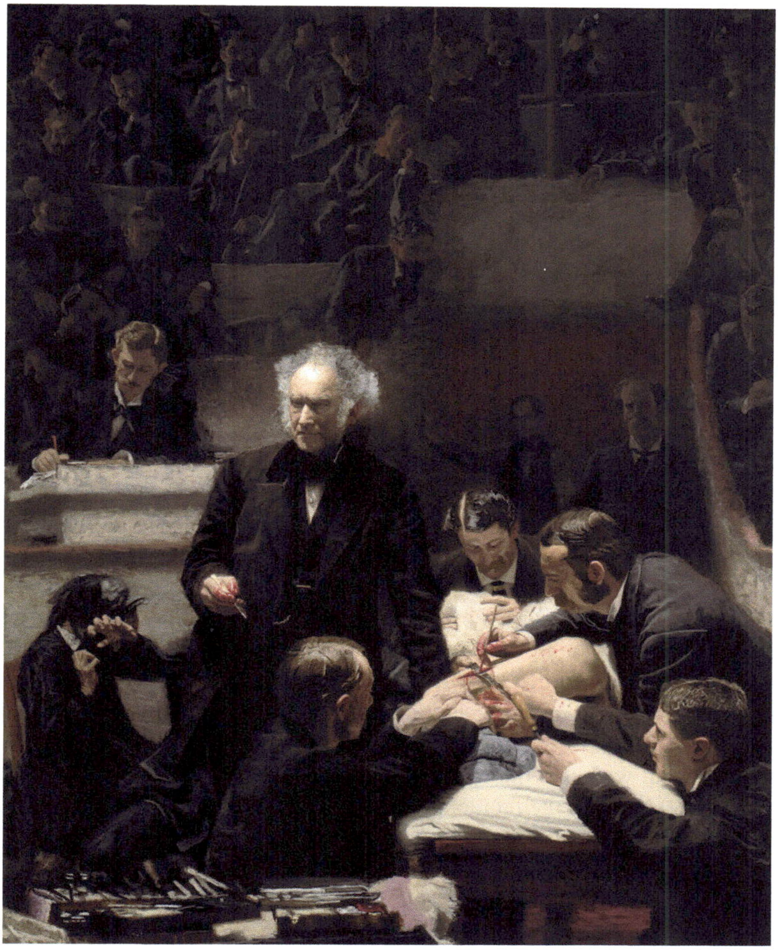

Fig. 1.2 "The Gross clinic", Thomas Eakins, 1875

He describes how skin infiltration appeared an average 14 months after a tumour is first detected, ulceration appears on average 6 months after that, fixation to the chest wall after a further 2 months and invasion of the other breast if the patient lived on average 32 months after the lump first appeared. The average time for the appearance of enlarged axillary nodes was 15 months in those few cases that presented with an "empty" axilla to start with. 25% of all these untreated cases exhibited obvious distant metastases within a year and another 25% after 3 years with only 5% surviving more than 5 years.

Since then a number of different series of untreated breast cancer have been reported. For example Greenwood in 1926 [4] described a 6 year follow up of 651 cases of untreated breast cancer with only 60 remaining alive at the end of this period. Daland in 1927[5] reported a series of 100 patients who were considered inoperable, unfit for surgery or who had refused the offer of surgery. The average duration of life was 40 months for the whole group, 43 months for those deemed operable at diagnosis and 29 months for those deemed inoperable.

The study that has attracted the most attention over the years was that of Julian Bloom published in 1968 [6]. His data came from the records of 250 women dying of breast cancer in the Middlesex Hospital Cancer ward between 1905 and 1933. Of this group 95% died of breast cancer but it should be noted that almost all of them presented with locally advanced or overt metastatic disease. The survival rates from the *alleged* onset of symptoms were 18% at 5 years and 0.8% at 15 years with a mean survival of about two and a half years. The reasons for withholding treatment are also worthy of note: old age or infirmity 35%, disease too advanced 30%, treatment refused 20% and early death the remainder.

Although of historical interest I can't really believe that these studies help to provide a baseline against which to judge the curative effect of modern treatment. Firstly, as with all retrospective uncontrolled series there has to be an element of selection. Why was treatment withheld? It is quite obvious that in the majority of these cases, with the exception of those refusing treatment, they all had an exceptionally poor prognosis to begin with. Secondly, they mostly represent women seeking medical attention at a time in the late nineteenth century or early twentieth century, when many women were content to co-exist with their lump in blissful ignorance until they died of old age or were knocked down by a Hansom cab!

Next the accuracy of the diagnosis might be called into question in the days before modern microscopy and the widespread adoption of the histological criteria of cancer.

Finally, for all we know the biological nature of the disease might have changed over the last 50 years as the incidence has increased following the major upheavals of demographic change and the widespread adoption of the oral contraceptive and HRT [7].

It would of course be inconceivable to suggest we study an untreated group today and the closest approximation we can find comes from a report of the Ontario cancer clinics between 1938 and 1956, just preceding the jump in breast cancer incidence in the developed world [8]. Close on 10,000 cases were analyzed accounting for 40% of all new cases arising in the province of Ontario during this period. Amongst this group were 145 well-documented cases who received no treatment of any kind. Although, yet again 100 of these cases were untreated because of late stage of presentation or poor general condition, the rest were unable or unwilling to attend for treatment. A careful note was made of the date the patient first became aware of the lump from which point survival rates were computed. The 5 year survival from first recorded symptom was 35% with a median survival of 47 months. The most surprising figure was a near 70% 5 year survival for the small group presenting with localized disease!

This then raises the inevitable question, is carcinoma of the breast inevitably a fatal disease if neglected? This question is almost impossible to answer with confidence although hinted at by anecdotal evidence. I have experience of four well-documented cases refusing treatment for 7, 10, 13 and 16 years respectively. One eventually died of stomach cancer with a still localized cancer within the breast weighing an estimated 2 kg. However, the best documented in the literature was reported by Steckler and Martin in 1973 [9]. They described a 38-year-old woman with histologically proven cancer who refused surgery and was then followed up for 20 years before consenting. We will never know how many of the cases we see in our daily practice carry such a favourable natural history.

1.2.4 The Influence of Surgery on the Natural History of Breast Cancer

From the popularization of the classical radical mastectomy at the very end of the nineteenth century [10] until about 1975 almost all patients with breast cancer, of a technically operable stage were treated with modifications of the radical mastectomy. To those without commitment to a prior hypothesis, this allowed for new insights about the nature of the malignant process. Before considering this matter it's worth revisiting the conceptual model that allowed the radical operation to reign supreme for 75 years.

Until the discovery of the microscope and the eventual correlation between cancer and its microscopic appearance in the late eighteenth and early nineteenth century, breast cancer was ascribed to an imbalance of the metaphysical "natural humours" first proposed by Aristotle in fifth century BC Athens and then elaborated upon by Galen in the Greco- Roman period of the second century AD [11]. It was asserted that the disease was an accumulation of black bile, "melancholia", in the breast. Support for this view was the fact that women with breast cancer were "melancholic" (one must question the direction of causality here) and that the disease was higher in frequency after the cessation of the menses which allowed "black bile" to accumulate. The therapeutic consequences of this belief involved bizarre diets, cupping, venesection and purgation with exotic enemas (some of these excesses are still practiced by the lunatic fringe of the alternative brigade).

In about 1840, Virchow described a revolutionary model of the disease building on the development of microscopy and post-mortem examinations of the cadavers of breast cancer victims [12]. He suggested that the disease started as a single focus within the breast, expanding with time and then migrating along lymphatic channels to the lymph glands in the axilla. These glands were said to act as a first line of defence filtering out the cancer cells. Once these filters became saturated the glands themselves acted as a nidus for tertiary spread to a second and then third line of defence like the curtain walls around a medieval citadel. Ultimately when all defences were exhausted the disease spread along tissue planes to the skeleton and vital organs.

The therapeutic consequences of this belief had to await the development of anaesthesia and antisepsis in the 1880s but were seized upon by Halsted in about 1895 with his complete experience being described in 1932 [13]. Armed with these insights, it seemed inevitable that patients would be cured by radical operations that cut away all of the breast, the overlying skin, the underlying muscles and as many lymph node groups compatible with survival.

So convincing were these arguments and so charismatic their chief proponent, the Halsted operation was adopted as default therapy all round the world.

At this perspective we are entitled to ask to what extent did the radical operation add to the curability of the disease and what can we learn about the nature of the beast by its behaviour following such mutilating surgery? We can also add a third question concerning human nature and our unwillingness to see facts "which almost slap us in the face" [14].

William Halsted operated at a time when the triumph of mechanistic principles was at its peak. The common man had begun enjoying the fruits of the Industrial Revolution. Naturally, Halsted's 'complete operation' was based on straightforward concepts about the behaviour of cancer, more mechanistic than biological.

His surgical expertise was remarkable, and for the first time, breast cancer seemed curable with recurrence rates (6% local +14% regional) at 3 years of follow-up, very low compared to the other series at that time. Unfortunately, only 23% of patients treated by Halsted survived 10 years [13].

The natural response to this failure was even more radical surgery. Internal mammary lymph nodes that received about 25% of the lymphatic drainage of the breast were not removed in the 'complete operation' but included in the super radical operations that followed or in the fields of radiation after surgery.

Retrospective studies indicated that more radical operations improved survival [15]. However, in randomized trials that followed later, no benefit could be demonstrated [16, 17]. Thus even when the tumour seemed to have been completely 'removed with its roots', the patients still developed distant metastases and succumbed: 30% of node negative and 75% of node-positive patients eventually dying of the disease over 10 years when they were treated by radical surgery alone [18] and with no evidence of "cure" if patients were followed up for 25 years [19]. In this latter seminal study by Brinkley and Haybittle, a group of over 700 breast cancer patients, treated by radical surgery alone and followed up for 25 years, continued to demonstrate an excess mortality compared to an aged matched population.

1.2.5 The Biological Revolution of the Late Twentieth Century

Prompted by the failures of radical operations to cure patients of breast cancer, Fisher proposed a revolutionary hypothesis that rejected the mechanistic models of the past [20]. He postulated that cancer spreads via the blood stream even before its clinical detection, with the outcome determined by the biology of tumor–host interactions. Based on this concept of 'biological predeterminism', he predicted the following:

(A) The extent of local treatment would not affect survival; and (B) systemic treatment of even seemingly localized tumours would be beneficial and might even offer a chance of cure.

Several pioneers in the field set up randomized clinical trials to test these hypotheses culminating in a series of world overviews [21]. Although the "Fisherian" doctrine is now taken as 'proven', we must accept that the proof is more in principle rather than in cure. The benefits from systemic therapy are modest, with a relative risk reduction in breast cancer mortality of about 25% overall, which translates to about 8–10% in absolute terms. As regards the extent of local treatment, many randomized trials have tested less versus more surgery with or without adjuvant radiotherapy.

A recent world overview of these trials [22] concluded that more radical local treatment; surgery or adjuvant radiotherapy does not have any influence on the appearance of distant disease and overall survival with one caveat (*vide infra)*. This is in spite of the increase in local recurrence rates with less radical local treatment, i.e. although radical surgery or postoperative radiotherapy had a substantial effect on reducing local recurrence rates, it did not improve overall or distant disease-free survival.

All the above can be taken as powerful corroboration of Fisher's theory that metastases of any importance have already occurred *before* the clinical or radiological detection in about 90% of all breast cancers.

1.2.6 Phenomena that Challenge the Existing Models

1.2.6.1 Local Treatment

Even in the world overview there is one finding that was not completely in keeping with Fisher's doctrine of biological predeterminism. Radiotherapy does actually reduce the breast cancer-specific deaths by about 3%—only to be counterbalanced by the increased mortality from late cardiac complications in those patients with cancer in the left breast because of radiation damage to the heart. More recently, two randomized-controlled trials evaluated the value of postoperative radiotherapy after mastectomy for tumours with a poor prognosis. The radiotherapy techniques in these two studies minimized the dose to the heart. Not surprisingly, there was a reduction in local recurrence rates, but there was also an improvement in the overall 10-year survival rates—9% [23] and 10% [24]. The most likely explanation for this large difference in survival rates could be a statistical quirk. Let us assume that radiotherapy does impart a small survival benefit. When several trials are conducted, the different magnitudes of effects seen are expected to follow a normal distribution. A sufficiently large trial would be highly likely to detect this small difference, whereas a small trial will rarely yield a positive result because of type II error. The effect in a small trial will need to be larger than the real effect (just by chance) for it to be detected at all, consequently small trials that are positive will usually be those which reveal a larger than real effect. Whatever the explanations for the magnitude of effect in these trials, it is clear that more extensive local treatment is not completely ineffective in improving survival. This could mean that local recurrence ***is*** a source of tertiary spread, although the metastases arising from the primary tumour at the point of diagnosis exert most of the prognostic influence or alternatively is merely a marker of a radio-resistant tumour with a poor prognosis; the local recurrence being an expression rather than a determinant of distant relapse.

1.2.7 Adjuvant Systemic Therapy Has Only a Modest Effect on Survival

The development of adjuvant systemic therapeutic regimens was based on the kinetics of tumour growth and its response to chemotherapy in animal models [25]. However, the early clinical trials predicted a large benefit and were consequently underpowered to detect the modest 'real' benefit. Consequently, there was considerable confusion, with the positive results of some of the early trials being contradicted by negative or equivocal results of others. The overview analysis, however, confirmed that adjuvant systemic therapy can in fact be beneficial [21]. It is the magnitude of benefit that is disappointingly modest—an absolute benefit of a maximum of 12% in high-risk premenopausal individuals and of 2% in equivalent-risk postmenopausal individuals is much smaller than anticipated from the experimental models.

The next step taken by medical oncologists was very similar in attitude to that taken by surgeons only a few decades ago, if a little doesn't work then try a lot!

This approach was bolstered by the excellent rate of long-term cure achieved in haematological malignancies. In addition, tumour cell lines showed a log–linear dose response when exposed to alkylating agents [26, 27].

Needless to say the high dose chemotherapy with bone marrow rescue was a failure and the least said about this sorry episode in the history of breast cancer the better, yet there may be lessons to learn from the failure of this approach.

1.2.8 When Does a Primary Tumour Seed Its Secondaries?

If we believe that once a primary tumour gains access to the vasculature it starts seeding metastases in a linear or exponential manner, it should be expected that because a larger tumour has been in the body for a longer time, and therefore has had access to the vasculature for longer than smaller tumours, a much higher percentage of patients with larger tumours should present with metastases. This is true to some extent with regard to lymphatic metastases, i.e. there is a correlation of number of involved lymph nodes with the size of the primary tumour. However, this relationship is far from linear. Thus there are small or even occult tumours that have several involved lymph nodes, while many large tumours are found not to have metastasized to the axilla. This discrepancy becomes even more apparent when we consider distant metastases. It would be expected that the proportion of patients presenting with distant metastases would be higher for those with larger tumours as opposed to those with smaller tumours. Nevertheless, in real life a patient presenting with a primary tumour along with distant metastases is uncommon, however large the tumour. In fact, the percentages of patients that present with symptomatic metastases is 0%, 3% and 7% in stages I, II and III of the primary tumour, respectively [28]. However, when you look at the incidence of metastases in these same groups 18 months after their primary diagnosis and therapy, there is a clear correlation of primary tumour size with the proportion of patients experiencing distant relapse. How can this be explained without challenging the linear model of breast cancer spread?

One explanation would be that although the number of metastases that are seeded by the primary tumour would be linearly related to the tumour size and biological aggressiveness, the *clinical* appearance of metastases is triggered *only* after the primary tumour has been disturbed or removed.

A modern theory that better explains tumour dormancy, would suggest that the micrometastases could remain *latent* for long periods of time with a potential to grow *or regress,* in response to some systemic trigger.

Judah Folkman [29] has demonstrated that the critical balance of factors stimulating and inhibiting angiogenesis are very important in maintaining the balance between proliferation and apoptosis. When this balance is disturbed, the metastases can either grow, or completely disappear according to whether the *microenvironment* favours proliferation or programmed cell death. One likely trigger for 'kick-starting' the growth of micro-metastases could be the act of surgery itself. After all in evolutionary terms an angiogenic response to trauma must facilitate healing in all sites of the body. Furthermore many tumours secrete anti-angiogenic factors that circulate in the body and inhibit angiogenesis in these latent metastases: an almost sinister evolutionary concept favouring the cancer—as if the primary tumour suppresses the outgrowth of micrometastases to keep its host alive!

Another way to examine this phenomenon is to consider the timing of recurrence and metastasis after primary therapy. This reveals a striking pattern that is usually expressed in terms of 'hazards'. Hazards are calculated by dividing the number of events in a particular time frame; say 6 months, by the number of patients at risk of having those events at the start of the period. In all clinical trials it is found that the hazards for metastasis rise sharply at 1–2 years after the primary diagnosis and then fall rising to a second peak at about 5–6 years [30]. It is extraordinary that this is true for any stage of the disease. The first peak occurs at the same time, whether the tumour was at stage I or stage III. It is only the amplitude of the peak that changes with stage, the later the stage the higher is the peak, but the timing of the signal remains the same.

These phenomena suggest a nonlinear dynamic model for breast cancer, which, like a chaotic system, is exquisitely sensitive to events around the time of diagnosis. It might even suggest that surgery could be responsible for accelerating the clinical appearance of metastatic disease. However, a randomized trial of surgery versus no surgery to prove this would no doubt be judged unethical in the absence of systemic therapy.

1.2.9 A new Model to Explain the Natural History of Breast Cancer

Taking all this into account I would like to develop a new model to explain the natural history of the disease which in addition to explaining the success of the Fisherian model of "biological predeterminism" also explains the clinical observations that fail to fit neatly into the contemporary paradigm.

First of all cancer should be seen as a process, not a morphological entity [31]. Individual cancers, while likely to originate from single cells, are constantly adapting to the local environment. There is no single substance or metabolic defect that is unique to cancer. Clonality, previously considered a hallmark of cancer, is neither always demonstrated in malignancy nor restricted to it [32]. The cancer cell is largely normal, both genetically and functionally.

The malignant properties are the result of a small number of genetic and/or environmental changes that have a profound effect on certain aspects of its behaviour. The three main processes of cancer, growth, invasion and metastasis, have their equivalents in normal tissues. Most cancers are diagnosed by virtue of their morphological or histological *similarity* to the tissue of origin. At the genetic level, with the exception of deletions, all necessary information is preserved, and the defective portion of DNA is small. The key processes of malignancy are genetically controlled by the under or over expression of normal genes and their products that normally serve essential cellular functions.

In addition, pathological and autopsy studies have suggested that most of the occult tumours in breast (and prostate cancers) may never reach clinical significance [33, 34].

Demicheli and colleagues [35] have also argued that a continuous growth model of breast cancer fails to explain the clinical data. The continuous growth model yielded tumour sizes too large to be missed at the preceding negative physical examinations, and required growth rates significantly lower than those consistent with clinical data. Furthermore the continuous growth model also fails to explain the biphasic recurrence pattern seen when hazards of recurrence are plotted for every year after diagnosis.

The new model is based on the concept of tumour dormancy/latency both in the preclinical phase within the breast and later with the micrometastases that seed in the early phase of the natural history of the disease, once the primary focus has developed its microvasculature. The latter remain dormant until some signal, perhaps the act of surgery or other adverse life event stimulates them into fast growth.

Groups of cells without angiogenic potential can grow but remain small (up to 10^5 or 10^6 cells). The metastatic focus may grow quickly if (i) a subset of these cell switches to an angiogenic phenotype and/or (ii) the inhibition of angiogenesis is removed. The model suggests that the metastatic development of unperturbed breast cancer is a sequential evolution from a non-angiogenic to an angiogenic state, with stochastic transitions from one state to the next.

This model may explain the early peak of hazard function for local and distant recurrences in resected cancer patients by combining with the *natural* metastatic development of unperturbed disease ("the Fisher effect") with the angiogenic signal following surgery ("the Folkman effect"). It also correlates well with the finding of a modest benefit after adjuvant systemic chemotherapy.

We can now add a new mathematical model to the biological model described above [36]. Breast cancer is like a complex organism existing in a state of dynamic equilibrium within the host, the equilibrium being very precarious and close to a chaotic boundary. Furthermore, the mathematics to describe the natural history of these "organisms" invokes nonlinear dynamics or chaos theory. This model is the first attempt to apply the new mathematics of complexity to make predictions about the factors influencing the natural history of breast cancer that might one day provide a therapeutic window.

Central to the understanding of this model is the pioneering work of Folkman on tumour angiogenesis [37]. As we know, solid tumours cannot grow beyond 10^6 cells or about 1–2 mm in diameter in the absence of a blood supply [40]. The initial prevascular phase of growth is followed by a vascular phase in which tumour-induced angiogenesis is the rate-limiting step for further growth and provides malignant cells direct access to the circulation [38].

In addition to the importance of the microvasculature, we can also visualize these microscopic foci as existing in a 'soup' of cytokines, endocrine polypeptides and steroids, with cells interacting with each other and with the surrounding stroma, interpreting competing signals directing the cancer cells in the direction of proliferation or apoptosis.

Such complexity cannot be modelled by linear dynamics, or even a full understanding of the complete catalogue of genetic mutations at the cellular level, because the critical events of multiple cell-to-cell interactions require a thorough understanding of epigenetic phenomena.

With my mathematically literate colleagues I have tried to model this complex system [36]. Our model, like other 'chaotic systems', produces beautiful fractal-like images that can be shown to be exquisitely sensitive to initial conditions (e.g., different concentrations or different gradients of the three biological variables). The three-dimensional vasculature of a tumour as simulated by these formulae is very similar to the vasculature of a breast tumour visualized using three-dimensional computerized tomography (CT) reconstruction [39].

There is ample scope for the addition of further complexity to the model, by incorporating more variables. The therapeutic consequences of the new models are almost self-evident. The intervention that suggests itself would be anti-angiogenic, and the timing of the intervention would be preoperative, so that at the time of surgery the system is primed to protect against sudden flooding with angiogenic signals. Indeed, some of the success attributed to adjuvant tamoxifen or chemotherapy might be a result of their anti-angiogenic potential rather than cytostatic/cytocidal effects [40, 41].

Assuming we can protect the subject from the first peak of metastatic outgrowth, we will then have to monitor her with extreme vigilance. By the time the metastases are clinically apparent it is perhaps too late, therefore monitoring the patient with tumour markers and reintroducing an anti-angiogenic strategy at the first rise in tumour markers might prove successful [42].

1.2.10 The Nature of Beauty and the Beauty of Nature

I wish to conclude this chapter by returning to my botanical model that I described at the start, but instead of celebrating the beauty of a rose I want to turn my attention to the weeping willow tree that recently was the inspiration for an essay I published in the New England Journal of Medicine [43]. If you look at the weeping willow tree in my front yard and measure its branches and feathery hanging leaf clusters by extending your arm, holding up a pencil, and squinting one eye, you will find that the ratio between the lengths of proximal and distal branches at each bifurcation is the same as that of the length of the trunk to the length of the first branches—approximately 1.62. That ratio also holds for second-, third-, and fourth-order branches. If you look closely, you can see that even the terminal leaf complexes repeat this beautiful symmetry. This repetition of this "golden ratio" is known as fractal geometry. It is but a small leap of imagination from botanical beauty to the idealized beauty of the human body. But what interests me more than surface beauty is the aesthetics of the internal anatomy of the human body both in sickness and in health. The obvious place to start is the aptly named bronchial tree, where once again we see perfect fractal geometry and golden ratios. The same applies to the vascular trees supplying most of the organs and the collecting systems of excretory or secretory glands. So what happens to this ubiquitous symmetry in disease?

Broccoli offers an almost perfect representation of the mammary ducts and glands at the time of lactation. The main difference, of course, is that the branches of the mammary gland are tubular. Imagine a tree-like tubular structure and then imagine taking transverse or random oblique cut sections and magnifying them. If the structure is perfectly symmetrical and the cuts are perfectly horizontal, you will see a plane scattered with symmetrically positioned circular structures. Of course, in real life the organs are not perfectly symmetrical and the pathologist's cut is not perfectly horizontal to the central tubes of the system. In fact, when you examine the breast carefully, you will find as many as 12 ducts opening at the nipple. Each of these is the mouth of a tree-like system for gathering milk at lactation from the glandular elements at the terminal ends of the system that look a little like the florets on the surface of broccoli. You can now picture what normal breast tissue looks like under the microscope—it appears as a collection of circles of varying diameter or as ellipses where the tubule has been cut obliquely. You will also see clusters of tightly packed cells representing the glandular elements that secrete milk.

If you increase the magnification, you can see the detail of the individual tubular structures. In health they are quite banal—one layer of simple cuboidal duct epithelial cells surrounded by a single layer of spindle-shaped myoepithelial cells. If you increase the power of the simple light microscope to its highest magnification, you will start seeing something of the extraordinary internal organization of these simple-looking cells. The cell is enclosed by a membrane that looks like simplicity itself until you begin envisaging the comings and goings of molecules and the recognitions of chemical signals by specific receptors on the cell surface that alert the interior mechanisms to speed up or slow down. Beyond all that, and even beyond the highest magnification of the electron microscope, we can try to imagine what's going on at the molecular level. What is remarkable is the near-perfect fidelity of these complex structures, retained through thousands of divisions of their cellular units and the sharing out of the genome between the two daughter cells at each event.

Surgeons and pathologists often describe breast cancers under the microscope as "ugly-looking lesions." When they're invaded by this ugliness, the duct and lobular epithelium lose their fractal geometry. When we grade these cancers, the severity of the patient's prognosis is directly proportionate to the ugliness of what we see. Could it possibly be that one of the first steps in malignant transformation is a mutation in the genes that control fractal geometry and some universal law that controls our appreciation of beauty? In other words, external symmetry might be a surrogate marker for internal symmetry, which is no doubt determined by sequences on the human genome that control fractal geometry. Loss of fractal geometry is associated with malignant transformation, but what is the direction of causality? Is the ugliness the cause or consequence of the malignant change, or is one a necessary but insufficient trigger for the other?

Some 20 years ago, I saw one of the first performances of Tom Stoppard's "Arcadia" at the National Theatre in London. In the third scene, set in a Georgian country house in 1809, Thomasina, a very precocious 16-year-old, asks her tutor, "God's truth, Septimus, if there is an equation for a curve like a bell, there must be an equation for one like a bluebell, and if a bluebell, why not a rose? Do we believe nature is written in numbers?" Perhaps Thomasina would have gone on to discover chaos theory if only the computer had been invented. As the story unfolded, I experienced a *eureka* moment—it suddenly seemed clear to me the natural history of breast cancer is unpredictable because we've been using the wrong mathematics all this time.

As already described [38], our group simulated oncogeneisis in a computer model and demonstrated a vasculature that had lost its fractal geometry. This now provides my link between the botanical world and the natural history of breast cancer as a result of a remarkable coincidence.

In the front yard of my house are two ornamental trees. One is *Salix caprea pendula*, the weeping willow described above, but the other is *Salix matsudama tortuosa*, the corkscrew willow. The former has beautiful fractal geometry, whereas the latter is a complete mess and reminds me of the vascular system of a cancer as generated by the Chaplain–Andersen model [38]. Searching the botanic literature, I found an interesting article suggesting that the mutant corkscrew phenotype was related to a dominant allele at a single locus and that this mutation is associated with vascular cell collapse [44]. Since then, I've speculated that loss of fractal geometry of the blood supply to human tissues might be an early step in oncogenesis, and perhaps many of the mutations we see in cancers might be the results rather than the cause of this early phenomenon. It has already been suggested that hypoxia leads to inflammation, loss of cell polarity, instability of the genome, and uncontrolled cell proliferation [45].

After publishing my essay in the New England Journal of Medicine [43]. I got into correspondence with a group of neuro-anatomists in Melbourne and learnt that I was not the first to make this connection. It appears that the fractal geometry of the neural network in the brain is controlled by a putative "fractogene" that controls the branching of neurones through a process known as "recursive genomics". This process involves methylation of DNA in the cytoplasm via a series of iterative steps linking a sequence of alleles on the genome as an epigenetic phenomenon [46]. They postulate that a point mutation in this "fractogene" might be the first step that triggers the genesis of a glioblastoma [47].

If this should be the case then we might have a complete model of the natural history of breast cancer from initiation to death from metastases that is dependant on chaos theory - the mathematics of nature, beauty and senescence. Armed with this knowledge a completely fresh approach to the prevention and treatment of breast cancer opens up with the aim of restoring the beauty of the internal structure of the human mammary gland that is often appreciated for its external symmetry.

References

1. Stewart I (1998) Life's other secret: the new mathematics of the living world. Allen Lane the Penguin Press, London
2. Braithwaite PA, Shugg D (1983) Rembrandt's Bathsheba: the dark shadow of the left breast. Ann R Coll Surg 65:337–339
3. Gross SW (1880) A practical treatise of tumours of the mammary gland. D. Appelton & Co., New York
4. Greenwood M (1926) A report on the natural duration of cancer: reports on public health and medical subjects, No. 33 H.M.S.O, London
5. Daland EM (1927) Untreated carcinoma of the breast. Surg Gynaecol Obstet 44:264–271
6. Bloom HJG (1968) Survival of women with untreated breast cancer-past and present. In: Forrest APM, Kunkler PB (eds) Prognostic factors in breast cancer. E&S Livingston Ltd, Edinburgh
7. Quinn MJ, Martinez-Garcia C, Berrino F (1998) Variations in survival from breast cancer in Europe by age and country, 1978-89. EUROCARE working group. Eur J Cancer 34:2204–2211
8. MacKay EN, Sellers AH (1965) Breast cancer at the Ontario Cancer Clinics, 1938–56: A statistical review. Medical statistics branch, Ontario department of health
9. Steckler RM, Martin RG (1973) Prolonged survival in untreated breast cancer. Am J Surg 126:111–119
10. Halsted WS (1894) The results of operations for the cure of cancer of the breast performed at the Johns Hopkins Hospital from June 1889 to January 1894. Johns Hopkins Hosp Rep 4:297–350
11. DeMoulin D (1983) A short history of cancer. Martinus Nyhoff Publishers, Boston
12. Virchow R (1863–1873) Die Krankhaften Geschwulste, vol 1. Hirshwald Publishers, Berlin
13. Lewis D, WFJ R (1932) A study of results of operations for the cure of cancer of the breast. Ann Surg 95:336

14. Halsted WS (1924) The training of the surgeon. In: Halsted WS (ed) Surgical papers, vol 2. The Johns Hopkins Press, Baltimore
15. Urban J (1978) Management of operable breast cancer: the surgeon's view. Cancer 42:2066
16. Meier P, Ferguson DJ, Karrison T (1985) A controlled trial of extended radical mastectomy. Cancer 55:880–891
17. Lacour J, Le M, Caceres E, Koszarowski T, Veronesi U, Hill C (1983) Radical mastectomy versus radical mastectomy plus internal mammary dissection. Ten year results of an international cooperative trial in breast cancer. Cancer 51:1941–1943
18. Brinkley D, Haybittle JL (1968) A 15 year follow up study of patients treated for carcinoma of the breast. Br J Radiol 41:215–221
19. Brinkley D, Haybittle JL (1975) The curability of breast cancer. Lancet 2:9–14
20. Fisher B (1980) Laboratory and clinical research in breast cancer: a personal adventure: the David a. Karnofsky memorial lecture. Cancer Res 40:3863–3874
21. Early Breast Cancer Trialists' Collaborative Group (1992) Systemic treatment of early breast cancer by hormonal, cytotoxic or immune therapy:133 randomized trials involving 31,000 recurrences and 24,000 deaths among 75,000 women. Lancet 339(1–15):71–85
22. Early Breast Cancer Trialists' Collaborative Group (1995) Effects of radiotherapy and surgery in early breast cancer. An overview of randomized trials. N Engl J Med 333:1444–1445
23. Overgaard M, Hansen PS, Overgaard J et al (1997) Postoperative radiotherapy in high-risk premenopausal women with breast cancer who receive adjuvant chemotherapy. Danish breast cancer cooperative group 82b trial. N Engl J Med 337:949–955
24. Ragaz J, Jackson SM, Le N et al (1997) Adjuvant radiotherapy and chemotherapy in node-positive premenopausal women with breast cancer. N Engl J Med 337:956–962
25. Skipper HE (1971) Kinetics of mammary tumor cell growth and implications for therapy. Cancer 28:1479–1499
26. Frei EIII, Teicher B, Holden SA, Cathart KNS, Wang Y (1988) Preclinical studies and clinical correlation of the effect of alkylating dose. Cancer Res 48:6417–6423
27. Frei EIII, Antman K, Teicher B, Eder P, Schnipper L (1989) Bone marrow autotransplantation for solid tumours—prospects. J Clin Oncol 7:515–526
28. Coleman RE, Rubens RD, Fogelman I (1988) Reappraisal of the baseline bone scan in breast cancer. J Nucl Med 29:1045–1049
29. Folkman J (1995) Angiogenesis in cancer, vascular, rheumatoid and other disease. Nat Med 1:27–31
30. Baum M, Badwe RA (1994) Does surgery influence the natural history of breast cancer? In: Wise H, Johnson HJ (eds) Breast cancer: controversies in management. Futura, Armonk, NY, pp 61–69
31. Schipper H, Turley EA, Baum M (1996) A new biological framework for cancer research. Lancet 348:1149–1151
32. Schipper H (1979) Historic milestones in cancer biology: a few that are important in cancer treatment. Semin Oncol 6:506–514
33. Baum M, Vaidya JS, Mittra I (1997) Multicentricity and recurrence of breast cancer. Lancet 349:208
34. Whitmore WFJ (1973) The natural history of prostate cancer. Cancer 32:1104–1112
35. Demicheli R, Retsky MW, Swartzendruber DE, Bonadonna G (1997) Proposal for a new model of breast cancer metastatic development. Ann Oncol 8:1075–1080
36. Baum M, Chaplain M, Anderson A, Douek M, Vaidya JS (1999) Does breast cancer exist in a state of chaos? Eur J Cancer 35:886–891
37. Folkman J (1971) Tumor angiogenesis: therapeutic implications. N Engl J Med 285:1182–1186
38. Folkman J, Watson K, Ingber D, Hanahan D (1989) Induction of angiogenesis during the transition from hyperplasia to neoplasia. Nature 339:58–61
39. Folkman J (1990) What is the evidence that tumors are angiogenesis dependent? [editorial]. J Natl Cancer Inst 82:4–6
40. Douek M, Davidson T, Hall-Craggs MA et al (1997) Contrast enhancement MRI and tumour angiogenesis in breast cancer. Br J Surg 84:1588

41. Haran E, Maretzek A, Goldberg I, Horowitz A, Degani H (1994) Tamoxifen enhances cell death in implanted MCF7 breast cancer by inhibiting endothelial growth. Cancer Res 54:5511–5514
42. Baum M, Benson JR (1996) Current and future roles of adjuvant endocrine therapy in management of early carcinoma of the breast. In: Senn HJ, Gelber RD, Goldhirsch A, Thurlimann B (eds) Recent results in cancer research—adjuvant therapy of breast cancer. Springer, Heidelberg, pp 215–226
43. Baum M (2015) Why does the weeping willow weep? Reconceptualizing oncogenesis in breast cancer. N Engl J Med 373(13):1267–1269
44. Lin J, Gunter LE, Harding SA et al (2007) Development of AFLP and RAPD markers linked to a locus associated with twisted growth in corkscrew willow (*Salix matsudana* 'Tortuosa'). Tree Physiol 27(11):1575–1583
45. Huang LE, Bindra RS, Glazer PM, Harris AL (2007) Hypoxia-induced genetic instability—a calculated mechanism underlying tumor progression. J Mol Med 85:139–148
46. Di Ieva A, Grizzi F, Jelinek H, Pellionisz AJ, Losa GA (2014) Fractals in the neurosciences, Part I: general principles and basic neurosciences. Neuroscientist 20(4):403–417
47. Di Ieva A, Esteban FJ, Grizzi F, Klonowski W, Martín-Landrove M (2015) Fractals in the neurosciences, Part II: clinical applications and future perspectives. Neuroscientist 21(1):30–43

Chapter 2
Perioperative Inflammation as Triggering Origin of Metastasis Development

Michael W. Retsky and Romano Demicheli

Abstract A multimodal pattern of hazard of relapse among early stage breast cancer patients has been identified in multiple databases from US, Europe and Asia. What began as a simple investigation of these anomalous data has taken the authors on a path through a diverse variety of clinical topics involving a number of medical specialties and now proposing a clinical trial in Nigeria. We have been studying these data to determine if this can lead to new ideas on how to prevent relapse in breast cancer. Using computer simulation and access to a very high quality database from Milan for patients treated with mastectomy, we proposed that relapses within 3 years of surgery are stimulated somehow by the surgical procedure. Most relapses in breast cancer are in this early category. Retrospective data from a Brussels anesthesiology group suggests a plausible mechanism. Use of ketorolac, a common NSAID analgesic used in surgery was associated with far superior disease-free survival in the first 5 years after surgery. The expected prominent early relapse events in months 9–18 are reduced fivefold. Transient systemic inflammation accompanying surgery (identified by IL-6 in serum) could facilitate angiogenesis of dormant micrometastases, proliferation of dormant single cells, and seeding of circulating cancer stem cells (perhaps in part released from bone marrow) resulting in early relapse and could have been effectively blocked by the perioperative anti-inflammatory agent. If this observation holds up to further scrutiny, it could mean that the simple use of this safe, inexpensive and effective anti-inflammatory agent at surgery might eliminate early relapses. We suggest this would be most effective for

---

Addressing the perioperative window in breast cancer; a 2000 year old unsolved problem in oncology.

Authors' note: Some figures and text are taken from our 2013 review [1] with kind permission from Bentham Science Publishers.

M.W. Retsky, PhD (✉)
Harvard TH Chan School of Public Health, Boston, MA, USA

University College London, London, UK
e-mail: michael.retsky@gmail.com

R. Demicheli
Istituto Nazionale Tumori di Milano, Fondazione IRCCS, Milan, Italy
e-mail: romano.demicheli@istitutotumori.mi.it

M.W. Retsky, R. Demicheli (eds.), *Perioperative Inflammation as Triggering Origin of Metastasis Development*, DOI 10.1007/978-3-319-57943-6_2

triple negative breast cancer and be especially valuable in low and middle income countries. Similar multimodal patterns have been identified in other cancers suggesting a general effect.

Keywords Breast cancer • Surgery • Inflammation • Bimodal relapse • Early relapse • Dormancy • Ketorolac • Triple negative breast cancer • High quality data • Computer simulation • Mammography • Racial disparity • Adjuvant chemotherapy • Nigeria

2.1 Introduction

The earliest known recorded description of breast cancer is from Imhotep in the Egyptian pyramid age of 3000–2500 BC. He wrote "*If thou examinest a man having tumors on his breast, (and) thou findest that swelling have spread over his breast*" and you place your hand upon his breast tumors and you find "*like touching a ball of wrappings, or they may be compared to the unripe hemat fruit, which is hard and cool to the touch*" they have no granulations; contain no fluid; give rise to no liquid discharge, "*thou shouldst say concerning him: One having tumors. An ailment against which I will fight.*" Imhotep describes an early differential diagnosis that rules out abscesses or inflammatory diseases. He further writes concerning treatment "There is no treatment." His comment regarding treatment remained accurate for many centuries. The earliest reports of successful treatment we could find are from Celsus (30 BC–38 AD) and Galen (131–203 AD) [2, 3].

Just as Imhotep described, the initial obvious presentation of breast cancer is usually a breast tumor. In modern times at least in developed countries, breast tumors are removed surgically. Surgeons are very good at removing the breast tumor and leaving no trace of cancer cells behind—at least in the breast. However that is not the end of the problem. The most serious sequential event is that it can return afterwards elsewhere in the body. This could happen any time in the next 15–20 years, yet with different time dependent probabilities. In breast cancer the common pathway from the original tumor to mortality from the disease is after metastatic relapse. Advances have been made but there is much room for improvement since 230,815 new cases of invasive breast cancer were diagnosed and 40,860 females died from breast cancer in the US in 2013 (latest data available from US Center for Disease Control) [4]. If a way could be found to prevent relapse from early stage cancer where the tumor is confined to the primary breast and resectable to late stage cancer where the tumor progresses to much less treatable sites such as liver, lung, bone, and brain, this would dramatically reduce the breast cancer problem. We are very impressed with recent exciting developments to treat metastatic cancer. However a far better solution in our opinion would be to prevent relapses rather than treat after they occur. We aim high in this project and intend to try to solve the problem upstream. Specifically, in this main chapter we will describe our studies that address the relapse problem that has been known for a very, very long time and we will propose a significant partial solution [1].

We have already mentioned in the Introduction and Baum chapter [5] how our investigation into this project began. In this main chapter, we will describe the research over the past 24 years that led us to narrowly studying what may be a simple, inexpensive and non-toxic method to reduce relapse and mortality by 25–50% in developed countries and perhaps more in developing countries. This therapy can be conducted anywhere in the world. In particular it can be done in low and middle income countries where they have 70% of the world's cancer burden and 5% of the resources [6].

We will make the case that this should be tested where the incidence of triple negative breast cancer (TNBC) is very high. That is where the benefit will appear best and where it is most needed.

2.2 Milan Data Showing Early Bimodal Relapse Pattern That Started This Investigation

Milan data are particularly well known for quality. Persons in Italy typically reside in the same towns and cities for generations so few are lost to follow-up and patients are known to be compliant with physician guidelines. The specific data from Milan that triggered this project were originally presented by Romano Demicheli. These data will be shown and discussed in detail but just as an overview, as shown in Table 2.1, there were 1173 patients treated well before the routine use of adjuvant chemotherapy and with long follow-up. There was a sharp peak in relapses at 18 months post surgery, a minimum at about 50 months and then a broad shallow peak with maximum at approximately 60 months and extending to 10 and more years. Once we knew what to look for, patterns very similar to this have now been identified in over 21 independent databases from Europe, US and Asia. There are more but we stopped counting at 21 [9].

Figure 2.1 shows Demicheli's Milan data for postmenopausal patients. The sharp peak is seen at 18 months, the minimum at approximately 50 months and broad shallow peak at about 60 months. That small bump at about 100 months is at present poorly understood due to the small number of events at that follow-up time.

Figure 2.2 shows equivalent data for the premenopausal patients. It can be seen that the 18 month peak now seems to have split into two peaks at 10 months and 30 months. There again is the minimum at 50 months and the shallow broad peak at

Table 2.1 Data presented in 1993 showing bimodal relapse patterns in breast cancer databases from Italy and UK [7, 8]

Milan data: 1173 early stage breast cancer patients with 16–20 year follow-up (mastectomy only)
Sharp peak in relapses at 18 months
Nadir at 50 months
Broad peak at 60–70 months with a long tail extending to 15–20 years
Now identified in 21 databases from US, Europe and Asia

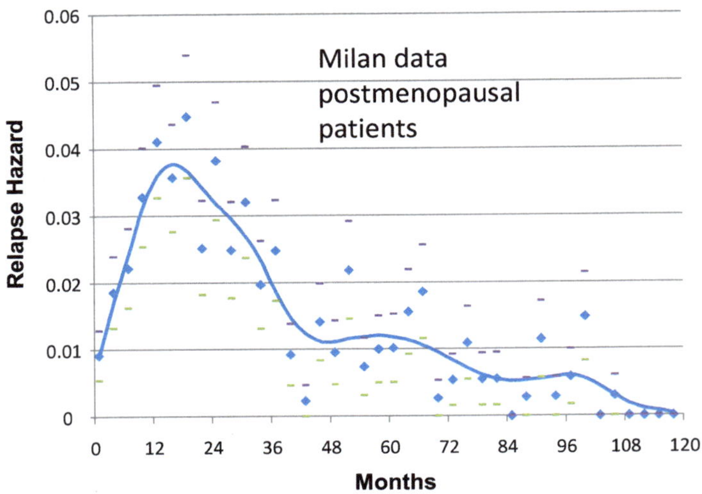

Fig. 2.1 Hazard of relapse for postmenopausal patients treated at *Istituto Nazionale Tumori* in Milan, Italy. Hazard is the number of events that occur in a time interval divided by the number of patients who enter that time as event free. Patients were treated by mastectomy well before the routine use of adjuvant therapy. The time interval in all hazard figures used here is 3 months. Average and standard deviations are indicated as *diamonds* and *bars*. The curve was obtained by a kernel-like smoothing procedure

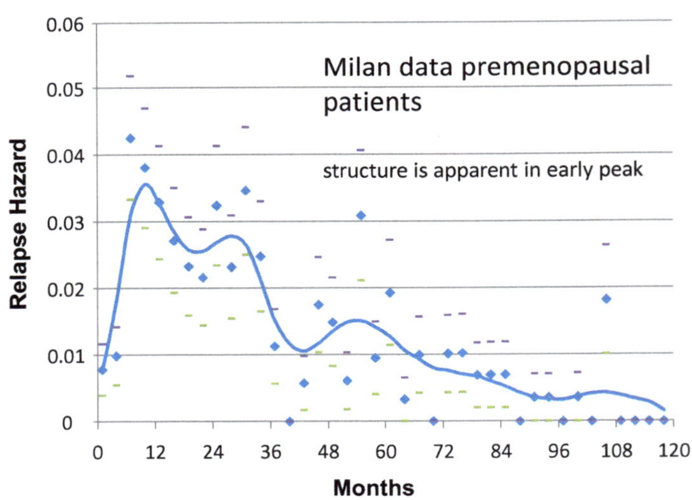

Fig. 2.2 Hazard of relapse for premenopausal patients treated at *Istituto Nazionale Tumori* in Milan, Italy. (Same as Fig. 2.1 except these are premenopausal patients)

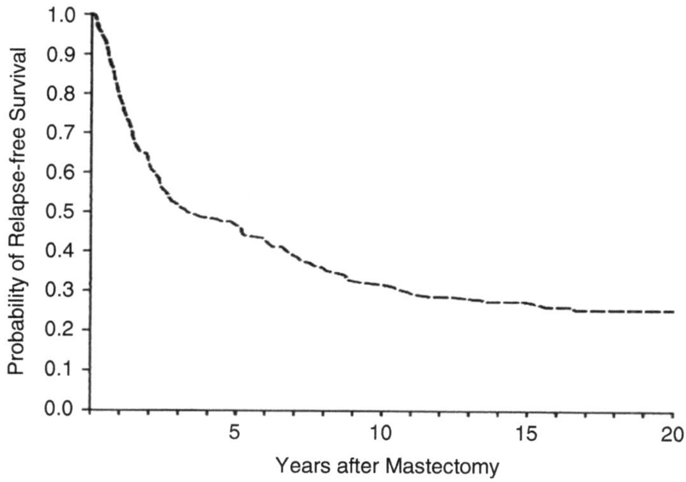

Fig. 2.3 Milan data for patients treated with mastectomy are presented in the more conventional format as disease free survival. The percentage disease free starts at 100% and rapidly drops until approximately 4 years where there seems to be a short plateau. Relapses start to happen again at about 5 years and slowly continue thereafter tapering off gradually at about 15 years. The plateau at 4 years corresponds to the end of the early relapses seen in Figs. 2.1 and 2.2. *Bonadonna, Valagussa et al. NEJM 1995*

60 or so months with a long tail extending to 10 years or more. It needs to be noted that the temporal resolution of these hazard data is 3 months while the more familiar disease-free survival presentation form is typically much longer. It should be emphasized that observing subtle structures of the recurrence dynamics needs large databases and accurate reporting of recurrence times.

Figure 2.3 shows these same Milan data but in the disease-free survival form. These data were previously published by Bonadonna et al. [10]. Bonadonna who unfortunately died in late 2015 was the clinician and the first person to use multiple drugs in adjuvant therapy to prevent relapse in breast cancer. Valagussa was the database manager since the study began. Retsky has had much good and bad experience with breast cancer databases [11]. He trust these Milan data and Pinuccia Valagussa is a major reason for that. As can be seen in this figure there is a rapid fall in disease-free survival in the first few years and then it seems to slow at 4 years before it abruptly begins to fall again extending to 10 and more years. That short plateau is not an artifact and corresponds to the minimum seen in Figs. 2.1 and 2.2.

Figure 2.4 is taken from Fisher et al. [12]. These data are also from the period before the routine use of adjuvant chemotherapy and thus consist of data from patients treated with mastectomy. Retsky was attending an American Society for Clinical Oncology (ASCO) conference after a period when he had been intensely studying the Milan data. Someone flashed this figure as part of a talk. Retsky could immediately identify the same bimodal relapse pattern. Let us explain. These Fisher et al. data are disease free survival grouped by nodes positive with zero nodes on the top and 12 and more nodes on the bottom. For the zero node population, surgery alone cures 80% of

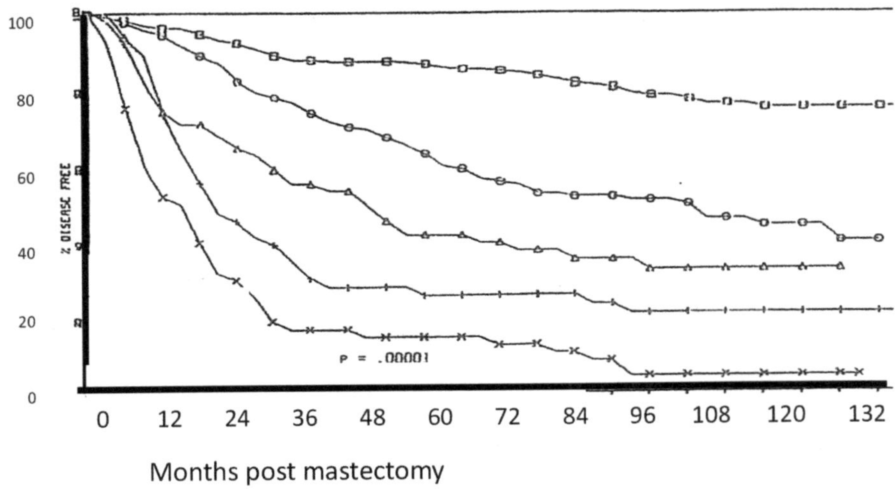

Fig. 2.4 Another well known and high-quality database is shown. Relapse-free survival for patients treated only with surgery. Grouped by nodal count. From top, nodes = 0, 1–3, 4–6, 7–12, >12. Bimodal pattern may be seen. *Fisher et al. Cancer 1984*

patients. Of the 20% who relapse, it can be seen that 10% are in the first 3 years and after a period with few if any relapses, the other 10% appear in the period after 50 or 60 months. For the 12 plus nodes population, it can be seen that essentially all patients eventually relapse. Of these, approximately 90% relapse in the first 3 years then there are few and afterwards the remainder relapse after 60 months. The timing of the relapses is equal from the zero node population to the 12 plus node population. It seems clear to us that similar early and late events are happening in the two groups but the early events are far more frequent for the 12 plus node group.

Something apparently happens to about 10% of the patients with zero nodes positive that results in relapse 1–3 years after surgery. For the patients with 12+ nodes, it seems that 90% of the patients undergo something identical. That apparently is the basic difference between the two populations of patients with widely different number of positive lymph nodes and prognosis. The magnitude of the early relapses is apparent in this figure. It seems that the label of poor prognosis is a result of the high number of early relapses and has far less to do with late relapses. This figure was published by Fisher et al. over 30 years ago but that it showed a bimodal relapse pattern was only known after we reported it as so a few years ago.

2.3 Multipeak Relapse Data Suggest Continuous Growth Is Not a Correct Description of Spontaneous Cancers

These multipeak relapse data are not consistent with the continuous Gompertzian or exponential growth model that has guided breast cancer therapy and early detection for many years [13–17]. The continuous growth model failed to explain growth dynamics of local recurrences after mastectomy suggesting the occurrence of tumor dormancy at clinical level [18]. These various peaks must indicate some clinically important and relevant biological activity but at the time we were unaware of what that was. Demicheli and Retsky began to collaborate.

Retsky visited the Milan National Cancer Institute in 1994. First, Pinuccia Valagussa put a computer disk containing the Milan data in his hand. Then Retsky sat in Demicheli's office who then described a simple model of tumor growth. Demicheli has both M.D. and Ph.D. degrees. In addition to knowledge of medical oncology, he did much research and published a number of papers on animal model growth. Demicheli then discussed what he considered to be a basic description of metastatic tumor growth. This will seem obvious now but 23 years ago that was definitely not the case. Demicheli said a cancer metastasis starts off as a single cell with malignant potential. It may remain in a non-dividing state for a variable period of time before it begins to divide. After this happens, it can grow to a size limited by lack of blood supply that corresponds to approximately one or a few mm in size. It can remain at this size for another variable period of time until angiogenesis occurs and then it can grow to a detectable size and is diagnosed as a metastatic lesion with lethal potential.

Retsky's task was to take Valagussa's data and Demicheli's model and try and understand what happened to cause the multimodal relapse patterns for pre- and postmenopausal patients treated with surgery only (Fig. 2.5).

Retsky obtained a small grant in 1995 to develop an expert system for clinical breast cancer based on these Milan data. Given his unusual background, Retsky was sufficiently experienced with using computer simulation and stochastic methods to

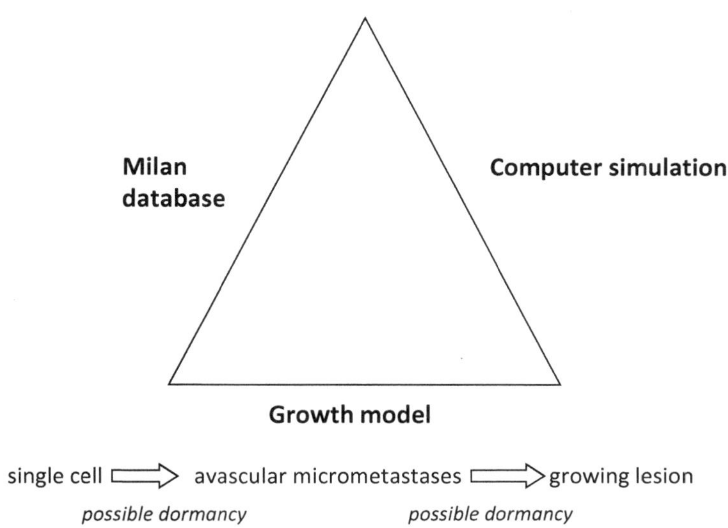

Fig. 2.5 Our strategy for this project. Fitting a simple growth model to Milan data. *Bonadonna, Valagussa et al. NEJM 1995* (Milan database); *Retsky et al BCR&T 1997* (computer simulation); *Demicheli et al. Ann Onc 1997* (growth model)

attempt such a project. At the time Retsky was at Harvard Medical School and on Judah Folkman's staff—another important advantage. Retsky arranged for Demicheli to visit the Folkman lab and speak with him and his staff during 1995. Although preliminary at that time, lab findings and clinical data showed a general agreement.

Retsky was more than willing to use Demicheli's model in the computer simulation but arrived at that viewpoint from a totally different perspective. Retsky did not have Demicheli's clinical viewpoint and experimental experience with animal models but the model was consistent with his prior research into the old literature.

2.4 Library Research at University of Texas–San Antonio

In 1989 while Retsky was Professor of Biology at University of Colorado–Colorado Springs he was invited to be Visiting Professor alternate weeks for 6 months in the Department of Oncology at University of Texas–San Antonio. This was in the department of William McGuire, M.D. who played a lead role in introducing estrogen and progesterone receptor values as prognostic markers in breast cancer [19]. They had a database of thousands of patients with receptor values and clinical outcome. McGuire had one of his staff two levels down extract a few columns from their data and provide it electronically to Retsky for his project. Retsky's task was to integrate these receptor values into a computer simulation he had previously developed and modify it to provide a relevant prognostic report for individual patients. This project did not work well at all. However as was discovered months later, the columns given to Retsky were mislabeled causing what appeared to be significant discrepancies between simulation results and actual clinical outcome. (It is interesting to compare this flawed data transfer process with Valagussa personally placing a computer disk with her Milan data in Retsky's hand.)

With the planned project results so discouraging, Retsky used his time in San Antonio to pursue other scientific interests. He then spent much time in the well equipped University of Texas Briscoe Medical Library reading papers from prior decades when tumors were not always immediately resected from patients and experimental tumors in animals were allowed to grow larger than in current times when animal rights are more respected. This was also at a time before libraries were digitized. Retsky could have ten volumes open on the table and look from one paper to another. He ended up writing a paper describing old published data on tumor growth in humans and animals [20]. Retsky was particularly interested in the mathematical description of tumor growth. Specifically did tumors grow continually according to the exponential or damped exponential Gompertzian equation as conventionally thought or did tumors grow with occasional periods of temporary dormancy as suggested in Retsky's first paper in cancer research in 1984? [21]. There are published clinical data reporting dormancy for periods of a year and more in primary breast, primary colon and metastatic pulmonary cancers. This Medical Hypotheses 1990 paper with much relevant information is available free open access.

2.5 Ingleby and Moore Data

One particular paper from 1956 [22] had what appeared to be very distinctive data showing dormancy followed by growth for an untreated primary breast cancer. A 78 year old patient had recently spent their family life savings on what proved to be futile treatment for her husband (carcinoma of the larynx) and stubbornly refused to have her recently discovered breast tumor resected. She did however allow occasional X-rays. Data reported by Ingleby and Moore based on X-ray shadows showed virtually no growth for 11 months (tumor grew from 7 to 8 cm^3 with volume doubling time of 20 years) followed by ordinary growth for another 11 months (tumor grew from 8 to 38 cm^3 which is a relatively normal 180 day volume doubling time). (1 cm^3 is approximately 10^9 cells.) There were skin changes during that period during which there was infinitesimal change in tumor dimensions. After this growth, the tumor was resected. Subsequent pathology report showed unremarkable adenocarcinoma. This was the only report Retsky could find in the literature showing more than two size measurements of an undisturbed primary breast tumor over a period of more than 1 year (there were 4 measurements taken over 22 months). It could not have grown with 20 year doubling time to the size when first measured. That would have been impossible since the tumor would have had to start growing before the patient was born. It must have grown faster previously and then reached a temporary dormant state for at least 11 months and then growth resumed.

These data were the subject of a polite but intense published argument with Larry Norton of Memorial Sloan Kettering Cancer Center who was the chief proponent of the Gompertzian equation as the general description of breast cancer growth [23, 24]. At least from our point of view, the Gompertzian growth model is clearly inconsistent with Ingleby and Moore data (Fig. 2.6).

By 1994 Retsky and Demicheli were kindred spirits when it came to possible dormancy in cancer growth—particularly for breast cancer.

The computer simulation went well but the results were unexpected. To summarize the results Fig. 2.7 is shown superimposed upon the Milan data for premenopausal women. The early dominant peak consists of two previously unreported mastectomy-induced relapse modes. Avascular micrometastases that were previously dormant are induced into angiogenesis and produce detectable size lesions at about 10 months post surgery. Also single dormant cells are induced into division and then stochastically undergo angiogenesis to produce relapses at about 30 months post surgery. Together these two relapse modes comprise about 50–80% of all relapses in breast cancer increasing with poor prognosis based on tumor size and the number of nodes positive. The mastectomy-induced angiogenesis mode is most prominent for young patients (premenopausal) with node positive status. The specific ratios are 5:1 node positive to node negative and 2:1 pre- to postmenopausal. Approximately 20% of premenopausal node positive patients experience surgery-induced angiogenesis. We speculated that the late peak with shallow maximum at about 60 months might represent what may be considered the natural history of metastatic growth with no stimulation of growth from surgery. The top of the late

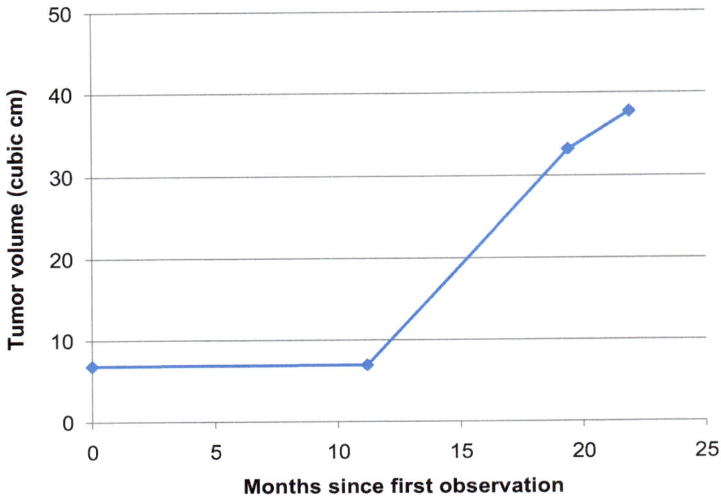

Fig. 2.6 Ingleby and Moore [22] tumor size data for an untreated primary breast tumor. Data were originally presented as area but converted to volume for this figure. Growth curve of untreated primary breast cancer

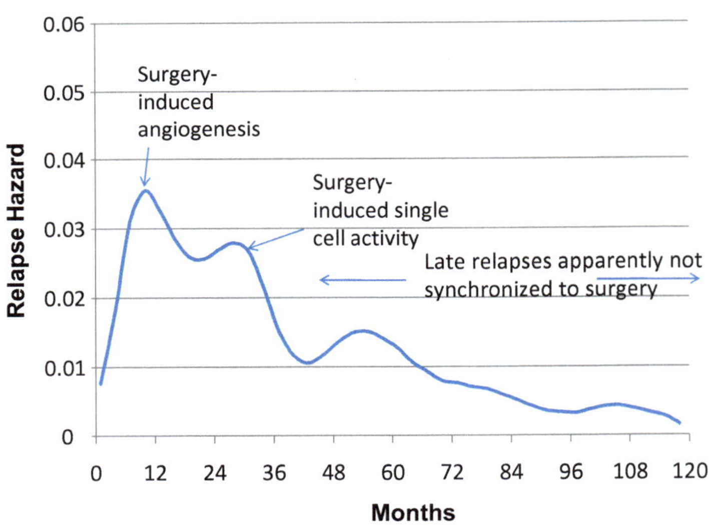

Fig. 2.7 Results of the computer simulation superimposed upon the Milan data for premenopausal patients. Interpretation from computer simulation superimposed upon premenopausal Milan data

shallow peak might indicate the point at which the benefit of surgery first appears. Without surgery, the relapses would continue rising instead of starting to decline at about 60 months. That implies the unstimulated metastatic pipeline is 5 years in duration but much shorter in the presence of intervention. These results were not well received. Nobody was pleased to see these findings.

A 2 day meeting was held in fall 1996 at the University of Colorado - Colorado Springs (UCCS) to discuss the counterintuitive results of this project. Attending were Robert Wardwell, Dr. Jack Speer, Douglas Swartzendruber, Paul Bame, Pinuccia Valagussa, Michael Retsky, and Romano Demicheli. At the time, Retsky was Professor of Biology and Swartzendruber was Dean of Letters, Arts and Sciences at UCCS. After the meeting Wardwell and Retsky took Valagussa and Demicheli on a driving tour to Taos, New Mexico where we spent some time exploring the Southwest US and American Indian culture. As one cultural highlight, Wardwell arranged a lunch meeting with a US citizen of Italian descent. This person was put through law school by the local Indians and lived among them for years. He was trained specifically to represent the Indian community in building and operating casinos on their land. Many questions were asked about the Indian culture. It was very educational.

During this trip Retsky became very impressed with Valagussa as having a perfect personality for a database manager. Valagussa has been a principle speaker at ASCO with several thousand oncologists in the audience so she is very knowledgeable about the subject. She would be the first person to know about a problem in a randomized controlled clinical trial. A classic example of such a problem would be more persons with positive nodes in the intervention arm than in the control arm of a mammography trial. Retsky had seen such a situation before and had met the (mild mannered) database manager. The problem did not get discussed until years after the trial was over when it was too late to do anything except argue about whether the trial was flawed against mammography [25, 26]. Valagussa would not be intimidated and be on the phone screaming to some physician in a distant city to fix their problem.

Retsky et al. [27] paper was published reporting the computer simulation results (with a cautionary label of "Hypothesis" inserted by the editor) and a parallel Demicheli et al. [28] paper was published describing the biological implication and relevance to breast cancer.

In November 1994 Retsky was diagnosed with Stage IIIc colon cancer. Overlapping this scientific investigation Retsky was diagnosed with stage IIIc colon cancer, the result of a routine colonoscopy. However based on his prior research in cancer growth, instead of the usual maximum tolerated adjuvant chemotherapy protocol, he used a previously untested low dose virtually non-toxic, long term (2.5 years) adjuvant chemotherapy that is now called metronomic chemotherapy. The therapy was designed by William Hrushesky, M.D. who is now one of our research colleagues. The reasoning behind this and other details have been described a number of times [29–31] including in a biography of Judah Folkman by Robert Cooke in 2001 [32] and an online report on ProPublica by Jake Bernstein in 2014 [33]. A more detailed discussion here would be a distraction from the main theme of the chapter. However it should be noted that the continuous growth Gompertzian kinetics that underlies the scientific basis of maximum tolerated chemotherapy can trace its roots to a mathematically flawed study from 1965 that includes data from only 18 rodents and one rabbit.

Ironically Retsky was under this treatment while conducting the computer simulation. Of note, there was no cognitive dysfunction or "chemo-brain" as it is commonly called by patients.

We have seen similar bimodal relapse patterns in other cancer sites. These include pancreatic, melanoma, non-small-cell lung cancer, prostate, bladder, esophageal, head and neck, osteosarcoma, and renal. This list includes combinations of large databases and case reports. A recent paper by Hamard et al. [34] addressed the possibility that glioblastoma might be another cancer site in which relapse is stimulated by surgery.

Demicheli was working with a group from Duke University and had access to their lung cancer database. He found a multipeak relapse pattern in non-small-cell lung cancer [35]. The timing was different from breast and there was a male to female difference but otherwise it looked very similar to breast. A paper by Maniwa et al. in 1998 shows what appears to be a clear clinical example of surgery induced angiogenesis in lung cancer [36]. Another clinical example of surgery induced angiogenesis can be seen in osteosarcoma (Fig. 2.4 in Retsky et al. Medical Hypotheses 1990) [20]. Data are from Smithers [37].

2.6 It Seems We Have Rediscovered a Problem That Was Known to Surgeons 2000 Years Ago

Remarkably physicians 2000 years ago were able to remove breast cancers without benefit of anesthesia and antibiotics and patients survived the treatment and some did not die from cancer. Celsus (30 BC–38 AD) wrote about cacoethes, carcinoma without ulcerations and then fungating ulcer as a staging sequence. He then wrote that only the cacoethes could be removed; all others are irritated by every method. The more violent the operation, the more angry they grow. Today we often hear about cancer as "angry". Galen (131–203 AD) wrote they have often cured the tumor growth disease when tumors were small but no one has successively treated it when tumors were large [2]. This information seems to have been overlooked or ignored since the time of Celsus and Galen. *We are apparently late-comers to a 2000 year old unsolved problem in oncology.*

2.7 Clinical Correlations to Suggested Surgery Induced Metastatic Activity

The surgery induced effects we describe are so large that they must be apparent in clinical cancer. Thus, looking for evidence of these effects we began to examine clinical breast cancer observations to see if and where they may appear. There are more [9, 11] but four such situations are presented below.

1. *Adjuvant chemotherapy*

   Adjuvant chemotherapy works best by far for premenopausal node positive patients. Indeed the curative benefit of adjuvant chemotherapy is approximately 12% for premenopausal node-positive patients and in the 2–6% range for all other categories [38]. This is consistent with our metastasis model. Surgery induces single cell activity that would produce a certain level of chemosensitivity for all patients. However, for premenopausal node positive patients, surgery induced angiogenesis produces very intense micrometastatic cancer growth just after surgery which corresponds to when the clinicians empirically found adjuvant chemotherapy is most effective. We published this hypothesis in 2004 [39]. Note the authors include Judah Folkman with 30 years experience in angiogenesis research and Gianni Bonadonna with 30 years experience in adjuvant chemotherapy research. Figure 2.8 shows Milan data for patients treated with the Bonadonna classic cyclophosphamide methotrexate 5-fluorouracil (CMF) chemotherapy compared to mastectomy only patients. It can be seen that the effect of adjuvant chemotherapy is mostly to reduce early relapses with far less effect on late relapses. That is consistent with our theory.
2. *Mammography paradox for women age 40–49*

   Very disturbing when initially reported, mammography works better for women age 50–59 than it does for women age 40–49. In the first few years of trials to measure the benefit of early detection, more women age 40–49 died of breast cancer in the intervention arm than in the control arm. This was apparent in large trials con-

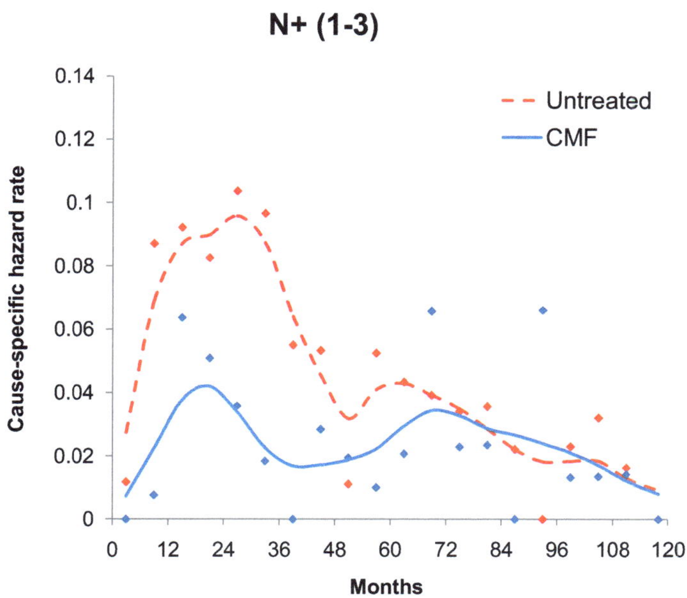

Fig. 2.8 Milan data for patients treated with the Bonadonna classic CMF chemotherapy compared to mastectomy only patients

ducted in US, UK and Sweden. We calculated that because of surgery induced angiogenesis 1/10,000 apparently healthy screened women age 40–49 in the screened population would relapse and die of metastatic breast cancer 3 years after the start of trials of early detection. (Relapse occurs approximately 1 year after detection and surgery and results in mortality 2 years later.) That is just what was found. Thus based on our analysis and Milan data, surgery induced angiogenesis for premenopausal node positive women could quantitatively explain the mammography paradox for young women. Data are shown in our prior publications [40].

Our studies suggest that early detection sometimes results in earlier recruitment of an unfavorable event. This is particularly the case for premenopausal women and even more so for those that have triple negative breast cancer (TNBC) and those that have early onset. We published papers from 2001 to 2013 on this subject. A paper in 2005 got some publicity in Wall Street Journal [41] and as a result we received some very helpful feedback that ultimately led to an explanation for the racial disparity in outcome. Isaac Gukas (who unfortunately died of cancer in 2013) was a surgeon in UK but was originally from Nigeria and practiced oncology there for over 10 years. Gukas reported in a letter to the editor that cancer of the breast commonly occurred in early age 40s in Nigeria and patients relapsed very soon after surgery. Thus Nigerian women would usually avoid surgery and see a traditional herbal therapist since they thought surgery "provoked" the cancer. Gukas coauthored several important papers with us over the next 6 years. His name as one of the authors of our papers was a major asset when we later presented our science in Nigeria.

3. *Racial disparity in outcome*

   This information from Gukas led us to propose an explanation for the racial disparity in outcome in the US. In the US there is a 1.5–2.2-fold excess mortality of Americans of African descent (AA) compared to Americans of European descent (EA). It turns out that breast cancer in AA appears at average age 46 while breast cancer in EA appears at average age 57. It is also apparent that there is an inversion in racial disparity outcome at age 57. That is, for AA of age less than 57 there is a racial disadvantage while for age greater than 57 there is a racial *advantage* according to a report by Jatoi et al. [42]. Thus it is hard to explain the racial disparity by considering reduced access to health care. We published a number of papers on this subject [43–45]. Demicheli et al. Cancer 2007 is perhaps the most pertinent [43].

   Since the average age of diagnosis of breast cancer in Nigeria is 42.7 years, this could also explain the very poor outcome in sub-Saharan Africa. It is shown that early relapses are highly associated with TNBC and especially with early onset breast cancer. These two factors that are very common in Nigeria could account for the very poor outcome in that country.

4. *"Aggressiveness" in young women*

   It is a commonly noted trait that breast cancer in young women is "aggressive". From our perspective this is a result of surgery induced angiogenesis and relapses at approximately 10 months post surgery. While this would appear to the cancer clinician as "aggressive", from our perspective it is clockwork relapse for premenopausal women at 10 months. Since this occurs in 20% of premenopausal node positive women, breast cancer would appear as "aggressive" for young women.

Summarizing results to this point, it is clear to us that something happens at or about the time of primary tumor surgical removal to induce two previously unreported modes of early relapse in mastectomy treated breast cancer. Surgery induced angiogenesis, most prominent for premenopausal node positive patients, occurs at approximately 10 months post surgery and surgery induced single cell division from dormancy is apparent at 30 months post surgery. These relapse modes comprise the majority of relapses and are most common for poor prognosis patients.

This is most likely a general effect and not just limited to breast cancer. It is more apparent for patients with markers for relapse such as tumor size and number of positive lymph nodes. Prior to 2010 we had a hypothesis to explain this but, compared to what was to follow, it was far less interesting [46].

2.8 Surprising Development from a Belgian Anesthesiology Group

A paper that led to an explanation of these data was published in 2010 by a Belgian anesthesiologist group. Forget et al. [47] retrospectively considered 327 consecutive breast cancer patients treated by mastectomy and conventional adjuvant therapy. The same surgeon conducted the mastectomies. This was done at a teaching hospital so they use a variety of analgesics to train the residents. The paper reported outcome for these patients grouped by what drug was given as anesthetic. One drug resulted in far fewer early relapses. That drug ketorolac was the only NSAID used. Forget et al. data are shown in Fig. 2.9 below.

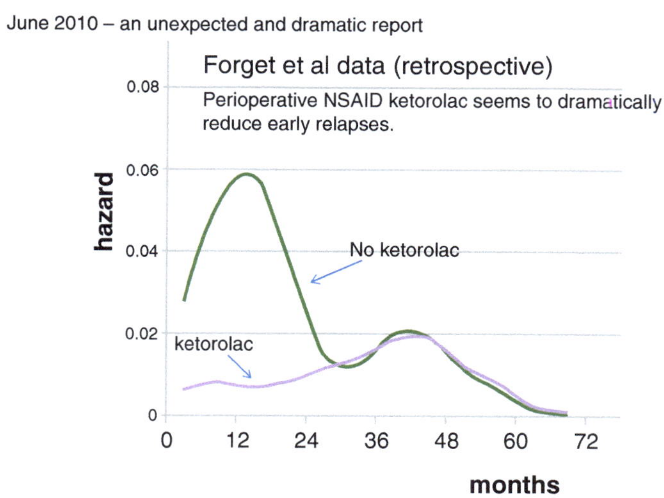

Fig. 2.9 Data from Forget et al. show disease free survival for patients given perioperative NSAID ketorolac vs. any other analgesic. Forget P, Vandenhende J, Berliere M, Machiels JP, Nussbaum B, Legrand C, De Kock M; Do intraoperative analgesics influence breast cancer recurrence after mastectomy? A retrospective analysis. Anesth Analg. 2010 Jun 1;110(6):1630–5

Demicheli and Retsky visited the hospital in Brussels. Presentations were made by both groups and their data were then updated by resident Sarah Amar and analyzed by Demicheli (Fig. 2.10). (Unfortunately we do not have access to these data to provide more current updates.)

What could explain the Forget et al. data (Table 2.2)?

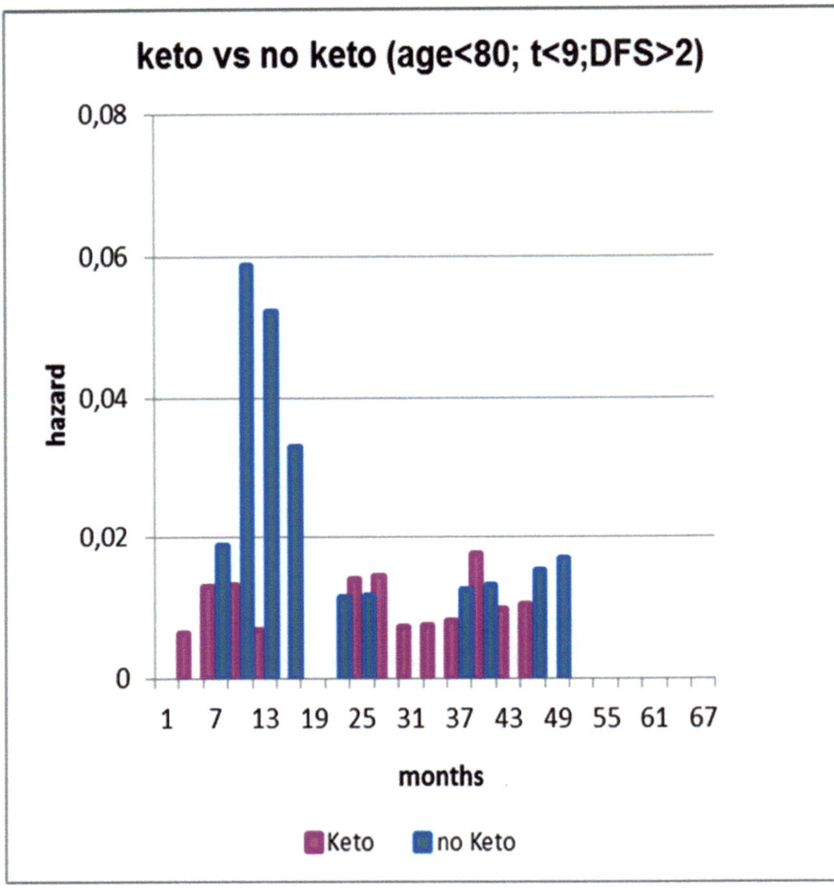

Months	0	6	12	18	24	30	36	42	48
Patients at risk	316	302	283	266	260	252	223	183	150
Keto group	175	168	162	157	155	151	140	115	99
No-Keto group	141	134	121	109	105	101	83	68	51

Fig. 2.10 As shown in this figure there is a fivefold reduction in relapse in months 9–18 for the NSAID treated patients. Forget et al data updated September 2011 by Sarah Amar and analyzed by Romano Demicheli. Fivefold reduction in relapses months 9–18. Three vs. 15 events

Table 2.2 What could explain the Forget et al. data?

We investigated the interactions among the following:
Surgery—It appears that cancer can take advantage of the primary tumor removal and/or the hard-wired wound healing process in humans
Inflammation—Transient systemic inflammation exists for about a week after surgery occurs as evidenced by IL-6 that is found in serum post-surgery
Angiogenesis—It is a main phase of the wound healing process as well as tumor progression. VEGF is increased in serum after breast cancer surgery (relative to this phenomenon, platelets actively sequester angioactive factors and degranulate in presence of inflammation and their counts are reduced by about 10% post surgery)
Circulating tumor cells (CTC)—are well known to be present in cancer patients and are correlated with outcome. It is also known that presurgical levels of CTCs are strongly correlated with early relapse in TNBC [48]. It is possible to consider that CTCs can get trapped in porous capillaries or venules as the result of inflammation
Immune system—is in some ways suppressed after surgery and it is considered that the immune system can prevent cancer growth. Thus when suppressed, it could release tumor growth
Cancer dormancy—is well accepted at the single cell level and at the avascular micrometastasis level

2.9 Our Attention Is Drawn to Inflammation

We were aware that some intervention that started before surgery would be necessary in order to prevent surgery-induced tumor activity but we were unaware of what could explain the data of Forget et al. A paper published along with the Forget et al. study by Gottschalk et al. [49] presented a long list of possible effects of surgery and the use of anesthesia that might impact tumor growth. These include immunosuppression, transfusion, pain, stress, hypothermia, inflammation and a few others. More recently Horowitz et al. [50] also discuss the perioperative influence on cancer growth. These are all possible however our interest was directed to inflammation as we knew there was a long historical and extensive literature correlating and connecting inflammation and cancer growth.

An earlier event also triggered our interest in inflammation. In 2005 a paper was submitted by El Saghir et al. [51] to Bio-Med-Central Cancer and Retsky was asked to review it. The paper was a case report of a 54 year old smoker from Lebanon who was diagnosed with non-resectable non-small-cell lung cancer. This patient was treated with radiation and while his prognosis was extremely poor, he was at least for a while able to function relatively normally. While driving his car, he bumped his head on the sun visor and within 30 days a 7 cm tumor grew at that spot. The paper was submitted and it was suggested that this might be a result of surgery-induced angiogenesis as we had reported in our papers. Having a quantitative understanding of surgery-induced growth, we were able to consider the numbers from the case report and quickly ruled out any possibility that surgery induced angiogenesis or anything that we have described as surgery induced tumor growth could explain this case. But then Retsky was at a loss and was wandering around the Folkman lab asking if anyone had any ideas on how to explain the case report. Taturo Udagawa suggested he look at inflammation and recommended a paper by Mina Bissell's group [52]. That paper described an avian model of virus-induced cancer. The curious thing was that tumor grew at any point where the bird was wounded and that this could be fully correlated with an anti-inflammatory intervention. If inflammation was prevented, tumor would not develop at the point of wounding and if inflammation was not so prevented, tumor would grow anywhere the bird was wounded. That could explain the El Saghir et al. paper. Retsky discussed this with Demicheli and then wrote in a published comment to the case report paper: "***The unusual isolated and exaggerated situation allowed El Saghir et al. to observe what may be a new and possibly important hematologic metastatic pathway: inflammation as a facilitating precursor to tumor*** [53]. *Metastasis is a very inefficient process. (Tens of thousands of viable) cancer cells might be found in a patient's blood but only a few metastases occur. The Martins-Green et al. discussion of an inflammation sequence would certainly increase metastatic efficiency since it bypasses extravasation through an intact vessel wall and it provides growth factors in the microenvironment. In the context of Paget's 1889 "seed and soil" metaphor* [54], *we have a situation here where many viable seeds and good fertilizer is applied in a large vacant field. The possible connection between inflammation and tumor growth might also help explain why anti-inflammatory drugs such as aspirin, prednisone and Celebrex are often used in cancer prevention and therapy.*"

Inflammation is a host response to insult of tissue. Damage to tissue either by pathogen or trauma from physical action triggers a cascade of complex events [55–57]. Inflammatory cells and associated complexes collaborate to reconstitute the extracellular matrix, clear debris, attack pathogens, and participate in the transfer and proliferation of healthy cells to the area insulted. This may be considered as a particular aspect of host homeostasis processes and the stability of tissues of the body. This is also considered the hard wired natural reaction to trauma and the resulting host repair process. Many factors including the host condition determine the extent, timing and magnitude of this process. Mast cells in particular can intensify the inflammatory response by releasing histamine which can increase capillary diameter thus increasing its permeability.

Balkwill et al. write that if genetic damage is the "match that lights the fire" of cancer, then inflammation is the "fuel that feeds the flames" and that the survival and proliferation of already initiated cancer cells is affected by inflammation [58]. Inflammation is known to be a significant component of the tumor microenvironment.

Inflammatory oncotaxis, a term used to describe tumor growth at a site of inflammation, has long been seen in persons with known or occult cancer and who have local trauma [59]. As an example, in 1914 when it was more common for persons to walk around with known cancer, Jones and Rous stated: "The localization of secondary tumors at points of injury has been so often remarked upon that it is unnecessary to cite specific instances. The cause for the phenomenon is unknown." [60].

Systemic inflammation can occur after surgery in which a primary tumor was resected for breast cancer and colon cancer. Regarding colon cancer, Pascual et al. [61] measured proinflammatory cytokine interleukin-6 (IL-6) in serum prior to open or laparoscopic colectomy to establish the baseline levels. To determine the temporal trends, the cytokine was measured again at 4, 12, 24 and 48 h and at 4 days after surgery. It appears that IL-6 level in serum was elevated in open surgery by a factor of 2 compared to laparoscopic surgery and would gradually return to baseline in a week or so. For breast cancer, there are data from Chow et al. [62] and from Perez-Rivas et al. [63] providing an association between primary tumor removal and inflammation that was transient for several days.

In their investigation of the effect of clarithromycin on transient inflammation post mastectomy, Chow et al. used three markers of inflammation that are found useful in predicting outcome in renal disease. These markers are IL-6, tumor necrosis factor-alpha (TNF-alpha) and C-reactive protein (CRP). With 54 patients, they measured inflammation in peripheral blood daily, starting the day prior to surgery and each day for 3 days after surgery. For both control and clarithromycin treated patients Chow et al. found no significant change in TNF-alpha but 60% increase in CRP and 50% increase in IL-6 for several days after surgery. Extrapolating their data it would seem that inflammation was elevated for approximately 1 week. In addition, platelets decreased by about 10% with the same temporal trends as CRP and IL-6.

In their study, Perez-Rivas et al. [63] compared serum markers before and after surgery for early stage breast cancer patients (56 with invasive disease and 7 with ductal carcinoma in situ) and healthy women (16 with benign fibroadenoma). Samples were collected 8 h before mastectomy or lumpectomy and 24 h after surgery. For the general population, they reported that concentration increased for Thrombospondin-2 (THSB2), Colony Stimulating Factor (CSF1), IL-6, IL-7, IL-16, Vascular Endothelial Growth Factor B (VEGF-B), Human Epidermal Growth Factor Receptor 2 (HER2), and Fas Ligand (FasL). These include markers of inflammation and angiogenesis promoters. For invasive breast cancer they report IL-16 and VEGF-A show high velocity after surgery and it is suggested that IL-16 is a factor in dormancy escape.

2.10 Possible Mechanisms for a Post-surgical Systemic Inflammatory Reaction to Drive Tumor Growth

In this following section we paraphrase and quote liberally from our 2013 review on possible mechanisms. A possible new mechanism involves mobile and attracted neutrophils and is described in the accompanying chapter by Bonnelykke-Behrndtz ML et al. [64]. This is possibly also related to discussion in the Forget and DeKock chapter [65] on the importance of neutrophil to lymphocyte ratio (NLR) and a report from Egawa et al. [66] on enhanced capillary leakage from vesicle in presence of inflammation. Such leakage increased to the extent that particles 2000 kDa could passage instead of only 70 kDa in absence of inflammation. Attention is made to the Schmidt et al. chapter and the Forget and DeKock chapter. At the time of writing this chapter we have not seen all submitted invited chapters so we will refrain from additional comments here (Fig. 2.11).

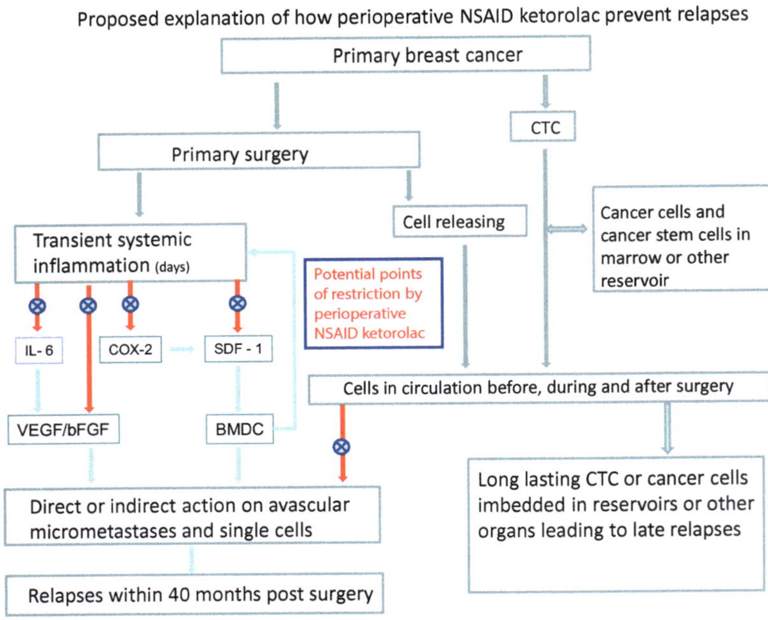

Fig. 2.11 Symbolic description of proposed explanations for Forget et al. data

Early relapses are assumed to be related, at least in part, to the inflammatory process due to primary tumor surgical removal, directly or indirectly eliciting peritumoral endothelial cell and single cell proliferation. A few possible mechanisms are explained. Angiogenic factors, like VEGF and bFGF, are directly released by degranulated platelets or even produced via IL-6. Bone marrow derived CXCR-4 positive cells, acting both on tumor foci and on the inflammatory process, are mobilized by SDF-1 directly released or even produced via COX-2. Perioperative ketorolac would restrict both endocrine and cellular pathways, thus impairing the metastatic process. CTC refers to circulating tumor cells.

The suggestion that inflammation can spur angiogenesis and tumor growth is supported by a number of reports [58, 67–70]. Inflammation could activate growth of dormant single cells or avascular micrometastases thus occasioning early recurrences. A reasonable hypothesis advocates that decrease of inflammatory response to the surgical maneuver may hamper the angiogenesis switch.

There are a few mechanisms that we can propose. At steady state conditions in adult mammals, the majority of endothelial cells are in a quiescent state and this is thought to play a role in the homeostasis of organs and the dormancy of tumors [71]. Inflammation may cause an upregulation possibly including the release of factors that stimulate endothelial cells to proliferate. Secretion of specific cytokines from endothelial cells could then support the regeneration of normal cells and malignant stem cells.

It appears that tumor stem cells like normal stem cells are able to change state from proliferation or quiescence with control of a supporting "niche", i.e., a specialized microenvironment including both cells and extra-cellular matrix (ECM). A metastatic "vascular niche", involving endothelial cells, where angiogenesis dependent dormancy could result from interaction between tumor cells and endothelial cells has been suggested, perhaps involving Notch signaling [72]. If so, it is reasonable to assume that the endothelial cells, under an angiogenic spike by the surgical approach to primary tumor, may contribute to dormancy interruption [73]. Thus, reducing inflammation could impair dormant foci awakening.

Additionally, an inflammatory stimulus could modify circulating tumor cell phenotype. When circulating tumor cell expression profile related to activation and ability to adhere, which is a prerequisite for metastasis formation, was analysed, changes in the expression of nanog, a sign of stem cell properties enabling the cells to self renew and grow, was observed. Moreover, EpCAM, HER2, and the adhesion molecule vimentin are risk factors of proliferation possibly influenced by inflammation [74, 75].

Mobilization of bone marrow derived cells that respond to chemo-attractant signals from various organs, undergo a homing process and release several chemokines was induced by tissue lesions [76]. This phenomenon is particularly marked during neovascularization of wounded tissues and is thought to result from direct or paracrine activity inducing capillary formation. Cell trafficking is a common basis of the above-mentioned processes [76]. Indeed, mobilization of normal stem cells from their natural niche and homing in a given tissue is regulated by definite signals. For example, hematopoietic stem cells express the chemokine receptor CXCR4 and selectively respond to SDF-1α. The SDF-1/CXCR4 axis is a main regulator of the normal cell trafficking underlying tissue homeostasis. It is also involved in tumor cell trafficking. CXCR4 overexpression has been detected in more than 20 human tumor types, including ovarian, prostate, esophageal, melanoma, neuroblastoma, and renal cell carcinoma [77]. Therefore, one could reasonably hypothesize that NSAIDs may interfere with SDF1 levels via the pathway COX-2 $\rightarrow$ PGE $\rightarrow$ SDF-1, thus impairing processes underlying metastasis development.

Even if an NSAID class effect is plausible, a specific effect of ketorolac remains possible. As already stated, whereas all NSAIDs act against the growth of tumors, they are probably not equivalent for this antitumoral effect [47]. Alternative targets, such as the tumor-associated NADH oxydase (tNOX), are possibly involved in this anticancer effect. The existence of tNOX explains the fact that some cancer cell lines lacking COX-2 respond to certain NSAIDs but not to others, suggestive of additional COX-2 independent antitumor activities [78].

Another possible explanation for the lack of surgery-induced angiogenesis when ketorolac is used involves inflammation induced platelet degranulation and that platelets are known to sequester angiogenesis regulating proteins including VEGF [79]. This is especially interesting in view of Chow et al. findings that platelets decrease by about 10% in the few days post-surgery. There is also a report that NSAIDs are antiangiogenic and another report that transcript of stem cell marker CD133 that is correlated with poor prognosis in a number of solid tumors was lower in patients treated preoperatively with NSAIDs [80, 81].

It is well established that many cancer patients have circulating tumor cells [82–84] and there are cells released as a result of surgery [85]. Camara et al. data show a surge in circulating epithelial cells after primary breast cancer surgery, but intriguingly, that surge occurs 3–7 days after surgery. Such a delayed increase in what may be circulating tumor cells after breast cancer surgery was also reported by Daskalakis et al. [86]. This phenomenon recalls the surge of CD34+ progenitor cells 3–5 days after tissue damage (e.g., myocardial infarction) [87]. Also it has been recently reported in an animal model, where mice with subcutaneous implantation of Lewis lung carcinoma were subjected to an operative injury, that surgery induced the release of cytokines/chemokines and mobilized bone marrow–derived cells (BMDC) [88]. These mobilized cells were then recruited into tumor tissue with concomitant enhancement of angiogenesis, thereby accelerating tumor growth. Furthermore, blocking recruitment of bone marrow stem cells by disrupting SDF/CXCR signals completely negated the accelerated tumor growth. Many questions arise. Are these surged cells reported by Camara [85] shed or spilled into circulation during surgery and if so why are they delayed by a few days? Or perhaps are these cells released from the bone marrow as part of the programmed wound healing process? Is this a connection to Dvorak's comment that cancer is "wound healing gone awry" [89]? What exactly controls this effect? Can a perioperative NSAID stop this process?

It further suggests that tumors may share physiological mechanisms with normal tissues and, moreover, that inhibiting the inflammatory process might reduce late metastases as well as can be seen in a recent report of daily use of aspirin [90]. Interestingly, the benefit of daily aspirin does not appear until after 2 years of use. This would be consistent with the possibility that late relapses are the result of a variety of inflammation driven events that induce single cell growth and that result in relapses approximately 30 months hence. If late relapses were the result of some type of induced angiogenesis, we would expect to see a benefit of daily aspirin at 10 or so months after starting.

Blood flow in capillaries is only 0.05 cm/s [91] which would make leaky capillary venules a relatively efficient way for circulating tumor cells to get trapped or enter tissue. It may be that what we previously called dormant single cells induced into metastatic growth were at least in some cases residing not at the site of eventual relapse. Rather, circulating tumor cells or BMDC released into circulation by a host response to surgery in an inflammatory environment extravasate, resulting months later in a metastatic tumor. It is thereby logical to expect that an effective perisurgical anti-inflammatory strategy may affect surgery-induced and possibly angiogenesis-mediated cancer spread.

The metastatic process is highly inefficient. A clonal malignant cell injected into the circulation has approximately 0.0001 probability to result in a growing metastatic site [92]. Inflammation bypasses the need for extravasation through an intact vessel wall and also provides growth factors to the microenvironment. We estimate using our computer simulation that the metastatic seeding process is amplified 100-fold during the few days after primary surgery.

This inflammation driven capillary leakage of CTCs theory has much appeal and seems to address all information presented above but there are other data that cannot be explained. In a 1984 paper Tarin et al. discussed 30 patients with peritoneovenous shunting for the alleviation of abdominal pain and distension in malignant ascites due to inoperable cancer [93]. This procedure returns the fluid to the circulation via a one way valved anastomosis between the peritoneum and the jugular vein. Surprisingly, although the patients treated with this technique receive direct infusions of malignant tumor cells into the blood, this study of 29 patients, 15 of whom came to autopsy, shows that they did not all develop metastases, some being completely free of such lesions despite long survival. Even when metastases do form, they are small and clinically asymptomatic, and the technique is therefore not hazardous. In some patients, inert tumor cells identifiable by natural markers were recognized in the tissues, but no growing metastases were observed. In others, the distribution of secondary deposits was unexpected in that metastases did not form in the organ containing the first capillary bed encountered, although hematogenous metastases had formed in other organs. Despite the fact that various factors such as (a) the small numbers of patients treated with the technique; (b) the sensitive nature of studies on terminally ill patients; and (c) the absence of consistency in the sample population with regard to factors such as length of survival and site of neoplasm, combine to reduce the number of suitable cases for study, the approach has unrivaled power and interest for those seeking to understand mechanisms underlying tumor metastasis in humans.

It is not known if the shunt insertion procedure produces systemic inflammation since the process is done under local anesthesia and there is no mention of inflammatory markers in serum such as IL-6. Nonetheless it appears that the Tarin et al. report does not support the conjecture that systemic inflammation in presence of CTCs leads to distant relapses within 3 years.

Are the missing early relapses in Forget et al. data never to happen or are they merely postponed to become late relapses? Whatever their source and shedding timing, cancer cells in circulation may have half-life of a few hours. Cancer cells are approximately 15 μm in diameter and capillaries are approximately 7 μm in diameter. A series of papers by Weiss et al. [94, 95] several decades ago discussed that the deformation to pass through the capillaries kills 80% or so of cancer cells each passage. The circulation period is several minutes so it is easy to understand why cancer cells have short half-life in the body. Unless injected into more hospitable surroundings such as tissue, these cells will likely harmlessly die off. These data and our analysis suggest that at least for some patients the early relapses apparently avoided in the Forget et al. data do not show up later.

Lastly, the reduced recurrence risk for patients receiving perioperative NSAID may be attributed, at least in part, to the reduced usage of opioids for pain management with ketorolac [96, 97]. It cannot be excluded that all the above mentioned mechanisms could act together impacting relapses within the subsequent few years.

2.11 TNBC and Early Relapses: Possibly an Ideal Group for Testing Perioperative Ketorolac

We now turn our attention to methods of testing this new hypothesis. Animal studies would be very important; however in view of the analyses and data presented we think this should be tested prospectively in a clinical trial. The next question that arises is what patient group would be a good candidate for a trial. Most breast cancer clinical trials, at least in the US, focus on distinct patient subgroups based on recurrence risk levels. The triple negative subgroup attracted our attention for several reasons [98]. Lacking markers for HER2, Estrogen or Progesterone receptors that strongly suggest that there is benefit of targeted therapy, triple negative breast cancer is looked upon by clinicians as a "bad tumor" with high recurrence rate in spite of adjuvant chemotherapy. That pessimistic viewpoint seems justified since TNBC has 12% incidence but accounts for approximately 20% of mortality in breast cancer.

We had access to a triple negative breast cancer data base from Milan that we analyzed with our hazard methods. The relapse hazard (Fig. 2.12 below) looks remarkably similar to the no-ketorolac group in the Forget et al. study shown in Fig. 2.9. Triple negative breast cancer therefore appears to be the ideal study group with which to test benefit of perioperative ketorolac in a clinical trial.

The incidence of TNBC is 12% in US population (as mentioned), 25% among African Americans, and 25–35% among patients from India and Korea [99–101]. In sub-Saharan Africa the TNBC incidence is apparently about 70%. (There may be other as yet unexamined groups also with high incidence of TNBC.) Locations with relatively high incidence of TNBC would be ideal places to conduct a clinical trial in order to make it easier to show an improvement in early relapse.

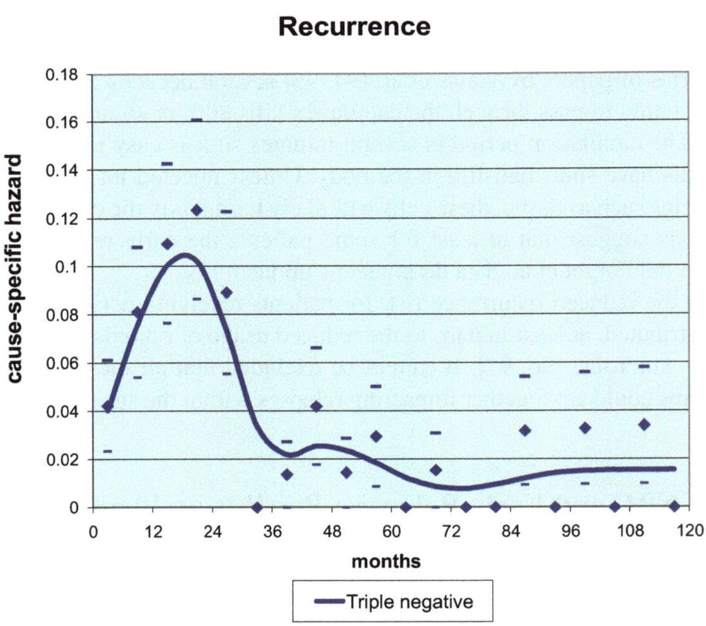

Fig. 2.12 Triple negative breast cancer data base from Milan that we analyzed with our hazard methods

As noted by Wallace et al., the racial disparity in breast cancer outcome is due primarily to deaths within the first few years after diagnosis providing an additional motivation to test at the earliest opportunity what we report here [102]. That would be consistent with the information just noted.

2.12 Current Activities

2.12.1 Focus on India and Nigeria

After speaking at an important conference on Challenging Dogma in Cancer in Mumbai, India at the Tata Memorial Centre in March 2016, Retsky was invited to visit a hospital in Surat, India. He gave the Tata presentation to the surgical staff and suggested a clinical trial is needed. The chief of surgery agreed and expressed intent to submit a proposal to their Institutional Review Board. They suggested including neighboring hospitals in such a trial. Ketorolac is already used in breast cancer for pain relief after mastectomy at the Surat Hospital so this would not be a major change for them. Health care is provided very inexpensively for all citizens by the government in India. The chief of surgery is now retired so a trial may not occur in that hospital but based on that discussion, it would seem reasonably feasible to conduct a trial of perioperative NSAID in India.

Retsky visited Abuja, Nigeria in September 2015 and May 2016. That is another good opportunity for a clinical trial of perioperative ketorolac. We knew that TNBC is very common in sub-Saharan Africa and particularly Nigeria. Considering our contacts in Nigeria, we were very interested in proposing a clinical trial there. However first we needed to recommend some means of recruiting patients with early stage breast cancer since we knew that most patients there present with locally advanced or late stage disease. What can we suggest as a method to increase women with breast lumps to seek medical care before it is too late for our therapy to make a difference? Before Retsky visited Nigeria in May 2016 to give an invited talk, our group had a very interesting discussion that lasted for about a week on email. A face to face meeting was not possible since we are scattered in four different countries. Retsky started the meeting with an email message to all. He said that Michael Baum is probably the world's authority on advantages and disadvantages of mammography. Should we recommend mammography to detect early stage breast cancer in Nigeria? They have essentially no infrastructure to conduct early detection. It is a blank slate. We knew from our collaboration with the late Isaac Gukas that women with a breast lump are reluctant to see a surgeon since it is common folklore that the cancer spreads after surgery or words to that effect. The word Isaac used was that the surgery "provoked" the cancer. Despite the known problem of over-diagnosis with use of mammography in US and Europe, Retsky was proposing to use mammography to detect early stage cancer in Nigeria. Baum argued instead that a country like Nigeria could not afford to train a new generation of radiologists and to purchase and maintain expensive mammography equipment. Perhaps there are other options. One of us found Corbex et al. and Devi et al. papers [103, 104]) and we immediately recognized that their description of what was done in Malaysia could be an excellent solution for Nigeria. The following abstract was written after our meeting. This was presented in Abuja, Nigeria in February 2016 and describes our current suggestion for Nigeria:

> Access to low cost treatment and team work among healthcare workers is key to the effective diagnosis and management of Cancers in Developing Countries. [105].
> Michael Retsky, Ph.D.
> Staff-Harvard TH Chan School of Public Health and Honorary Faculty—University College London.
> Breast cancer is a major health concern in many countries in the world. My research is based in US and UK and while we share a serious breast cancer problem with Nigeria, there are differences that may help us propose methods to improve outcome in general. The US has a multi-racial population and we know, while the incidence is lower, there is a racial disparity in outcome for African Americans (AA) compared to European Americans (EA) of 1.5–2.2-fold. However this racial disparity inverts as age of diagnosis increases. That is, AA present at average age 46 while EA present at average age 57. However AA who happen to present at or above age 57 have superior outcome compared to EA. Thus there must be a biological explanation to racial disparity likely related to age at onset rather than reduced access to quality medical care as one might suspect. It is easier to solve a biological problem than a socioeconomic problem. What is biologically different about breast cancer in AA compared to EA? The main differences are that breast cancer in AA presents early, is typically triple negative (TNBC) and metastatic relapses occur within a few years of surgery. There are no known biological receptors for TNBC that would indicate the effectiveness of any known targeted therapy. The only therapy that is used in treating TNBC is conventional chemotherapy. These drugs have been available for decades, are toxic and are only slightly effective.
> As would be expected, breast cancer in Nigeria is very similar to AA, diagnosed at average age 43 years, is very commonly TNBC, and relapses occur shortly after tumor removal.
> My colleagues and I have proposed that the surgery to remove a primary breast cancer causes a systemic inflammatory response in the host that initiates early metastatic activity. We think this is most common in young women and could be prevented if there was a method to prevent inflammation from surgery. Based on a retrospective study by my Belgian colleague, ketorolac, a very low cost non-toxic common non-steroidal anti-inflammatory drug (NSAID) that is sometimes used just before surgery to prevent pain seems to prevent early relapses. Nigeria would be an ideal place to confirm this result. If it works as we suspect, it could be used anywhere. A protocol for a clinical trial in Nigeria was written by Demicheli [106].

We think this perioperative NSAID therapy needs to be used in patients before the cancer is locally advanced. However, more often than not, breast cancer patients in Nigeria first see a physician only after the cancer has already become locally advanced (inoperable). This same late presentation problem has been dramatically reduced in Malaysia by reducing the time between first abnormal breast appearance and seeing a physician [103, 104]. This clinical down-staging program covering a population of 1.1 million women managed to reduce late presentation from 60 to 35% in less than 5 years. The program consisted of training by a teaching team (3 medical staff and 6 nurses) and about 400 first line health staff throughout the state and cost less than US $34,000. To conduct a clinical trial of perioperative NSAID in Nigeria as we propose, something similar needs to be conducted here.

See Osaro Nelson's chapter on breast cancer in Nigeria [107] and we coauthored a book on treatment of breast cancer in Nigeria [108]. As mentioned, a protocol was published for treating patients with perioperative NSAID ketorolac in Nigeria. There are two key features that should be noted. First the anti-cancer action of perioperative ketorolac has been separated from the analgesic process. That is, ketorolac is used to try preventing relapses, with other standard measures to prevent pain from the primary surgery. The second is that ketorolac is scheduled to be used perioperatively as expected but additionally continued every 8 h for the 3 days post surgery to expand its anti-inflammatory action within its appropriate use. Despite the many concerns fully documented by the Erhabor et al. chapter, we find Nigeria to be an excellent place to conduct a clinical trial of perioperative ketorolac.

2.13 Analysis of Data from Norway on Relapse Hazard After Delayed Reconstruction

Demicheli and coauthors analyzed data on 312 patients who had reconstruction after mastectomy but the reconstruction was delayed (median time to reconstruction 33 months after original mastectomy). Thus they could look at relapse hazard counting time either from the day of mastectomy or from the day of reconstruction. Both ways of setting the clock to zero produced the same two waves of relapses. In each case, the first wave was at 18 months and the second wave was at 50–60 months. The magnitude of the 18 month peak was related to the extent of surgery. For simple implant the peak was not large but for the more extensive Tram-Flap procedure, the magnitude was large. The conclusion was that a surgical maneuver seems to be the initiating step in the metastatic activity from dormancy. It seems that this eliminates the possibility of cancer cells physically released during the incision as a cause of early relapse—at least in this situation (acknowledgement to Robert Weinberg for this observation). The notion that gives a minor role, if any, to CTCs released by primary tumor is in keeping with the above reported findings on pre-surgical CTC detection and on peritoneovenous shunting for malignant ascites [109].

2.14 Concerns About Bleeding Complications

One of the issues related to the perioperative use of ketorolac has been concern about bleeding complications. There are mixed reports of excessive bleeding with use of perioperative ketorolac [110]. In our opinion, these concerns, while real, pale in significance compared to the concerns about surgery induced inflammation that can lead to over half of all relapses in breast cancer.

2.15 Summary

Careful analysis of breast cancer recurrences suggests a paradigm where early recurrences, i.e. the majority of adverse events resulting in poor prognosis, are induced by angiogenic switching of avascular micrometastases and single cell activation. Both events are triggered by primary tumor surgical removal.

Results reported by Forget et al. analysis of retrospective data, suggesting perioperative NSAID ketorolac significantly reduces early relapses, may be deciphered in the light of this model. Indeed, post-surgical transient systemic inflammation might be the precipitating factor and common denominator for early relapses. In particular, inflammation would be important for angiogenesis induction of avascular distant micrometastases.

A few points need further investigations. First, the Forget et al. findings need to be confirmed in randomized clinical trials. Such investigations are imperative not only from the scientific point of view but more so for their possible clinical consequences, resulting from the fact that breast cancer mortality could be reduced by 25 to over 50% at low cost and toxicity. A subset of patients for a randomized clinical trial should be characterized by unfavorable prognostic factors resulting in early recurrences covering the first 2–3 years. We suggest that the best breast cancer population for such a trial may be triple negative breast cancer and particularly when onset is early as exists in sub-Saharan Africa.

In spite of the fact that breast cancer is known as a disease that runs its course in a decade or more, most of the relevant events resulting in recurrences apparently occur shortly after primary surgery. Investigations focused on events occurring during the first few days and weeks following primary tumor removal are strongly warranted.

There have been very exciting recent developments in methods to prolong life with metastatic cancer. That is welcome news indeed. We are proposing upstream improvements in cancer care that together with the downstream improvements should result in major reductions in the worldwide cancer problem. The new path outlined here could be a revolutionary break ("Something for nothing" rarely if ever happened in cancer therapy) from the past and should also be explored in other neoplasias. High priority should be given to test this hypothesis as it is implementable regardless of state of socio-economic development because of its low cost.

Table 2.3

1. Early relapses in breast cancer which comprise the majority of relapses consist of surges of angiogenesis and single cell activation from dormant states. These events are triggered by primary surgery
2. Forget et al. retrospective data suggest perioperative NSAID ketorolac reduces early relapses fivefold. *While we are cautiously optimistic, this still needs to be confirmed.* If confirmed, this may reduce breast cancer mortality by 25–50% at low cost and toxicity. As the only possible adverse effects, there are the usual risks associated with NSAIDs
3. These data suggest transient systemic inflammation is the precipitating factor resulting in angiogenesis and single cell growth from dormancy. We do not claim to know all the relevant processes but it does seem that systemic inflammation is an initiating event
4. Breast cancer runs its course in over a decade but relevant events leading to relapse seem to occur in the week after surgery.
5. Based on computations using our simulation, this suggests metastatic progression is amplified by perhaps 100-fold during the week post primary surgery
6. A small trial is underway in Belgium and we have identified India and especially sub-Saharan Africa as excellent places to conduct a clinical trial (high incidence of TNBC & early onset). Protocol is published [106]. Retsky visited Nigeria July 2015 and May 2016
7. As ketorolac is about $2, used at most a few times per patient and there are approximately two million new breast cancer cases discovered every year, an expenditure of $10 million could reduce the breast cancer problem by 25–50% in the world. (That is both the good news and the bad news.)

2.16 Conclusions

To be clear, we are discussing an *unsolved 2000 year old problem in oncology to which we are late-comers* (Table 2.3).

Acknowledgements Many people other than the authors have participated in this project. Contributions were made by Robert Wardwell, Jack Speer, Douglas Swartzendruber, Victor Petrosky, Paul Bame, Vikas Sukhatme, Patrice Forget, Rick Rogers, Katherina Pachmann, Marc DeKock, Gianni Bonadonna, Judah Folkman, Pinuccia Valagussa, Isaac Gukas, Jayant Vaidya, and Michael Baum. The authors wish to acknowledge the seminal work of friends and mentors Judah Folkman and Bernard Fisher. Much of this work was supported by a grant from The Komen Foundation 2010-2014. An SBIR grant from NIH in 1995 was used to develop the computer simulation reported in 1997. A number of figures and several sections of text were taken from Retsky et al. CMC 2013 [1] with permission of Bentham Science Publishers.

Conflicts of interest Michael Retsky is on the board of directors of the Colon Cancer Alliance. No other COIs to report.

References

1. Retsky M, Demicheli R, Hrushesky WJ, Forget P, De Kock M, Gukas I, Rogers RA, Baum M, Sukhatme V, Vaidya JS (2013) Reduction of breast cancer relapses with perioperative non-steroidal anti-inflammatory drugs: new findings and a review. Curr Med Chem 20(33):4163–4176. Review. PubMed PMID: 23992307; PubMed Central PMCID: PMC3831877. https://www.ncbi.nlm.nih.gov/pmc/articles/PMC3831877/

2. Ariel I (1994) A historical review of breast cancer treatment. In: Johnson H, Wise L (eds) Breast cancer: controversies in management. Futura, Armonk
3. University of Chicago Oriental Institute. https://oi.uchicago.edu/research/publications/oip/edwin-smith-surgical-papyrus-volume-1-hieroglyphic-transliteration
4. US Center for Disease Control. https://www.cdc.gov/cancer/breast/statistics
5. Retsky M, Demicheli R (2017) Introduction. Springer, New York, p xvii
6. Sikora K (1999) Developing a global strategy for cancer. Eur J Cancer 35:1870–1877
7. Demicheli R, Abbattista A, Miceli R, Valagussa P, Bonadonna G (1996) Time distribution of the recurrence risk for breast cancer patients undergoing mastectomy: further support about the concept of tumor dormancy. Breast Cancer Res Treat 41(2):177–185. PubMed PMID: 8944336
8. Baum M (1996) Does surgery disseminate or accelerate cancer? Lancet 347(8996):260. PubMed PMID: 8551898
9. Retsky MW, Demicheli R, Hrushesky WJ, Baum M, Gukas ID (2008) Dormancy and surgery-driven escape from dormancy help explain some clinical features of breast cancer. APMIS 116(7–8):730–741. doi:10.1111/j.1600-0463.2008.00990.x. Review. PubMed PMID: 18834415
10. Bonadonna G, Valagussa P, Moliterni A, Zambetti M, Brambilla C (1995) Adjuvant cyclophosphamide, methotrexate, and fluorouracil in node-positive breast cancer: the results of 20 years of follow-up. N Engl J Med 332(14):901–906. PubMed PMID: 7877646
11. Retsky M, Demicheli R, Hrushesky W, Baum M, Gukas I (2010) Surgery triggers outgrowth of latent distant disease in breast cancer: an inconvenient truth? Cancers (Basel) 2(2):305–337. doi:10.3390/cancers2020305. PubMed PMID: 24281072; PubMed Central PMCID: PMC3835080
12. Fisher ER, Sass R, Fisher B (1984) Pathologic findings from the National Surgical Adjuvant Project for breast cancers (protocol no. 4). X. Discriminants for tenth year treatment failure. Cancer 53:712–723
13. Laird AK (1965) Dynamics of tumour growth: comparison of growth rates and extrapolation of growth curve to one cell. Br J Cancer 19:278–291
14. Laird AK (1969) Dynamics of growth in tumors and in normal organisms. Natl Cancer Inst Monogr 30:15–28. PubMed PMID: 5351826
15. Pittello RF, Schabel FM, Skipper HE (1970) The "sensitivity" of resting and dividing cells. Cancer Chemother Rep Part 1 54(3):137–142
16. Norton L (1988) A Gompertzian model of human breast cancer growth. Cancer Res 48(24 Pt 1):7067–7071. PubMed PMID: 3191483
17. Norton L. Cancer log-kill revisited. Am Soc Clin Oncol Educ Book 2014:3–7. doi:10.14694/EdBook_AM.2014.34.3. Review. PubMed PMID: 24857052
18. Demicheli R et al (1994) Local recurrences following mastectomy: support for the concept of tumor dormancy. J Natl Cancer Inst 86:45–48
19. Sunderland MC, McGuire WL (1990) Prognostic indicators in invasive breast cancer. Surg Clin North Am 70(5):989–1004. Review. PubMed PMID: 2218829
20. Retsky MW, Swartzendruber DE, Wardwell RH, Bame PD (1990) Is Gompertzian or exponential kinetics a valid description of individual human cancer growth? Med Hypotheses 33(2):95–106. PubMed PMID: 2259298. https://www.researchgate.net/publication/20897370_Is_Gompertzian_kinetics_a_valid_description_of_individual_tumor_growth
21. Speer J, Petrosky V, Retsky M, Wardwell R (1984) A stochastic numerical model of breast cancer growth that simulates clinical data. Cancer Res 44:4124–4130
22. Ingleby H, Moore L (1956) Periodic roentgenographic studies of a growing human mammary cancer. Cancer 9(4):749–752. PubMed PMID: 13356257
23. Norton L, Simon R (1986) The Norton-Simon hypothesis revisited. Cancer Treat Rep 70:163–169
24. Retsky M, Swartzendruber D, Wardwell R, Bame P (1989) Petrosky V Correspondence re: Larry Norton, a Gompertzian model of human breast cancer growth. Cancer Res 49:6443–6444. Cancer Res 1988 48:7067–7071

25. Fletcher SW (1997) Whither scientific deliberation in health policy recommendations? Alice in the wonderland of breast-cancer screening. N Engl J Med 336(16):1180–1183. PubMed PMID: 9099666
26. Retsky M, Demicheli R, Hrushesky W (2001) Breast cancer screening for women aged 40-49 years: screening may not be the benign process usually thought. J Natl Cancer Inst 93(20):1572. PubMed PMID: 11604483
27. Retsky MW, Demicheli R, Swartzendruber DE, Bame PD, Wardwell RH, Bonadonna G, Speer JF, Valagussa P (1997) Computer simulation of a breast cancer metastasis model. Breast Cancer Res Treat 45(2):193–202. PubMed PMID: 9342444
28. Demicheli R, Retsky MW, Swartzendruber DE, Bonadonna G (1997) Proposal for a new model of breast cancer metastatic development. Ann Oncol 8(11):1075–1080. Review. PubMed PMID: 9426326
29. Retsky M (2011) Metronomic chemotherapy was originally designed and first used in 1994 for early stage cancer—why is it taking so long to proceed? J Bioequiv Availab 3: 00i–0iv doi:10.4172/jbb.100000e6. https://dash.harvard.edu/bitstream/handle/1/5111470/Retsky_MetronomicChemotherapy.pdf?sequence=1
30. Retsky M (2013) How long should adjuvant chemotherapy be given in early stage colon cancer? J Clin Exp Pathol 3(1):136. doi:10.4172/2161- 0681.1000136. https://dash.harvard.edu/bitstream/handle/1/12559516/Retsky_HowLong.pdf?sequence=1
31. Retsky MW et al (2014) Ecancermedicalscience 8:ed38
32. Cooke R (2001) Dr. Folkman's war—angiogenesis and the struggle to defeat cancer. Random House, New York, pp 346–348
33. Bernstein J. MIA in the war on cancer: where are the low-cost treatments? http://www.propublica.org/article/where-are-the-low-cost-cancer-treatments
34. Hamard L, Ratel D, Selek L, Berger F, van der Sanden B, Wion D (2016) The brain tissue response to surgical injury and its possible contribution to glioma recurrence. J Neurooncol 128(1):1–8. doi:10.1007/s11060-016-2096-y. Epub 2016 Mar 9. Review. PubMed PMID: 26961772.
35. Demicheli R, Fornili M, Ambrogi F, Higgins K, Boyd JA, Biganzoli E, Kelsey CR (2012) Recurrence dynamics for non-small cell lung cancer: effect of surgery on the development of metastases. J Thorac Oncol 7(4):723–730
36. Maniwa Y, Okada M, Ishii N, Kiyooka K (1998) Vascular endothelial growth factor increased by pulmonary surgery accelerates the growth of micrometastases in metastatic lung cancer. Chest 114(6):1668–1675. PubMed PMID: 9872204
37. Smithers DW (1968) Clinical assessment of growth-rate in human tumors. Clin Radiol 19:113
38. Bergh J, Jönsson PE, Glimelius B, Nygren P, SBU-Group (2001) Swedish council of technology assessment in health care a systematic overview of chemotherapy effects in breast cancer. Acta Oncol 40:253–281
39. Retsky M, Bonadonna G, Demicheli R, Folkman J, Hrushesky W, Valagussa P (2004) Hypothesis: induced angiogenesis after surgery in premenopausal node-positive breast cancer patients is a major underlying reason why adjuvant chemotherapy works particularly well for those patients. Breast Cancer Res 6(4):R372-4. PubMed PMID: 15217504; PubMed Central PMCID: PMC468653
40. Retsky M, Demicheli R, Hrushesky W (2001) Premenopausal status accelerates relapse in node positive breast cancer: hypothesis links angiogenesis, screening controversy. Breast Cancer Res Treat 65:217–224
41. Amy Dockser Marcus, The Wall Street Journal, September 13, 2005; Page D1 probing surgery's link to cancer recurrence. Some researchers say removing a tumor can trigger a process that leads to new growth
42. Jatoi I, Anderson WF, Rao SR, Devesa SS (2005) Breast cancer trends among black and white women in the United States. J Clin Oncol 23:7836–7841
43. Demicheli R, Retsky MW, Hrushesky WJ, Baum M, Gukas ID, Jatoi I (2007) Racial disparities in breast cancer outcome: insights into host-tumor interactions. Cancer 110:1880–1888

44. Retsky M, Demicheli R, Gukas I, Hrushesky W (2007) Enhanced surgery-induced angiogenesis among premenopausal women may partially explain the breast cancer excess mortality of blacks compared to whites. Int J Surg 5:300–304
45. Gukas I, Jatoi I, Demicheli R, Retsky M, Hrushesky W, Baum M (2009) Complex interplay between race and breast cancer: should this affect breast cancer diagnostic and therapeutic strategies? Curr Med Literature 21:1–8
46. Retsky MW, Hrushesky WJ, Gukas ID (2009) Hypothesis: primary antiangiogenic method proposed to treat early stage breast cancer. BMC Cancer 9:7. PubMed PMID: 19133151; PMCID: PMC2633344
47. Forget P, Vandenhende J, Berliere M, Machiels JP, Nussbaum B, Legrand C, De Kock M (2010) Do intraoperative analgesics influence breast cancer recurrence after mastectomy? A retrospective analysis. Anesth Analg 110(6):1630–1635. http://www.ncbi.nlm.nih.gov/pubmed/20435950
48. Karhade M, Hall C, Mishra P, Anderson A, Kuerer H, Bedrosian I, Krishnamurthy S, Lucci A (2014) Circulating tumor cells in non-metastatic triple-negative breast cancer. Breast Cancer Res Treat 147(2):325–333. doi:10.1007/s10549-014-3103-7. PubMed PMID: 25164970; PubMed Central PMCID:PMC4149877
49. Gottschalk A, Sharma S, Ford J, Durieux ME, Tiouririne M (2010) Review article: the role of the perioperative period in recurrence after cancer surgery. Anesth Analg 110(6): 1636–1643
50. Horowitz M, Neemna E, Ben Eliyahu S (2015) Nat Rev Clin Oncol 12:213–226; published online 20 January 2015. doi:10.1038/nrclinonc.2014.224
51. El Saghir NS, Elhajj II, Geara FB, Hourani MH (2005) Trauma associated growth of suspected dormant micrometastasis. BMC Cancer 5:94
52. Martins-Green M, Boudreau N, Bissell MJ (1994) Inflammation is responsible for the development of wound-induced tumors in chickens infected with Rous sarcoma virus. Cancer Res 54(16):4334–4341. [PubMed]
53. Retsky M (2005) Comment—what would explain the sudden growth of lung cancer after minor trauma reported by El Saghir et al? BMC Cancer 5:94. https://bmccancer.biomedcentral.com/articles/10.1186/1471-2407-5-94/comments
54. Paget S (1889) The distribution of secondary growth in cancer of the breast. Lancet 1:571–573
55. Martin P, Parkhurst SM (2004) Parallels between tissue repair and embryo morphogenesis. Development 131:3021–3034
56. Werner S, Grose R (2003) Regulation of wound healing by growth factors and cytokines. Physiol Rev 83:835–870
57. Badiavas EV, Abedi M, Butmarc J, Falanga V, Quesenberry P (2003) Participation of bone marrow derived cells in cutaneous wound healing. J Cell Physiol 196:245–250
58. Balkwill F, Mantovani A (2001) Inflammation and cancer: back to Virchow? Lancet 357(9255):539–545. [PubMed]
59. Walter ND, Rice PL, Redente EF, Kauvar EF, Lemond L, Aly T, Wanebo K, Chan ED (2011) Wound healing after trauma may predispose to lung cancer metastasis: review of potential mechanisms. Am J Respir Cell Mol Biol 44(5):591–596. [PubMed]
60. Jones FS, Rous P (1914) On the cause of the localization of secondary tumors at points of injury. J Exp Med 20(4):404–412. [PMC free article] [PubMed]
61. Pascual M, Alonso S, Parés D, Courtier R, Gil MJ, Grande L, Pera M (2011) Randomized clinical trial comparing inflammatory and angiogenic response after open versus laparoscopic curative resection for colonic cancer. Br J Surg 98(1):50–59. [PubMed]
62. Chow LW, Yuen KY, Woo PC, Wei WI (2000) Clarithromycin attenuates mastectomy-induced acute inflammatory response. Clin Diagn Lab Immunol 7(6):925–931. [PMC free article] [PubMed]
63. Perez-Rivas LG, Jerez JM, Fernandez-De Sousa CE, de Luque V, Quero C, Pajares B, Franco L, Sanchez-Muñoz A, Ribelles N, Alba E (2012) Serum protein levels following surgery in breast cancer patients: a protein microarray approach. Int J Oncol 41(6):2200–2206. [PubMed]

64. Bonnelykke-Behrndtz ML et al (2017) The impact of wound inflammation on cancer progression; studies in fish and patients. Springer, New York
65. Forget P, DeKock M (2017) Long term consequences of acute inflammation in cancer surgery: new findings and perspectives. Springer, New York
66. Egawa G, Nakamizo S, Natsuaki Y, Doi H, Miyachi Y, Kabashima K (2013) Intravital analysis of vascular permeability in mice using two-photon microscopy. Sci Rep 3:1932. doi:10.1038/srep01932. PubMed PMID: 23732999; PubMed Central PMCID: PMC3671357
67. Keibel A, Singh V, Sharma MC (2009) Inflammation, microenvironment, and the immune system in cancer progression. Curr Pharm Des 15(17):1949–1955. [PubMed]
68. McAllister SS, Weinberg RA (2014) The tumour-induced systemic environment as a critical regulator of cancer progression and metastasis. Nat Cell Biol 16(8):717–727. doi:10.1038/ncb3015. Review. PubMed PMID: 25082194
69. Allavena P, Mantovani A (2012) Immunology in the clinic review series; focus on cancer: tumour-associated macrophages: undisputed stars of the inflammatory tumour microenvironment. Clin Exp Immunol 167(2):195–205. [PMC free article] [PubMed]
70. Mantovani A, Marchesi F, Porta C, Sica A, Allavena P (2007) Inflammation and cancer: breast cancer as a prototype. Breast 16(Suppl 2):S27–S33. [PubMed]
71. Carmeliet P, Jain RK (2000) Angiogenesis in cancer and other tissues. Nature 407:249–257. [PubMed]
72. Favaro E, Amadori A, Indraccolo S (2008) Cellular interaction in the vascular niche: implications in the regulation of tumour dormancy. APMIS 116:648–659. [PubMed]
73. Butler JM, Kobayashi H, Rafii S (2010) Instructive role of the vascular niche in promoting tumour growth and tissue repair by angiocrine factors. Nat Rev Cancer 10(2):138–146. [PMC free article] [PubMed]
74. Bao B, Ahmad A, Kong D, Ali S, Azmi AS, Li Y, Banerjee S, Padhye S, Sarkar FH (2012) Hypoxia induced aggressiveness of prostate cancer cells is linked with deregulated expression of VEGF, IL-6 and miRNAs that are attenuated by CDF. PLoS One 7(8):e43726. [PMC free article] [PubMed]
75. Tveito S, Andersen K, Kåresen R, Fodstad Ø (2011) Analysis of EpCAM positive cells isolated from sentinel lymph nodes of breast cancer patients identifies subpopulations of cells with distinct transcription profiles. Breast Cancer Res. 13(4):R75. [PMC free article] [PubMed]
76. Kavanagh DP, Kalia N (2011) Hematopoietic stem cell homing to injured tissues. Stem Cell Rev 7(3):672–682. [PubMed]
77. Domanska UM, Kruizinga RC, Nagengast WB, Timmer-Bosscha H, Huls G, de Vries EGE, Walenkamp AME (2013) A review on CXCR4/CXCL12 axis in oncology: no place to hide. Eur J Cancer 49(1):219–230. http://dx.doi.org/10.1016/j.ejca.2012.05.005. [PubMed]
78. Morré DJ, Morre DM (2006) tNOX, an alternative target to COX-2 to explain the anticancer activities of non-steroidal anti-inflammatory drugs (NSAIDS). Mol Cell Biochem 283(1–2):159–167. [PubMed]
79. Klement GL, Yip TT, Cassiola F, Kikuchi L, Cervi D, Podust V, Italiano JE, Wheatley E, Abou-Slaybi A, Bender E, Almog N, Kieran MW, Folkman J (2009) Platelets actively sequester angiogenesis regulators. Blood 113(12):2835–2842. [PMC free article] [PubMed]
80. Pakneshan P, Birsner AE, Adini I, Becker CM, D'Amato RJ (2008) Differential suppression of vascular permeability and corneal angiogenesis by nonsteroidal anti-inflammatory drugs. Invest Ophthalmol Vis Sci 49(9):3909–3913. [PubMed]
81. Lönnroth C, Andersson M, Nordgren S, Lundholm K (2012) Downregulation of Prominin 1/CD133 expression in colorectal cancer by NSAIDs following short-term preoperative treatment. Int J Oncol 41(1):15–23. [PubMed]
82. Krebs MG, Hou JM, Ward TH, Blackhall FH, Dive C (2010) Circulating tumour cells: their utility in cancer management and predicting outcomes. Ther Adv Med Oncol 2(6):351–365. [PMC free article] [PubMed]
83. Zhe X, Cher ML, Bonfil RD (2011) Circulating tumor cells: finding the needle in the haystack. Am J Can Res 1(6):740–751. [PMC free article] [PubMed]

84. Meng S, Tripathy D, Frenkel EP, Shete S, Naftalis EZ, Huth JF, Beitsch PD, Leitch M, Hoover S, Euhus D, Haley B, Morrison L, Fleming TP, Herlyn D, Terstappen LW, Fehm T, Tucker TF, Lane N, Wang J, Uhr JW (2004) Circulating tumor cells in patients with breast cancer dormancy. Clin Cancer Res 10(24):8152–8162. [PubMed]
85. Camara O, Kavallaris A, Nöschel H, Rengsberger M, Jörke C, Pachmann K (2006) Seeding of epithelial cells into circulation during surgery for breast cancer: the fate of malignant and benign mobilized cells. World J Surg Oncol 4:67. [PMC free article] [PubMed]
86. Daskalakis M, Mavroudis D, Sanidas E, Apostolaki S, Askoxylakis I, de Bree E, Georgoulias V, Melissas J (2011) Assessment of the effect of surgery on the kinetics of circulating tumour cells in patients with operable breast cancer based on cytokeratin-19 mRNA detection. Eur J Surg Oncol 37(5):404–410. [PubMed]
87. GrØgaard HK, Solheim S, Landsverk KS, Seljeflot I, Hoffmann P, Arnesen H, Ilebekk A (2011) Circulating CD34+ progenitor cells and growth factors in patients treated with PCI for acute myocardial infarction or stable angina pectoris. Scand J Clin Lab Invest 71:322–329. [PubMed]
88. Takemoto Y, Li TS, Kubo M, Ohshima M, Ueda K, Harada E, Enoki T, Okamoto M, Mizukami Y, Murata T, Hamano K (2011) Operative injury accelerates tumor growth by inducing mobilization and recruitment of bone marrow-derived stem cells. Surgery 149(6):792–800. [PubMed]
89. Dvorak HF (1986) Tumors: wounds that do not heal. Similarities between tumor stroma generation and wound healing. N Engl J Med 315(26):1650–1659. [PubMed]
90. Rothwell PM, Wilson M, Price J, Belch JF, Meade TW, Mehta Z (2012) Effect of daily aspirin on risk of cancer metastasis: a study of incident cancers during randomised controlled trials. Lancet 379(9826):1591–1601. [PubMed]
91. Stucker M, Baier V, Reuther T, Hoffmann K, Kellam K, Altmeyer P (1996) Capillary blood velocity in human skin capillaries located perpendicularly to the skin surface: measured by a new laser Doppler anemometer. Microvasc Res 52:188–192. [PubMed]
92. Mehlen P, Puisieux A (2006) Metastasis: a question of life or death. Nat Rev Cancer 6(6):449–458. Review. PubMed PMID: 16723991. [PubMed]
93. Tarin D, Price JE, Kettlewell MG, Souter RG, Vass AC, Crossley B (1984) Mechanisms of human tumor metastasis studied in patients with peritoneovenous shunts. Cancer Res 44(8):3584–3592
94. Barbera-Guillem E, Weiss L (1993) Cancer-cell traffic in the liver. III lethal deformation of B16 melanoma cells in liver sinusoids. Int J Cancer 54(5):880–884. PubMed PMID: 8325713
95. Barbera-Guillem E, Smith I, Weiss L (1993) Cancer-cell traffic in the liver. II. Arrest, transit and death of B16F10 and M5076 cells in the sinusoids. Int J Cancer 53(2):298–301. PubMed PMID: 8425768
96. Burke JP, Pestotnik SL, Classen DC, Lloyd JF (1996) Evaluation of the financial impact of ketorolac tromethamine therapy in hospitalized patients. Clin Ther 18(1):197–211. [PubMed]
97. Gach K, Wyrębska A, Fichna J, Janecka A (2011) The role of morphine in regulation of cancer cell growth. Naunyn Schmiedebergs Arch Pharmacol 384(3):221–230. [PMC free article] [PubMed]
98. Elias, A,D (2010) Triple-negative breast cancer: a short review. Am J Clin Oncol 33(6): 637–645
99. Manjunath S, Prabhu JS, Kaluve R, Correa M, Sridhar TS (2011) Estrogen receptor negative breast cancer in India: do we really have higher burden of this subtype? Indian J Surg Oncol 2(2):122–125
100. Keam B, Im SA, Kim HJ, Oh DY, Kim JH, Lee SH, Chie EK, Han W, Kim DW, Moon WK, Kim TY, Park IA, Noh DY, Heo DS, Ha SW, Bang YJ (2007) Prognostic impact of clinic pathologic parameters in stage II/III breast cancer treated with neoadjuvant docetaxel and doxorubicin chemotherapy: paradoxical features of the triple negative breast cancer. BMC Cancer 7:203
101. Patil VW, Singhai R, Patil V, Gurav PD (2011) Triple-negative (ER, PgR, HER-2/neu) breast cancer in Indian women. Breast Cancer 3:9–19

102. Wallace TA, Martin DN, Ambs S (2011) Interactions among genes, tumor biology and the environment in cancer health disparities: examining the evidence on a national and global scale. Carcinogenesis 32(8):1107–1121
103. Corbex M, Burton R, Sancho-Garnier H (2012) Breast cancer early detection methods for low and middle income countries, a review of the evidence. Breast 21(4):428–434. doi:10.1016/j.breast.2012.01.002. Epub 2012 Jan 30. Review. PubMed PMID: 22289154
104. Devi BC, Tang TS, Corbex M (2007) Reducing by half the percentage of late-stage presentation for breast and cervix cancer over 4 years: a pilot study of clinical downstaging in Sarawak, Malaysia. Ann Oncol 18(7):1172–1176. Epub 2007 Apr 13
105. Retsky M (2016) Abuja, Nigeria
106. Demicheli R, Osaro E, Retsky M, Patrice F, Vaidya JS, Bello SO (2016) Protocol for a randomised, multicentre, double blinded phase iii study of perioperative ketorolac in women of African descent with operable breast cancer. J Intern Med 2(1):017. http://internalmedicine.jacobspublishers.com/images/Internal_Med/J_J_Intern_Medicine_2_1_017.pdf
107. Osaro E (2017) Randomized clinical trials on breast cancer in Nigeria and other developing countries—challenges and constraints. Springer, New York
108. Challenges associated with the diagnosis and management of breast cancer in Nigeria—the need for affordable and accessible care, Erhabor O, Abdulrahaman Y, Retsky M, Forget P, Vaidya JS, Bello O, Adias TC, Dagana A, Egenti BN, Mainasara AS, Sahabi SM, Rilwanu TI, Ahmed Y, Hassan M, Ifedayo A, Okara GC, Lori J, Ibiang L. AuthorHouse™ UK 1663 Liberty Drive Bloomington, IN 47403 USA. www.authorhouse.co.uk
109. Dillekås H, Demicheli R, Ardoino I, Jensen SA, Biganzoli E, Straume O (2016) The recurrence pattern following delayed breast reconstruction after mastectomy for breast cancer suggests a systemic effect of surgery on occult dormant micrometastases. Breast Cancer Res Treat 158:169–178
110. Gobble RM, Hoang HL, Kachniarz B, Orgill DP. Ketorolac does not increase perioperative bleeding: a meta-analysis of randomized controlled trials. Plast Reconstr Surg. 2014 Mar;133(3):741-55. doi: 10.1097/01.prs.0000438459.60474.b5. PubMed PMID: 24572864 http://www.druglib.com/abstract/go/gobble-rm1_plast-reconstr-surg_20140000.html

Chapter 3
Peri-operative Shift in Angiogenesis-Related Factors in Breast Cancer Patients

Georgios K. Georgiou and Evangelos Briasoulis

Abstract Surgery still remains the cornerstone of breast cancer treatment but in some cases it has been implicated for stimulating early locoregional recurrence or even distant metastatic spread. There is evidence that angiogenesis, initiated by the surgical wounding itself during the process of healing, could offer valuable answers in such matters as well as enable a more profound understanding of the mechanisms of carcinogenesis in general. In our study, we investigated the impact of breast surgery on circulating angiogenesis-related factors in the peripheral blood. We used plasma samples from ten female patients with biopsy-proven breast cancer (Ca group) and six other females with fibroadenoma (Control group) before surgery (PRO) and post-operatively on days 3 (D3) and 7 (D7, only for breast cancer patients). These samples were analyzed for circulating levels of vascular endothelial growth factor A (VEGF-A), Interleukin-8 (IL-8) and fibroblast growth factor 2 (FGF2/bFGF) using ELISA. Moreover, 84 angiogenesis-associated mRNA transcripts were also assessed using quantitative RT-PCR arrays at the same time points. We were able to find a different angiogenic profile between breast cancer patients and those with benign breast disease (fibroadenoma). The effect of surgery on the mechanism of new blood vessel formation was found to be more robust and far more prolonged in women suffering from malignancy of the breast, than those operated for fibroadenoma. Mastectomy provoked a transient increase in VEGF-A plasma levels and altered the expression of many angiogenesis-related circulating gene transcripts.

Keywords Angiogenesis • mRNA transcripts • Breast cancer • PCR arrays • ELISA

G.K. Georgiou, M.D., M.Sc., Ph.D. (✉)
Department of Surgery, University of Ioannina Medical School, Ioannina, Greece
e-mail: georgmd7@gmail.com

E. Briasoulis, M.D., Ph.D.
Department of Haematology, University of Ioannina Medical School, Ioannina, Greece

M.W. Retsky, R. Demicheli (eds.), *Perioperative Inflammation as Triggering Origin of Metastasis Development*, DOI 10.1007/978-3-319-57943-6_3

3.1 Study Outline

We studied ten female patients with core-biopsy proven adenocarcinoma of the mammary gland (either left or right), with or without axillary lymph node involvement. Metastatic disease was excluded during standard diagnostic imaging workup. Patients forming this group of the study (Study Group/Group A) were randomly selected and not according to their disease stage (by means of TNM classification), specific histological subtype, grade or hormonal receptor status. We also included both pre- and post-menopausal women of all ages. This was done in order to study breast cancer patients as a whole and acquire a more general picture of the patients' angiogenic profile, which we thought would be more appropriate if a universal diagnostic biomarker is to be discovered. Moreover, we aimed not at correlating our measurements with clinicopathological patient data (as the number of subjects involved is indeed small), but rather focused on the shift in kinetics of factors studied as a result of surgery.

We solely applied a number of exclusion criteria in an effort to avoid unwanted parallel neo-angiogenesis stimulation due to other causes, since it is already known that certain pathological circumstances can also initiate neo-angiogenesis in adults, whose vascular network normally rests in a quiescent state (except for female endometrium during the menstrual cycle). For example, patients suffering from diabetes mellitus present with microangiopathy and often have microvessel formation [1]. Other pathological entities in which neo-angiogenesis may be triggered are chronic inflammatory diseases and autoimmune diseases (rheumatoid arthritis, inflammatory bowel disease etc.), perhaps in the context of robust expression of inflammatory mediators (IL-1, IL-8, TNF, etc.) which are also involved in angiogenesis [2–4]. Recent trauma or major surgical (or interventional) procedures also promote neo-angiogenesis in the context of wound healing [5, 6]. In addition, a recent history of myocardial infarction or other any major "vascular" event (cerebrovascular ischemia, limb ischemia, etc.) has been shown to promote the angiogenetic process through HIF-1α secretion [3, 7], as also does gross acute systematic inflammation [2, 8]. Finally, erythropoietin administration has been linked with VEGF promotion and making cancer cells less susceptible to ischemia, thus linked with unfavorable prognosis in some studies [9, 10]. Thus we only included patients whose medical history and physical examination was devoid of the above mentioned situations.

These ten breast cancer patients were not studied against healthy individuals but against another group of six females with benign breast disease (imaging-based diagnosis of fibroadenoma). There exist many studies where angiogenesis-related factors are measured in healthy individuals and breast cancer patients for subsequent comparison. However, since our aim was to investigate the longitudinal effect of surgery on angiogenesis, we selected patients that would also undergo breast surgery as Control Group (Group B). Analytic demographic data of all patients involved in the study are presented in Table 3.1.

We first sought to determine the angiogenic profile of each group to see if any differences exist between women with benign and malignant disease. We studied

Table 3.1 Patient demographics

Patient	Age (years)	Disease	Surgical procedure	TNM staging	Grade	Hormonal receptors	HER-2
1	47	Fibroadenoma	Excisional biopsy				
2	41	Fibroadenoma	Excisional biopsy				
3	28	Fibroadenoma	Excisional biopsy				
4	43	Fibroadenoma	Excisional biopsy				
5	32	Fibroadenoma	Excisional biopsy				
6	36	Fibroadenoma	Excisional biopsy				
7	58	Ductal invasive BC (right)	WLE + ALND	$T_{1c}N_1$	2	ER+, PR+	2+
8	60	Ductal invasive BC (left)	MRM + ALND	T_2N_0	2	ER+, PR+	0+
9	50	Ductal invasive BC (right)	MRM + ALND	$T_{1c}N_0$	2	ER+, PR+	2+
10	41	Ductal invasive BC (right)	WLE + ALND	$T_{1b}N_0$	2	ER+, PR+	0+
11	58	Ductal invasive BC (right)	WLE + ALND	T_2N_2	2	ER+, PR+	1+
12	76	Ductal invasive BC (right)	MRM + ALND	T_2N_0	2	ER+, PR+	0+
13	52	Ductal invasive BC (right)	MRM + ALND	T_2N_0	2	ER+, PR+	2+
14	39	Ductal invasive BC (left)	WLE + ALND	$T_{1c}N_1$	3	ER+, PR+	1+
15	55	Ductal invasive BC (right)	MRM + ALND	T_2N_1	2	ER+, PR+	0+
16	43	Ductal invasive BC (left)	WLE + ALND	$T_{1b}N_0$	2	ER+, PR+	2+

WLE + ALND wide local excision and axillary lymph node dissection, *MRM + ALND* modified radical mastectomy and axillary lymph node dissection, *BC* breast adenocarcinoma, *ER+* estrogen receptor positive, *PR+* progesterone receptor positive. Patients No 2, 3, 4, 5, 6, 10, 14 and 16 were premenopausal

the protein expression of three angiogenesis-related molecules, VEGF, IL-8 and bFGF. Then we studied the effect of surgery in these angiogenesis-related factors in both groups, to find any possible alterations in the kinetics of these molecules as a result of the surgery per se. Then we took our study one step backwards, trying to find if these changes were also apparent in the level of gene transcription. We chose to examine a panel of 84 genes, some of which are well-known, others less well-studied or even some that are simply "suspicious" of somehow affecting angiogenesis. Blood samples from the two groups of subjects were taken at the same time-point before and after surgery and at the same time of day each time.

3.2 Special Considerations Regarding Study Design

A common problem when trying to 'monitor' angiogenesis through measuring of circulating angiogenesis-related factors is that tissue wounding itself cannot be easily (if at all) quantified. Performing an excisional biopsy for fibroadenoma with a maximum diameter of 2–3 cm certainly results in not as much tissue trauma as when performing a wide local excision (not to mention modified radical mastectomy) plus axillary lymph node dissection for malignant lesions. In the first case it is rational to think that the wound healing process and angiogenic effects are local, while systematic inflammatory response stimulation is minimal. On the other hand, when performing proper breast cancer surgery the areas traumatized are significantly bigger and result in greater mobilization of the healing mechanisms. So is this comparison justified? At some point yes, if we accept that there can never be two patients undertaking an identical surgical procedure by means of tissue loss, blood loss, operative time, number of sutures applied, etc. Moreover, excising a 3-cm large fibroadenoma from a large breast may be as equal in terms of tissue trauma as performing wide local excision in a woman with a small breast.

Patients in Group A had their malignancy diagnosed by means of performing core-biopsy due to a clinically or radiologically detected suspicious lesion. We were aware that this minor trauma in the breast could also initiate angiogenesis and thus interfere with our baseline (pre-operative) measurements in these patients. Thus we allowed for a substantial period of time (at least 20 days) to elapse between the biopsy procedure and the definite surgery. This "artificial delay" was not done as a means of controlling the data in our study (which could be even regarded as unethical), but it was necessary for acquiring the biopsy results, performing proper disease staging (computed tomography of the brain, lungs and abdomen or bone scan) and preparing the patient for the surgery (anaesthesiologic assessment, adjusting certain drug doses, etc.).

Another important issue in our study is the fact that we chose to conduct our analyses using plasma samples rather than serum, since there is an ongoing debate as to which of the two specimens is most suitable [11]. We used BD Vacutainer® tubes (BD Diagnostics®, NJ USA), containing K2ethylenediaminetetraacetic acid (EDTA) at a concentration of 3.6 mg/ml, which were filled with an additional 2 ml of patient's venous blood for each measurement. What we do know is that platelets (but also leukocytes to some extent) are carriers of preshaped VEGF molecules inside their granules [12, 13]. They may also contain other angiogenesis-related factors (either promoters or inhibitors), which they release in the circulation when they become activated and start to clot, such as in cases of tissue trauma, endothelial cell damage etc. [14, 15]. Thus when measuring VEGF serum levels we calculate both the real circulating levels of the factor and those released from coagulated platelets inside the blood collection tube [16, 17]. However, when we acquire plasma samples we can estimate the exact VEGF levels in the peripheral blood, which are inevitably found to be significantly lower than those measured in serum samples [16, 18].

We performed measurements of circulating angiogenesis-related factors using commercially available ELISA kits (Quantikine ELISA kit, R&D Systems Inc., Minneapolis, MN, USA), as it is a well-described and vastly used low-cost method for measuring levels of proteins in the circulating blood. However, older as well as recent studies have questioned the accuracy and reproducibility of this method [19, 20]. Some assays may measure only certain (out of the numerous) isoforms of VEGF, while others may not be able to identify the portion of VEGF that is protein-bound ($VEGF_{121}$ and $VEGF_{165}$ are the only freely soluble isoforms) [19]. Moreover, it's not uncommon to see significantly different measurements of the same samples when analyzed in different laboratories [20]. This is a reason why it may be quite difficult to find similar values among existing studies even if they have used the same ELISA kit, the same specimen (e.g. plasma sample) and similar groups of patients (e.g. post-menopausal women with stage II breast cancer). Perhaps there should be a well-organized universal effort towards standardizing the method of sampling, handling and analyzing of specimens for possible biomarkers.

On the other hand, real-time PCR is a valuable tool for studying gene expression. It is technically somewhat more demanding, surely more expensive, but enables the simultaneous analysis of a large number of target genes. Our study was the first to assess such a great number of angiogenesis-related genes in different time points before and after surgery for malignant and benign breast disease [21].

3.2.1 VEGF (Vascular Endothelial Growth Factor)

VEGF is one of the most studied angiogenesis-related factors. It was discovered in 1983 and was initially named Vascular Permeability Factor (VPF) [22, 23]. In fact, we have to deal with a superfamily of proteins consisting of VEGF-A, VEGF-B, VEGF-C and VEGF-D, with a molecular weight in the range of 20–45 kDa [24, 25]. VEGF-A, also known as Placental Growth Factor (PlGF), is the main member of this family (in fact when we generally refer to VEGF it is VEGF-A that we're talking about). It acts through binding to three receptors (Receptor Tyrosine Kinases, RTKs), named VEGFR1 (or Flt-1), VEGFR2 (or KDR/Flk-1) and VEGFR3 (or Flt-4), as well as two other non-RTK receptors; neuropilin-1 (NRP-1) and neuropilin-2 (NRP-2) [23, 26, 27]. Moreover, there seem to be numerous different isoforms of

Table 3.2 VEGF-A plasma values of all patients expressed in pg/ml

VEGF-A	PRO	D3	D7
Control-1	13.98	32.07	
Control-2	36.90	60.40	
Control-3	18.76	22.78	
Control-4	10.09	32.88	
Control-5	19.11	20.11	
Control-6	28.00	40.99	
Ca-1	45.06	65.06	52.91
Ca-2	64.66	114.77	71.20
Ca-3	20.09	107.86	22.67
Ca-4	18.07	37.47	25.06
Ca-5	108.54	84.49	285.69
Ca-6	59.71	17.72	16.45
Ca-7	62.76	99.10	70.88
Ca-8	30.12	107.11	40.66
Ca-9	48.00	78.99	60.88
Ca-10	24.71	30.87	31.10

PRO baseline levels (before surgery), *D3* on post-operative day 3, *D7* on post-operative day 7. *Control* patient with fibroadenoma (Control Group), *Ca* breast cancer patient (Study Group)

VEGF-A through alternative splicing, with VEGF-A_{121} and VEGF-A_{165} being the most frequently encountered ones [11].

Under normal circumstances, VEGF-A promotes the proliferation, migration and differentiation of endothelial cells, possesses neurotrophic and neuroprotective properties, while also being necessary for haemopoiesis [27–29]. VEGF-A plays a key-role in the process of angiogenesis as well, a fact that has been well documented both in laboratory and clinical studies. Increased VEGF-A levels have been found in the peripheral blood of patients suffering from myocardial infarction, trauma or different types of cancer, that of breast included [8, 28, 30]. VEGF-A is produced and secreted from cancer cells as a result of stimulation by the hypoxia (or other less known events), binding to hypoxia-inducible factor 1 (HIF-1) and starting the cascade of events that lead to new blood vessel formation [26]. As for VEGF-C and VEGF-D, there is sufficient evidence to involve them in the process of lymphangiogenesis, acting through the receptor VEGFR-3, while their role in angiogenesis seems to be much less important [23, 31, 32].

Several researchers have attempted to investigate the potential role of VEGF-A as a biomarker for breast cancer. Some studies report increased levels of this factor in the circulation of breast cancer patients in comparison to healthy controls [8, 25, 33]. Moreover, there seems to be a positive correlation between circulating levels of VEGF-A and cancer stage, since women with locoregionally advanced disease or metastatic disease exhibit greater levels of this factor in their blood [8, 33–36]. In addition, certain immunohistochemical studies have linked the expression of VEGF-A in surgical specimens of breast cancer patients with disease prognosis [30, 37–40]. Others compare tissue expression of VEGF-A with its circulating levels, in

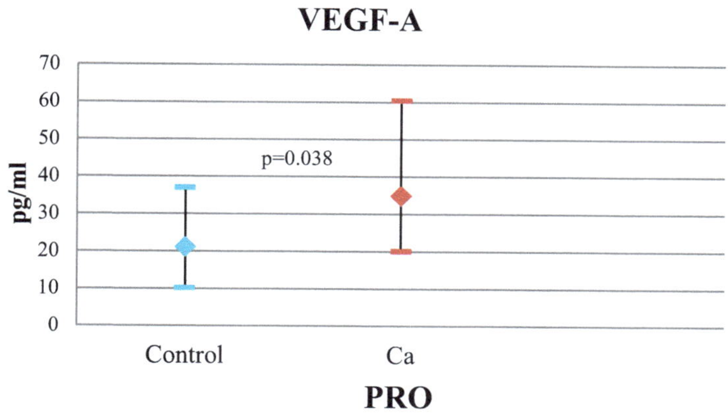

Fig. 3.1 Comparison of baseline (PRO) VEGF-A levels between the two groups

order to investigate the factor's action both regionally and systematically [41–43]. Levels of VEGF-A have also been studied in wound drains and compared to systematic circulation [44, 45].

In our study, we firstly investigated the comparative expression of VEGF in female patients with malignancy of the breast (adenocarcinoma) versus females with non-malignant disease (fibroadenoma). Since angiogenesis is regarded as a crucial step in tumor development, we speculated that women with biopsy-proven breast cancer would exhibit higher levels of this pro-angiogenic factor in the peripheral blood, when compared to healthy non-tumor bearing women. Results can be seen in Table 3.2. This assay has a sensitivity of 9 pg/ml and a detection range of 31.2-2000 pg/ml [46].

Indeed, we found a statistically significant difference (p = *0.038*) in VEGF plasma levels between the two groups, since patients with fibroadenoma had VEGF plasma levels in the range of 10–36.9 pg/ml (mean 21.145 pg/ml), while breast cancer patients VEGF between 18 and 108.54 pg/ml (mean 48.17 pg/ml) (Fig. 3.1).

Similar values have been reported by other investigators as well [14, 47, 48]. Some prefer to measure VEGF levels in serum samples [8, 49–51], while others in plasma [43, 47, 52]. Although our study included a small number of patients in each group, without any kind of stratification according to disease stage, it still provides evidence that breast cancer patients have elevated circulating levels of VEGF, which could be attributed to the adoption of an angiogenic phenotype. Other investigators also confirm the finding of increased circulating VEGF levels in breast cancer patients versus non-cancer patients [35, 48].

Another issue that we set out to investigate was how the surgical wounding could affect the angiogenic mechanism. We tried to answer this question by monitoring VEGF levels and reporting respective changes at certain crucial time-points after surgery. We chose to conduct our measurements on the third and seventh post-operative day for breast cancer patients and on the third post-operative day in the group of patients with fibroadenoma, since existing literature showed those to be the most important time-points for changes in the levels of angiogenic factors [53–56].

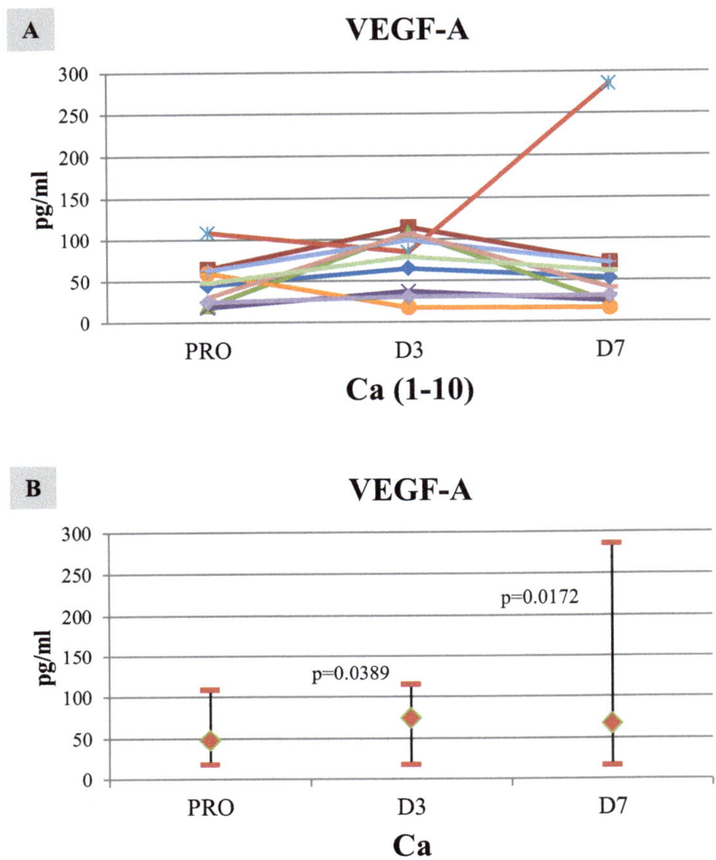

Fig. 3.2 (**a**) Aligned plot of repeated measures of vascular endothelial growth factor A (VEGF-A) with matched values stacked in subcolumns. The outlier (on D7) refers to a patient with locally advanced disease (T2N2) who eventually relapsed. (**b**) Also mean values and statistical significance are depicted

As we can see in Fig. 3.2, breast cancer patients' VEGF levels seem to increase on post-operative day 3 (D3) as compared to pre-operative (PRO) values and then gradually tend to decrease towards post-operative day (D7), while still remaining higher than the PRO (baseline) levels.

This initial post-operative increase was also seen in the patients operated on for fibroadenoma, whose levels also increased on D3 versus PRO ($p = 0.008$). This early post-operative increase in VEGF levels has been documented in other studies as well [56]. It is believed that VEGF plays a crucial role in the initial stages of wound healing (mostly triggered by HIF-1a secretion, which is also an early event) while later on it becomes less important, as other factors take over and complete the process. Thus we can expect that patients with benign disease undergoing a surgical procedure may anticipate their VEGF levels to return to normal (pre-operative values) soon after the wound healing process has successfully concluded [53]. However, breast cancer patients have already initiated angiogenic activity and in these patients the process ensues far beyond the completion of wound healing [57]. This fact may be responsible for the triggering of occult ('dormant' until that time) micrometastatic foci, which in this rich-in-angiogenesis mediators environment turn the 'angiogenic switch' on and initiate neo-angiogenesis [58, 59].

Another fact that was of particular interest in our study was that the greatest VEGF values were seen in the patient with the most advanced clinical stage (T_2N_2) (Fig. 3.2). Moreover, 1 week after the operation she continued having high VEGF values. During routine follow-up she was diagnosed with locoregional recurrence at the axilla 34 months after the initial wide local excision (plus axillary lymph node dissection) and was treated with re-operation (modified radical mastectomy plus axillary revision). We did not attempt to correlate VEGF levels with disease stage, menopausal status and other clinical features, as others have done [33]. Our aim was to document serial measurements of this angiogenic factor at different time points. Although we are talking about findings from a single patient, thus we are not allowed to draw general conclusions, we may be seeing a trend towards elevated VEGF levels in patients with more aggressive disease. Besides, certain studies have also investigated the prognostic value of circulating VEGF levels in breast cancer patients, but we are still far from establishing VEGF as a prognostic biomarker [47].

Moreover, some studies have failed to document increased VEGF levels in the systematic circulation after breast surgery, while discovering a temporary increase locoregionally, as seen in the high VEGF levels coming from fluid samples from the drain tubes [45, 54]. A special barrier mechanism has been proposed between the area of the wound and the systematic circulation, which allows for a locally rich angiogenic environment (necessary for wound healing) while at the same time excluding the rest of the body from the (perhaps negative?) action of VEGF [44, 56].

3.2.2 IL-8 (Interleukin-8)

IL-8, also known as CXCL8, is a small diluted peptide with molecular weight of 8–10 kDa, belonging to the superfamily of CXC-chemokines [60]. It is produced by many cell types, including mononuclears, neutrophils, macrophages, fibroblasts, epithelial, endothelial and cancer cells [61]. The corresponding gene (SCYB8) is located on the 4q12-q21 chromosome [61]. It starts with encoding of a 99-amino-acid long protein, which later on is processed so as to become biologically active with 72 (produced from mononuclears and macrophages) or 77 amino-acids (produced from non-immune cells) [60, 62].

IL-8 is produced and secreted in response to a number of stimuli, such as the activation of the systematic inflammatory response (triggered by TNF-a, IL-1, etc.), stress, hypoxia, sex hormones (androgens, estrogens, etc.) [62]. It acts through 2 G-protein surface receptors, CXCR1 and CXCR2, promoting and altering the expression of a series of transcriptional factors [63, 64]. IL-8 is chemotactic for all

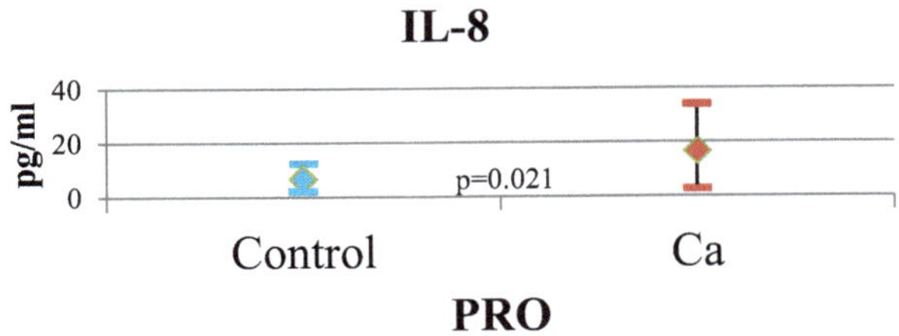

Fig. 3.3 Comparison between plasma IL-8 levels between Control Group and Study Group (Ca)

cells of the immune system, while also possessing the unique feature of polymorphonuclear neutrophils activation [61]. It is a pro-inflammatory cytokine which participates in the process of inflammation and wound healing by stimulating fibroblasts and promoting angiogenesis [61]. On the other hand, there are implications that it is responsible for certain abnormal situations where a pathological immune system is involved, such as cystic fibrosis, asthma, chronic obstructive pulmonary disease and adult respiratory distress syndrome [12, 65–67].

IL-8 seems to be a key-player in oncogenesis and tumor development, even though the exact mechanism for these actions has not yet been fully elucidated [68, 69]. Increased IL-8 levels have been found in the blood vessels that collect the blood from sites of colorectal cancer [70]. In addition, IL-8 seems to interfere in certain crucial steps in the evolution of non-small cell lung cancer [71] or melanoma [72, 73]. Moreover, some cancer types (such as that of the prostate or the ovary) exhibit production of substantial amounts of IL-8, either coming directly from the cancer cells themselves or from elements of the surrounding stroma [61]. As for breast cancer, IL-8 has been shown to have a robust expression in malignant tissue when compared to the normal mammary gland [74]. Moreover, the receptors CXCR1 and CXCR2 also express more strongly in specimens coming from patients suffering from breast cancer than from normal subjects [75]. Regarding angiogenesis, during the last two decades several experimental studies have shown a role for IL-8 in the promotion of new blood vessel formation [76–79]. IL-8 induces the proliferation, chemotaxis and survival of endothelial cells [60]. VEGF-A and hypoxia are major stimulating factors for IL-8 production and secretion [69, 80].

Our study showed that IL-8 plasma levels were significantly raised in breast cancer patients in comparison to women with fibroadenoma ($p = 0.021$) (Fig. 3.3).

Out of the six patients with benign breast disease, three had IL-8 values lower than the detection limit of the ELISA method used and in two of the six the values were slightly above the limit of detection (sensitivity: 7.5 pg/ml, detection range: 31.2–2000 pg/ml) [81] (Table 3.3).

Most researchers report similar results for IL-8 levels, either measured in serum [68, 82–85] or plasma [86, 87]. However, Pusztai et al. failed to detect any significant changes in IL-8 plasma levels between 70 breast cancer patients and 15 healthy controls [88]. Derin et al. also could not detect significant differences between 48 women with breast malignancy and 21 healthy women [89]. However, none of these studies incorporated a control group of women with non-malignant breast disease, as we did.

Peri-operative IL-8 kinetics in plasma of breast cancer patients showed a slight increase on D3 ($p = 0.22$ versus PRO), followed by a sharp decrease towards D7, on

Table 3.3 IL-8 plasma values of all patients expressed in pg/ml

IL-8	PRO	D3	D7
Control-1	7.99	1.09	
Control-2	12.30	22.22	
Control-3	2.00	6.99	
Control-4	1.88	2.99	
Control-5	6.99	6.09	
Control-6	8.01	4.99	
Ca-1	2.59	4.77	6.98
Ca-2	15.10	29.17	23.29
Ca-3	24.59	11.64	14.51
Ca-4	12.71	30.02	1.62
Ca-5	17.67	51.41	10.50
Ca-6	33.71	1.87	2.08
Ca-7	9.89	15.00	5.77
Ca-8	15.99	32.77	7.99
Ca-9	10.09	12.99	3.99
Ca-10	21.00	19.11	2.99

PRO baseline levels (before surgery), *D3* on post-operative day 3, *D7* on post-operative day 7. *Control* patient with fibroadenoma (Control Group), *Ca* breast cancer patient (Study Group)

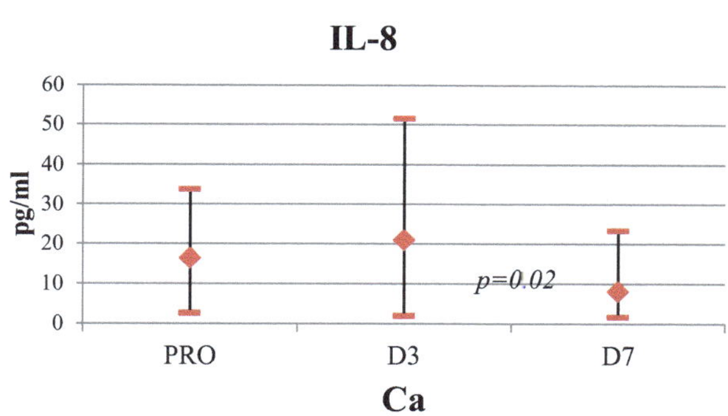

Fig. 3.4 Initial insignificant increase in IL-8 plasma levels on D3, followed by a significant drop below the baseline levels on D7

which IL-8 levels were even lower than the baseline (PRO) ones ($p = 0.02$) (Fig. 3.4). As for the Control Group, changes before and after the procedure were insignificant ($p = 0.368$).

3.2.3 *bFGF (Basic Fibroblast Growth Factor)*

Basic Fibroblast Growth Factor (bFGF) or FGF-2, is a 18 kDa protein encoded by a specific gene located on chromosome 4 and belongs to the FGF superfamily which consists of more than 20 different molecules [90]. They possess pleotropic biological actions (chemotaxis, mitogenic activity, angiogenetic proportions, etc.) since they connect to a number of receptors on different types of cell populations. Apart from the typical RTK-type FGF-ligands of the FGF family (FGFR1, FGFR2, FGFR3 and FGFR4), they also bind to integrins, gangliosides and heparan sulfate proteoglycans [90, 91]. Together with the acidic Fibroblast Growth Factor (aFGF) or FGF-1, they comprise the most important and well-studied molecules of the FGF superfamily.

FGFs participate in certain physiological functions, including the proliferation and migration of several cell types (fibroblasts, smooth muscle fibres, endothelial cells, etc.), while at the same time acting as anti-apoptotic factors promoting cell survival [90, 92, 93]. They are also incorporated in wound healing and organogenesis of heart, lungs, neural system as well as the development of prostate and mammary gland [90, 93]. As for angiogenesis, FGF-1, FGF-2, FGF-4, FGF-5 and FGF-8 are key molecules, influencing the signaling of other factors such as VEGF and cytokines [91, 94].

The exact role for FGFs in carcinogenesis is still unclear. It seems as these factors are excreted by cancer cells or by the surrounding stroma [93]. Experimental studies have shown that it possesses promoting properties regarding the proliferation, survival and invasiveness of cancer cells [95, 96]. Moreover, increased levels of aFGF and its receptor FGFR1 have been found in specimens from breast cancer patients in comparison to healthy controls [97]. Especially in breast cancer, in around 10% of patients there is a significant amplification of the genetic epitope for FGFR1 which is located on the chromosomal region of 8p11-12, a fact that has been linked to poor prognosis in these group of patients [98, 99].

Speaking strictly for aFGF, its presence has been confirmed in different types of tissues and organs, including the kidneys, the brain, as well as all the blood vessels of the human body, in whose layer this factor is in abundance [100]. bFGF was the first angiogenic factor to be isolated in its pure form almost three decades ago, but more recently aFGF is also considered to possess significant angiogenic properties [101, 102]. In particular, aFGF stimulates the migration of endothelial cells and the formation of blood vessels [92, 100]. It acts synergistically with VEGF both during the phase of tissue healing and during the phase of neo-angiogenesis that is seen in cancer [103, 104]. Nevertheless, the exact mechanism of this factors production and secretion remains largely unknown.

FGF-2 over-expression has been documented in some cases of triple-negative breast cancer, a highly-aggressive subtype of this malignant adenocarcinoma of the mammary gland that does not express receptors for estrogen, progesterone or HER-2 (Human EGFR 2/ErbB2) [105]. Certain studies report over-expression of bFGF in the stroma of hormone-dependent (hormone-receptor positive) patients with breast cancer [106]. Most studies report increased expression of bFGF in surgical specimens from women with malignancy when compared to specimens from healthy women [107–109]. However, other researchers found the opposite when using other methodology [108]. As for circulating bFGF, there are only a few studies addressing this issue [110, 111]. Hewala et al. found increased levels of this factor in the blood of breast cancer patients when compared to the control group [111]. Sliutz et al. evaluated bFGF as a ‘surrogate biomarker’ for monitoring

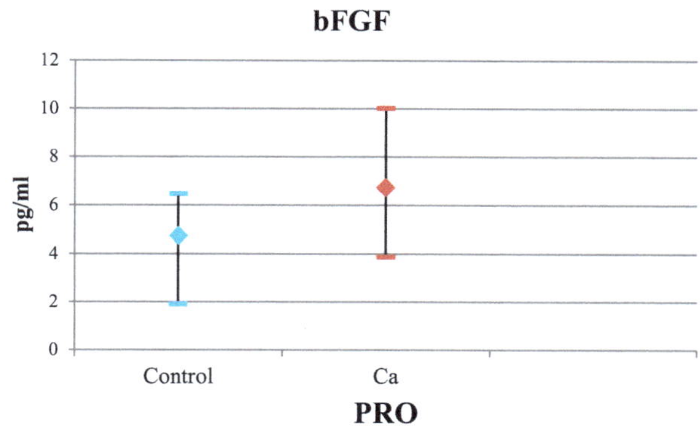

Fig. 3.5 No significant differences in baseline levels of bFGF between the two groups

Table 3.4 All patients bFGF values

bFGF	PRO	D3	D7
Control-1	5.21	7.45	
Control-2	6.12	10.10	
Control-3	3.87	5.00	
Control-4	4.89	4.88	
Control-5	1.90	3.88	
Control-6	6.48	9.11	
Ca-1	1.26	1.16	9.70
Ca-2	1.11	5.33	13.85
Ca-3	3.13	14.78	11.15
Ca-4	1.25	6.13	10.73
Ca-5	4.95	9.26	2.20
Ca-6	23.82	19.96	30.92
Ca-7	3.77	4.00	5.01
Ca-8	7.00	5.59	10.11
Ca-9	1.22	4.11	4.90
Ca-10	4.88	6.99	8.88

response to treatment and detecting recurrences in a small group of patients [112]. Finally, Curigliano et al. reported differences in peri-operative bFGF kinetics depending on the type and the extent of the procedure performed in female breast cancer patients [54]. A few studies also performed similar studies using plasma samples [113–115].

We could not find any statistically significant difference between circulating bFGF levels between breast cancer patients and women with fibroadenoma (Fig. 3.5).

Moreover, in many circumstances reported values were below the detection limit of the assay (sensitivity: 3 pg/ml, detection range: 10–640 pg/ml) [116] (Table 3.4).

Larsson et al. included 80 healthy volunteers in their study and also found bFGF levels in their plasma samples to be less than 6.4 ng/l (the equivalent of 6.4 pg/ml), a fact that we also noticed in our study concerning the control group [114]. These

Fig. 3.6 Peri-operative kinetics in the Study Group

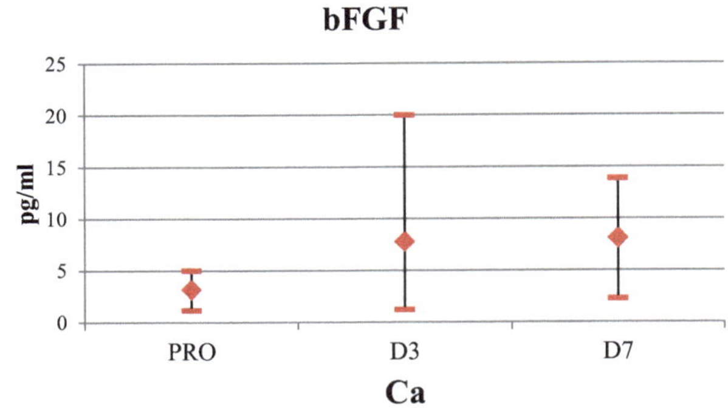

patients exhibited a robust increase in bFGF levels on D3, perhaps in the context of wound healing. As for the group of study (with malignancy) they also had raised levels on D3 and this trend could be seen until D7, but far from statistically significance in any of these time points (Fig. 3.6). Thus, perioperative kinetics of bFGF were different from those seen with VEGF and IL-8. Perhaps extending the study to more distant time points from the operation (e.g. 15th and 30th post-operative days) could bring more light to the question whether the ongoing raised bFGF levels are due to the healing wound process or the neo-angiogenesis process.

3.3 Comparative Analysis of Angiogenesis-Related Genes Between Patients with Breast Cancer and Fibroadenoma Using Quantitative Real Time PCR

We studied 84 genes that are related to angiogenesis through detecting the presence of their mRNA transcripts in the peripheral blood of patients.

3.3.1 Study Group vs Control Group Before Surgery (PRO)

Patients with breast cancer exhibit overexpression of the following well-known pro-angiogenic genes (Fig. 3.7): Epidermal Growth Factor (EGF), Fibroblast Growth Factor 1 (FGF-1 or aFGF), Interleukin 8 (IL-8), Vascular Endothelial Growth Factor C (VEGF-C) and Thrombospondin 1 (THBS1). Moreover, other less known factors were also found to be over-expressed in the Study Group: Neuropilin 1 (NRP1), Ephrin B2 (EFNB2) and Ephrin A3 (EFNA3), Chemokine ligand 11 (CCL11) etc.

The gene encoding Sphingosine kinase 1 (SPHK1) was the one with the greatest magnification (×12), whilst the only gene to be underexpressed was that of Chemokine ligand 10 (CXCL10). SPHK1 is one of the two (together with Sphingosine kinase 2, SPHK2) enzymes that stimulate through phosphorylization

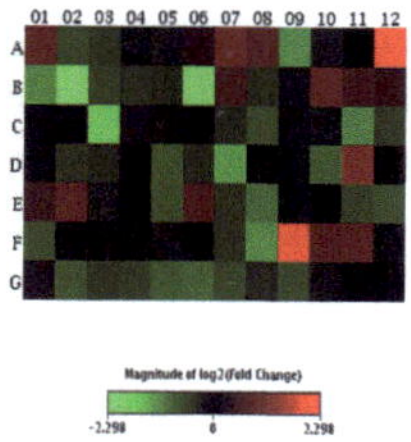

Layout	01	02	03	04	05	06	07	08	09	10	11	12
A	AKT1 1.79	ANGPT1 -1.59	ANGPT2 -1.43	ANGPTL3 -1.15	ANPTL4 -1.18	ANPEP 1.29	BAI1 2.00	CCL11 1.67	CCL2 -2.44	CDH5 -1.18	COL18A1 -1.07	COL4A3 4.65
B	CXCL1 -2.32	CXCL10 -4.49	CXCL3 -1.50	CXCL5 -1.35	CXCL6 -1.30	CXCL9 -4.86	TYMP 1.49	S1PR1 -1.34	EFNA1 1.16	EFNA3 1.90	EFNB2 1.46	EGF 1.36
C	ENG 1.07	EPHB4 1.05	EREG -3.56	FGF1 1.22	FGF2 -1.14	FGFR3 -1.05	FIGF -1.30	FLT1 -1.68	HAND2 1.13	HGF -1.17	HIF1A -2.30	HPSE -1.45
D	ID1 -1.09	ID3 -1.37	IFNA1 -1.29	IFNB1 1.08	IFNG -1.75	IGF1 -1.31	IL1B -2.61	IL6 -1.01	IL8 -1.11	ITGAV -1.88	ITGB3 2.33	JAG1 -1.05
E	KDR 1.36	LAMA5 1.76	LECT1 -1.20	LEP -1.02	MDK -1.68	MMP2 1.60	MMP9 -1.37	NOTCH4 -2.00	NRP1 -1.09	NRP2 1.07	PDGFA -1.53	PECAM1 -1.72
F	PF4 -1.61	PGF -1.04	PLAU 1.05	PLG -1.06	PLXDC1 -1.16	PROK2 -1.06	PTGS1 -1.35	SERPINF1 -2.43	SPHK1 4.92	STAB1 1.68	TEK 1.77	TGFA -1.13
G	TGFB1 1.18	TGFB2 -1.71	TGFBR1 -1.38	THBS1 -1.46	THBS2 -1.80	TIMP1 -1.91	TIMP2 -1.57	TIMP3 -1.26	TNF -1.58	TNFAIP2 -1.17	VEGFA 1.07	VEGFC 1.12

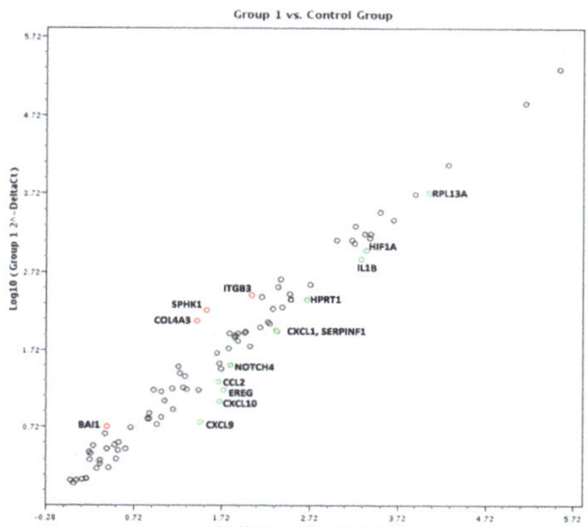

Gene symbol	*Description*	*Fold-regulation*
	GENES UP-REGULATED	
SPHK1	Sphingosine kinase 1	4.9189
COL4A3	Collagen, type IV, alpha 3 (Goodpasture antigen)	4.6536
BAI1	Brain-specific angiogenesis inhibitor 1	2.0023
ITGB3	Integrin, beta 3 (platelet glycoprotein IIIa, antigen CD61)	2.3349
	GENES DOWN-REGULATED	
EREG	Epiregulin	-3.5595
SERPINF1	Serpin peptidase inhibitor, clade F (alpha-2 antiplasmin, pigment epithelium derived factor), member 1	-2.4256
CXCL9	Chemokine (C-X-C motif) ligand 9	-4.8568
CXCL10	Chemokine (C-X-C motif) ligand 10	-4.4898
IL1B	Interleukin 1, beta	-2.6147
CCL2	Chemokine (C-C motif) ligand 2	-2.4425
CXCL1	Chemokine (C-X-C motif) ligand 1 (melanoma growth stimulating activity, alpha)	-2.3161
HIF1A	Hypoxia inducible factor 1, alpha subunit (basic helix-loop-helix transcription factor)	-2.3001
NOTCH4	Notch 4	-2.0023

Fig. 3.7 Scatter plot analysis and heat map of all patient samples preoperatively. The heat map demonstrates comparative expression of all 84 genes. Significantly upregulated genes (for example, SPHK1) are depicted in a more intense *red color* (F09), while significantly downregulated genes are shown with a more intense *green colour* (for example, CXCL10 in B02). The graph below plots the log10 of normalized gene expression levels between the control group (x-axis) and the breast cancer group (y-axis). Genes with a more than twofold upregulation in the breast cancer group are depicted in the upper left corner with *red dots*, while genes which are more than twofold downregulated are represented in the lower right section with *green dots* (these genes are analytically listed in the adjacent table)

the molecule of sphingosine 1, which is an active metabolite of sphingolipids that are essential elements of the cellular membrane [117]. Under normal circumstances it is produced by a variety of cell types (red blood cells, endothelial cells, etc.) and participates in cellular development and survival, inflammation and apoptosis [118]. During the last decade a number of studies have recognized a substantial role for sphingosine's stimulated molecule (Sphingosine 1 phosphate, S1P) both in the process of carcinogenesis [119] and that of neo-angiogenesis and lymphangiogenesis [120, 121]. It appears that this molecule is produced by cancer cells themselves and acts in the extracellular component through a series of highly-specialized receptors (S1P receptors 1–5), acting in an endocrine, autocrine and paracrine manner [118]. It is now believed that the overexpression of SPHK1 that is seen in certain types of cancers (that of breast included [122, 123]), is the result of hypoxia and the release of HIF1a [124, 125]. Moreover, SPHK1 levels have been linked to breast cancer prognosis in some studies [126].

The role of IL-8 has been discussed earlier. FGF-1/aFGF is another well-studied pro-angiogenic factor [100, 127]. It is a 155 amino-acid-long protein molecule that participates in multiple normal functions such as organogenesis and development, inflammation and wound healing [93]. In one of the first studies regarding FGF-1, Bansal et al. used RT-PCR and found significantly lower levels of both the mRNA for FGF-1 and the final biologically active product (FGF-1) in breast cancer patients biopsy tissue samples versus biopsies from women with non-malignant disease [128]. Penault-Llorca et al. found overexpression of the encoding gene for FGF-1 (and FGF2) in specimens from breast cancer [98]. Similar results were also reported by Yoshimura et al. [97]. Jaakkola et al. discovered that the gene for FGFR4 (the most specialized out of the four receptors for FGF-1) is most robustly expressed in patients suffering from malignancy in the mammary gland or the other reproductive organs [129]. However, overexpression of FGF-1 and FGFR4 has also been found in fibroadenoma tissue samples, rendering the whole subject more complex [130].

Another overexpressed gene in breast cancer patients is that for VEGF-C. VEGF-C belongs to the family of endothelial growth factors, acts through its receptors VEGFR2 (for neo-angiogenesis) and VEGFR3 (for lymphangiogenesis), that is expressed solely in lymphatic vessels [131]. The presence of VEGF-C has been recognized in specimens from breast cancer patients [132, 133]. In addition, there seems to be a positive correlation between its presence and positive lymph nodes [134], while some studies have evaluated VEGF-C as a prognostic biomarker [131, 135].

Epidermal growth factor (EGF) is one of the multiple molecules (others being TGF-α, AREG, NRG1, TDGF-1 etc.) that connect with ErbB type I tyrosine kinase receptors (RTKs), which also includes ErbB1 (EGFR, HER1), ErbB2 (Neu, HER2), ErbB3 (HER3) and ErbB4 (HER4) [136]. These receptors have the ability to alter the development of the mammary gland and may often be overexpressed or show mutations in cases of breast cancer [137, 138]. Moreover, it seems that VEGF and EGFR share common signaling pathways, while EGF is also incorporated in VEGF expression [139].

Apart from the above mentioned overexpressed proangiogenic genes, there were two angiogenesis inhibitors also overexpressed. TIMP3 belongs to tissue inhibitors of metalloproteinase (TIMP), a family of low molecular weight proteins that suppress the action of metalloproteinases, the latter being responsible for degeneration and remodelling of extracellular matrix [140]. As for TIMP3, it has been shown that it inhibits binding of VEGF to VEGFR-2, thus putting a halt to the series of reactions that would emerge from this connection [141]. Increased circulating mRNA levels for TIMP3 have been reported for patients with positive axillary lymph nodes due to breast cancer metastasis [142]. In addition, certain genetic polymorphisms may be responsible for giving proangiogenic TIMPs properties [143].

Thrombospondin 1 (THBS1 or TSP-1) is a low molecular weight glycoprotein (450 kDa) that is stored in the extracellular matrix but also present in the a-granules of platelets [144, 145]. Its role in inflammation and wound healing has long ago been recognized [144, 145]. As for angiogenesis, it seems to have an inhibitory effect [127]. It acts both directly upon the endothelial cells and indirectly (through other cell types) affecting their mobility and survival [91, 146]. Nevertheless,

Clezardin et al. reported increased mRNA levels for TSP-1 in breast cancer biopsy samples against tissues from normal or hyperplastic glands [147, 148]. Moreover, in vitro studies have proposed that TSP-1 may be linked to the adoption of metastatic potential from cancer cells [146].

3.4 Comparative Analysis of Angiogenesis-Related Genes in Patients with Breast Cancer (Study Group) Before Surgery (PRO) and on Post-operative Day 3 (D3)

Women suffering from breast cancer showed an over-expression of SPHK1, COL4A3, BAI1 and ITGB3 on D3 (Fig. 3.8).

SPHK1, as already discussed above, is induced by HIF-1α as a result of compromised tissue oxygenation and participates in inflammatory response, however,

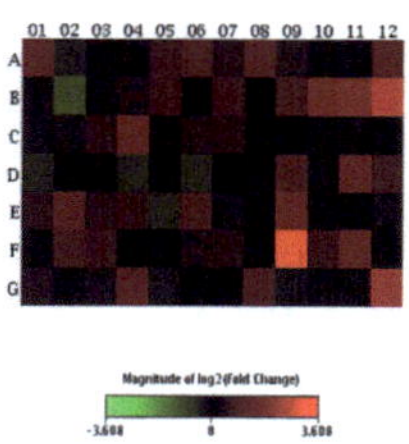

Layout	01	02	03	04	05	06	07	08	09	10	11	12
A	AKT1 2.24	ANGPT1 -1.34	ANGPT2 1.02	ANGPTL3 1.03	ANPTL4 1.64	ANPEP 1.97	BAI1 1.45	CCL11 2.18	CCL2 1.98	CDH5 -1.00	COL18A1 1.06	COL4A3 2.15
B	CXCL1 1.22	CXCL10 -2.01	CXCL3 1.17	CXCL5 1.38	CXCL6 1.64	CXCL9 1.06	TYMP 1.64	S1PR1 -1.01	EFNA1 1.86	EFNA3 3.39	EFNB2 3.69	EGF 5.86
C	ENG 1.23	EPHB4 1.27	EREG 1.50	FGF1 2.87	FGF2 1.14	FGFR3 1.43	FIGF 1.46	FLT1 1.02	HAND2 1.08	HGF -1.17	HIF1A -1.12	HPSE 1.05
D	ID1 -1.39	ID3 -1.02	IFNA1 1.08	IFNB1 -1.42	IFNG -1.08	IGF1 -1.45	IL1B 1.01	IL6 1.08	IL8 2.04	ITGAV -1.13	ITGB3 2.72	JAG1 1.65
E	KDR 1.48	LAMA5 2.28	LECT1 1.48	LEP 1.56	MDK -1.42	MMP2 1.96	MMP9 1.27	NOTCH4 -1.06	NRP1 2.98	NRP2 1.14	PDGFA 1.03	PECAM1 1.22
F	PF4 1.08	PGF 1.82	PLAU 1.63	PLG 1.16	PLXDC1 1.11	PROK2 1.41	PTGS1 1.44	SERPINF1 -1.00	SPHK1 12.20	STAB1 1.62	TEK 2.83	TGFA 1.13
G	TGFB1 1.38	TGFB2 1.01	TGFBR1 1.29	THBS1 2.21	THBS2 -1.26	TIMP1 1.12	TIMP2 1.08	TIMP3 2.00	TNF -1.28	TNFAIP2 -1.05	VEGFA 1.13	VEGFC 4.94

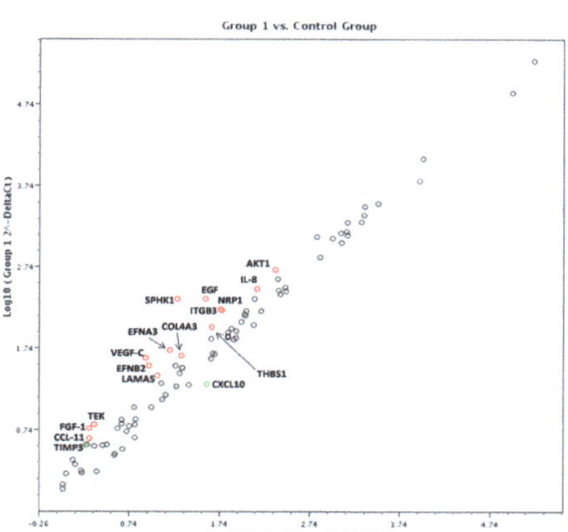

Gene symbol	Description	Fold-regulation
GENES UP-REGULATED		
SPHK1	Sphingosine kinase 1	12.196
EGF	Epidermal growth factor	5.8563
VEGFC	Vascular Endothelial Growth Factor-C	4.9417
NRP1	Neuropilin 1	2.9214
FGF1	Fibroblast growth factor	2.8712
LAMA5	Laminin, alpha 5	2.2842
COL4A3	Collagen, type IV, alpha 3 (Goodpasture antigen)	2.1485
IL8	Interleukin-8	2.035
EFNB2	Ephrin-B2	3.6893
EFNA3	Ephrin-A3	3.3909
TEK	TEK tyrosine kinase, endothelial	2.835
ITGB3	Integrin, beta 3 (platelet glycoprotein IIIa, antigen CD61)	2.7195
AKT1	V-akt murine thymoma viral oncogene homolog 1	2.2372
THBS1	Thrombospondin 1	2.2064
CCL11	Chemokine (C-C motif) ligand 11	2.1785
TIMP3	TIMP metallopeptidase inhibitor 3	2
GENES DOWN-REGULATED		
CXCL10	Chemokine (C-X-C motif) ligand 10	-2.0139

Fig. 3.8 Scatter plot analysis and heat map of all patient samples on postoperative day 3. Significantly upregulated genes (for example, SPHK1) are depicted in a more intense *red color* (F09), while significantly downregulated genes are shown with a more intense *green color* (for example, CXCL10 in B02). The graph below plots the log10 of normalized gene expression levels between the control group (x-axis) and the breast cancer group (y-axis). Genes with more than twofold upregulation in the breast cancer group are depicted in the upper left corner with *red dots*, while genes which are more than twofold downregulated are represented in the lower right section with *green dots* (these genes are analytically listed in the adjacent table)

existing data are insufficient for attributing a specific role for SPHK1 in angiogenesis and tumor development. COL4A3 (collagen type IV alpha3 or Goodpasture antigen) is a cytokine whose role in Alport syndrome and Goodpasture syndrome has well been described [149]. Moreover, current evidence supports a correlation with certain types of malignancy, such as lung cancer [150] or gastric cancer [151]. It participates in the formation of basal membrane and plays a distinct role in wound healing [149]. Its post-operative over-expression could be explained by the process of basal membrane remodelling after tissue trauma.

On the other hand, several factors were found to be under-expressed after surgery. Such factors were: Epiregulin (EREG), Serpin peptidase inhibitor 1 (SERPINF1), Interleukin1β (IL1β), chemokines CXCL1, CXCL9, CXCL10 and CCL2, Hypoxia inducible factor 1 alpha (HIF-1α) and NOTCH4. As for IL1, studies report significant increase in its levels (either as IL-1α or IL-1β) in breast cancer specimens [152], while it has been shown that it promotes both VEGF and VEGFR2 expression [153]. For this purpose it can sometimes express a synergistic effect with the factor NOTCH4, another pro-angiogenic molecule that has been correlated with poor disease prognosis [153]. Its subsequent decrease towards D3 could be attributed to the surgical removal of the primary tumor site, which is a great source of angiogenesis enhancers.

Other factors under-expressed were HIF1A, SERPINF1 and cytokines CXCL1, CCL2 and CXCL9. SERPINF1 is not a well-studied molecule. Existing evidence supports an anti-angiogenic role for this factor [154]. Finally, HIF1A is a key-player in the process of angiogenesis, a factor incorporated early on the whole process, initiating the cascade of events towards new blood vessel formation in response to tissue hypoxia [155].

3.5 Comparative Analysis of Angiogenesis-Related Genes in Patients with Breast Cancer (Study Group) Between Post-operative Day 3 (D3) and Post-operative Day 7 (D7)

On D7 there was an increase in CXCL9 expression, which had shown a trend towards decreasing from baseline towards D3 (Fig. 3.9). The exact opposite trend was documented with COL4A3, which on D3 was under-expressed as compared to its baseline levels, but started to increase on D7. A comparative over-expression was also seen on D7 for FGF-1 and TEK, as well as for TIMP3 (Table 3.5). These factors have already been discussed.

Angiopoietin 1 (ANGPT1) is an important protein in blood vessel formation but in neo-angiogenesis that is seen in cancer as well. It binds to Tie-2 receptor, which is a TKR controlling certain interactions between endothelial cells and extracellular matrix components, which are necessary for the stabilization and maturation of vascular endothelium [156]. ANGPT1 is regarded as a pro-angiogenic molecule in con-

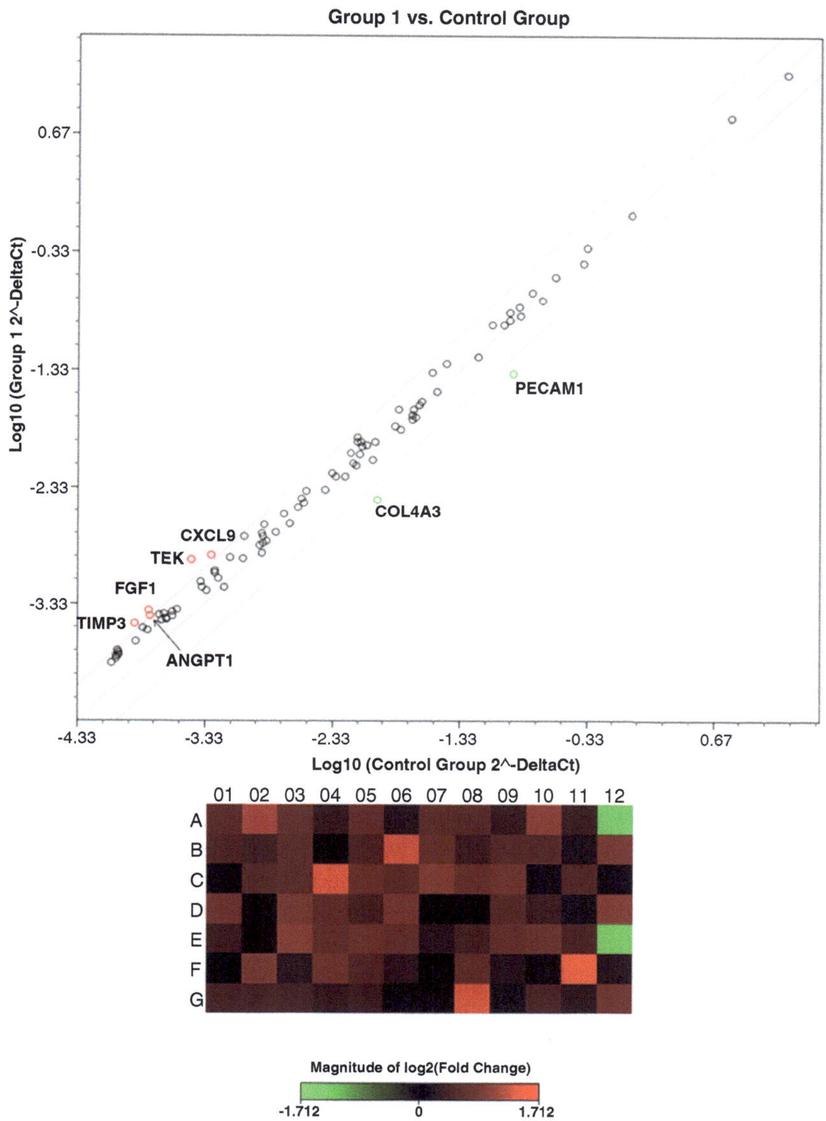

Fig. 3.9 Scatter plot and heat map of all patient samples on D7

trast to ANGPT2, which is thought to be an angiogenesis inhibitor [127]. The triggering of the "angiogenic switch" has been linked to the predominance of ANGPT2 over ANGPT1 [157]. Lastly, Platelet/Endothelial Cell Adhesion Molecule 1 (PECAM1), which is encoded by the corresponding gene, comes with a series of actions that are important for the functionality of normal vascular endothelium, but also participates in neo-angiogenesis [158].

Table 3.5 List of all genes with expression changes

Gene symbol	Gene description	Fold change
Upregulated genes		
ANGPT1	ANGPT1 angiopoietin 1	2.07
CXCL9	Chemokine (C-X-C motif) ligand 9	2.34
FGF1	Fibroblast growth factor 1	2.41
TEK	TEK tyrosine kinase, endothelial	3.01
TIMP3	TIMP metallopeptidase inhibitor 3	2.36
Downregulated genes		
COL4A3	Collagen, type IV, alpha 3 (Goodpasture antigen)	−2.83
PECAM1	PECAM1 platelet/endothelial cell adhesion molecule 1	−2.77

3.6 Conclusions

Breast cancer patients seem to have a different angiogenic profile, when compared to those with benign breast disease (fibroadenoma). VEGF-A and IL-8 plasma levels were found to be significantly increased in female patients with malignancy, regardless of disease stage or histological type. This could be possibly attributed to the early onset of angiogenesis even in patients with locoregional disease, as the ones included in our study. Our findings are in agreement with the existing literature which attributes a crucial role to these proteins in the mechanisms of new blood vessel formation. However, complex interactions between a great number of factors involved in this process does not allow yet the establishment of specific biomarkers.

Moreover, the effect of surgery on the mechanism of new blood vessel formation was found to be more robust and far more prolonged in women suffering from malignancy of the breast, than those operated for fibroadenoma. Surgery still remains the cornerstone of breast cancer treatment, but in some cases it has been implicated for initiating early locoregional recurrence or even distant metastatic spread. Perhaps this could be explained as a result of angiogenesis triggering by the surgical wounding itself, since a large number of proteins are circulating in the operating site and the systematic circulation as well, both during and after surgery. We were able to demonstrate that several genes are overexpressed in breast cancer patients after the operation. These interactions need further investigation since they could prove extremely useful in decision making regarding the timing of adjuvant therapy, the potential use of anti-angiogenic drugs or the establishment of prognostic biomarkers in breast cancer.

References

1. Adamis AP, Miller JW, Bernal MT et al (1994) Increased vascular endothelial growth factor levels in the vitreous of eyes with proliferative diabetic retinopathy. Am J Ophthalmol 118:445–450

2. Balkwill F, Mantovani A (2001) Inflammation and cancer: back to Virchow? Lancet 357:539–545
3. Folkman J (1995) Angiogenesis in cancer, vascular, rheumatoid and other disease. Nat Med 1:27–31
4. Folkman J (2003) Angiogenesis in arthritis. In: Smolen JS, Lipsky PE (eds) Targeted therapies in rheumatology. Martin Dunitz, London, pp 111–131
5. van der Bilt JD, Borel Rinkes IH (2004) Surgery and angiogenesis. Biochim Biophys Acta 1654:95–104
6. Hofer SO, Molema G, Hermens RA et al (1999) The effect of surgical wounding on tumour development. Eur J Surg Oncol 25:231–243
7. Schaper W, Schaper J (eds) (1993) Collateral circulation; heart, brain, kidney, limbs. Kluwer Academic, Boston
8. Kraft A, Weindel K, Ochs A et al (1999) Vascular endothelial growth factor in the sera and effusions of patients with malignant and nonmalignant disease. Cancer 85:178–187
9. Cao Y (2013) Erythropoietin in cancer: a dilemma in risk therapy. Trends Endocrinol Metab 24:190–199
10. Acs G, Acs P, Beckwith SM et al (2001) Erythropoietin and erythropoietin receptor expression in human cancer. Cancer Res 61:3561–3565
11. Murukesh N, Dive C, Jayson GC (2010) Biomarkers of angiogenesis and their role in the development of VEGF inhibitors. Br J Cancer 102:8–18
12. Italiano JE Jr, Richardson JL, Patel-Hett S et al (2008) Angiogenesis is regulated by a novel mechanism: pro- and antiangiogenic proteins are organized into separate platelet alpha granules and differentially released. Blood 111:1227–1233
13. Klement GL, Yip TT, Cassiola F et al (2009) Platelets actively sequester angiogenesis regulators. Blood 113:2835–2842
14. Salven P, Orpana A, Joensuu H (1999) Leukocytes and platelets of patients with cancer contain high levels of vascular endothelial growth factor. Clin Cancer Res 5:487–491
15. George ML, Eccles SA, Tutton MG et al (2000) Correlation of plasma and serum vascular endothelial growth factor levels with platelet count in colorectal cancer: clinical evidence of platelet scavenging? Clin Cancer Res 6:3147–3152
16. McIlhenny C, George WD, Doughty JC (2002) A comparison of serum and plasma levels of vascular endothelial growth factor during the menstrual cycle in healthy female volunteers. Br J Cancer 86:1786–1789
17. Salgado R, Benoy I, Bogers J et al (2001) Platelets and vascular endothelial growth factor (VEGF): a morphological and functional study. Angiogenesis 4:37–43
18. Arisato T, Hashiguchi T, Sarker KP et al (2003) Highly accumulated platelet vascular endothelial growth factor in coagulant thrombotic region. J Thromb Haemost 1: 2589–2593
19. Jelkmann W (2001) Pitfalls in the measurement of circulating vascular endothelial growth factor. Clin Chem 47:617–623
20. Thomeas V, Chow S, Gutierrez JO et al (2014) Technical considerations in the development of circulating peptides as pharmacodynamic biomarkers for angiogenesis inhibitors. J Clin Pharmacol 54:682–687
21. Georgiou GK, Igglezou M, Sainis I et al (2013) Impact of breast cancer surgery on angiogenesis circulating biomarkers: a prospective longitudinal study. World J Surg Oncol 11:213
22. Senger DR, Galli SJ, Dvorak AM et al (1983) Tumor cells secrete a vascular permeability factor that promotes accumulation of ascites fluid. Science 219:983–985
23. Byrne AM, Bouchier-Hayes DJ, Harmey JH (2005) Angiogenic and cell survival functions of vascular endothelial growth factor (VEGF). J Cell Mol Med 9:777–794
24. Holmes DI, Zachary I (2005) The vascular endothelial growth factor (VEGF) family: angiogenic factors in health and disease. Genome Biol 6:209
25. Pande D, Negi R, Khanna S et al (2011) Vascular endothelial growth factor levels in relation to oxidative damage and antioxidant status in patients with breast cancer. J Breast Cancer 14:181–184

26. Ferrara N, Gerber HP, LeCouter J (2003) The biology of VEGF and its receptors. Nat Med 9:669–676
27. Yamazaki Y, Morita T (2006) Molecular and functional diversity of vascular endothelial growth factors. Mol Divers 10:515–527
28. Kut C, Mac Gabhann F, Popel AS (2007) Where is VEGF in the body? A meta-analysis of VEGF distribution in cancer. Br J Cancer 97:978–985
29. Dvorak HF (2005) Angiogenesis: update 2005. J Thromb Haemost 3:1835–1842
30. Bando H, Weich HA, Brokelmann M et al (2005) Association between intratumoral free and total VEGF, soluble VEGFR-1, VEGFR-2 and prognosis in breast cancer. Br J Cancer 92:553–561
31. Makinen T, Veikkola T, Mustjoki S et al (2001) Isolated lymphatic endothelial cells transduce growth, survival and migratory signals via the VEGF-C/D receptor VEGFR-3. EMBO J 20:4762–4773
32. Cao R, Eriksson A, Kubo H et al (2004) Comparative evaluation of FGF-2-, VEGF-A-, and VEGF-C-induced angiogenesis, lymphangiogenesis, vascular fenestrations, and permeability. Circ Res 94:664–670
33. Thielemann A, Baszczuk A, Kopczynski Z et al (2013) Clinical usefulness of assessing VEGF and soluble receptors sVEGFR-1 and sVEGFR-2 in women with breast cancer. Ann Agric Environ Med 20:293–297
34. Gasparini G (2000) Prognostic value of vascular endothelial growth factor in breast cancer. Oncologist 5(Suppl 1):37–44
35. Nishimura R, Nagao K, Miyayama H et al (2003) Higher plasma vascular endothelial growth factor levels correlate with menopause, overexpression of p53, and recurrence of breast cancer. Breast Cancer 10:120–128
36. Zhao J, Yan F, Ju H et al (2004) Correlation between serum vascular endothelial growth factor and endostatin levels in patients with breast cancer. Cancer Lett 204:87–95
37. Gasparini G, Toi M, Gion M et al (1997) Prognostic significance of vascular endothelial growth factor protein in node-negative breast carcinoma. J Natl Cancer Inst 89:139–147
38. Gasparini G, Harris AL (1995) Clinical importance of the determination of tumor angiogenesis in breast carcinoma: much more than a new prognostic tool. J Clin Oncol 13:765–782
39. Nicolini A, Campani D, Miccoli P et al (2004) Vascular endothelial growth factor (VEGF) and other common tissue prognostic indicators in breast cancer: a case-control study. Int J Biol Markers 19:275–281
40. Moran MS, Yang Q, Goyal S et al (2011) Evaluation of vascular endothelial growth factor as a prognostic marker for local relapse in early-stage breast cancer patients treated with breast-conserving therapy. Int J Radiat Oncol Biol Phys 81:1236–1243
41. Balsari A, Maier JA, Colnaghi MI, Menard S (1999) Correlation between tumor vascularity, vascular endothelial growth factor production by tumor cells, serum vascular endothelial growth factor levels, and serum angiogenic activity in patients with breast carcinoma. Lab Investig 79:897–902
42. Garvin S, Dabrosin C (2008) In vivo measurement of tumor estradiol and vascular endothelial growth factor in breast cancer patients. BMC Cancer 8:73
43. Caine GJ, Lip G, Zanetto U et al (2007) A comparison of plasma versus histologic indices of angiogenic markers in breast cancer. Appl Immunohistochem Mol Morphol 15:382–388
44. Karayiannakis AJ, Zbar A, Polychronidis A, Simopoulos C (2003) Serum and drainage fluid vascular endothelial growth factor levels in early surgical wounds. Eur Surg Res 35:492–496
45. Wu FP, Hoekman K, Meijer S, Cuesta MA (2003) VEGF and endostatin levels in wound fluid and plasma after breast surgery. Angiogenesis 6:255–257
46. www.rndsystems.com/products/human-vegf-quantikine-elisa-kit_dve00. In Edition
47. Adams J, Carder PJ, Downey S et al (2000) Vascular endothelial growth factor (VEGF) in breast cancer: comparison of plasma, serum, and tissue VEGF and microvessel density and effects of tamoxifen. Cancer Res 60:2898–2905
48. Benoy I, Salgado R, Colpaert C et al (2002) Serum interleukin 6, plasma VEGF, serum VEGF, and VEGF platelet load in breast cancer patients. Clin Breast Cancer 2:311–315

49. Rykala J, Przybylowska K, Majsterek I et al (2011) Angiogenesis markers quantification in breast cancer and their correlation with clinicopathological prognostic variables. Pathol Oncol Res 17:809–817
50. Konukoglu D, Turhan MS, Celik V, Turna H (2007) Relation of serum vascular endothelial growth factor as an angiogenesis biomarker with nitric oxide & urokinase-type plasminogen activator in breast cancer patients. Indian J Med Res 125:747–751
51. Yamamoto Y, Toi M, Kondo S et al (1996) Concentrations of vascular endothelial growth factor in the sera of normal controls and cancer patients. Clin Cancer Res 2:821–826
52. Caine GJ, Blann AD, Stonelake PS et al (2003) Plasma angiopoietin-1, angiopoietin-2 and Tie-2 in breast and prostate cancer: a comparison with VEGF and Flt-1. Eur J Clin Investig 33:883–890
53. Bondestam J, Salven P, Jaaskela-Saari H et al (2000) Major surgery increases serum levels of vascular endothelial growth factor only temporarily. Am J Surg 179:57–59
54. Curigliano G, Petit JY, Bertolini F et al (2005) Systemic effects of surgery: quantitative analysis of circulating basic fibroblast growth factor (bFGF), vascular endothelial growth factor (VEGF) and transforming growth factor beta (TGF-beta) in patients with breast cancer who underwent limited or extended surgery. Breast Cancer Res Treat 93:35–40
55. Belizon A, Balik E, Feingold DL et al (2006) Major abdominal surgery increases plasma levels of vascular endothelial growth factor: open more so than minimally invasive methods. Ann Surg 244:792–798
56. Hormbrey E, Han C, Roberts A et al (2003) The relationship of human wound vascular endothelial growth factor (VEGF) after breast cancer surgery to circulating VEGF and angiogenesis. Clin Cancer Res 9:4332–4339
57. Caine GJ, Stonelake PS, Lip GY, Blann AD (2007) Changes in plasma vascular endothelial growth factor, angiopoietins, and their receptors following surgery for breast cancer. Cancer Lett 248:131–136
58. Baum M, Demicheli R, Hrushesky W, Retsky M (2005) Does surgery unfavourably perturb the "natural history" of early breast cancer by accelerating the appearance of distant metastases? Eur J Cancer 41:508–515
59. Retsky MW, Demicheli R, Hrushesky WJ et al (2008) Dormancy and surgery-driven escape from dormancy help explain some clinical features of breast cancer. APMIS 116:730–741
60. Brat DJ, Bellail AC, Van Meir EG (2005) The role of interleukin-8 and its receptors in gliomagenesis and tumoral angiogenesis. Neuro Oncol 7:122–133
61. Qazi BS, Tang K, Qazi A (2011) Recent advances in underlying pathologies provide insight into interleukin-8 expression-mediated inflammation and angiogenesis. Int J Inflam 2011:908468
62. Waugh DJ, Wilson C (2008) The interleukin-8 pathway in cancer. Clin Cancer Res 14:6735–6741
63. Holmes WE, Lee J, Kuang WJ et al (1991) Structure and functional expression of a human interleukin-8 receptor. Science 253:1278–1280
64. Murphy PM, Tiffany HL (1991) Cloning of complementary DNA encoding a functional human interleukin-8 receptor. Science 253:1280–1283
65. Donnelly SC, Strieter RM, Kunkel SL et al (1993) Interleukin-8 and development of adult respiratory distress syndrome in at-risk patient groups. Lancet 341:643–647
66. Nakamura H, Yoshimura K, McElvaney NG, Crystal RG (1992) Neutrophil elastase in respiratory epithelial lining fluid of individuals with cystic fibrosis induces interleukin-8 gene expression in a human bronchial epithelial cell line. J Clin Invest 89:1478–1484
67. Mattoli S, Marini M, Fasoli A (1992) Expression of the potent inflammatory cytokines, GM-CSF, IL6, and IL8, in bronchial epithelial cells of asthmatic patients. Chest 101:27S–29S
68. Benoy IH, Salgado R, Van Dam P et al (2004) Increased serum interleukin-8 in patients with early and metastatic breast cancer correlates with early dissemination and survival. Clin Cancer Res 10:7157–7162
69. Xie K (2001) Interleukin-8 and human cancer biology. Cytokine Growth Factor Rev 12:375–391

70. Haraguchi M, Komuta K, Akashi A et al (2002) Elevated IL-8 levels in the drainage vein of resectable Dukes' C colorectal cancer indicate high risk for developing hepatic metastasis. Oncol Rep 9:159–165
71. Yuan A, Yu CJ, Luh KT et al (2002) Aberrant p53 expression correlates with expression of vascular endothelial growth factor mRNA and interleukin-8 mRNA and neoangiogenesis in non-small-cell lung cancer. J Clin Oncol 20:900–910
72. Ugurel S, Rappl G, Tilgen W, Reinhold U (2001) Increased serum concentration of angiogenic factors in malignant melanoma patients correlates with tumor progression and survival. J Clin Oncol 19:577–583
73. Huang S, Mills L, Mian B et al (2002) Fully humanized neutralizing antibodies to interleukin-8 (ABX-IL8) inhibit angiogenesis, tumor growth, and metastasis of human melanoma. Am J Pathol 161:125–134
74. Green AR, Green VL, White MC, Speirs V (1997) Expression of cytokine messenger RNA in normal and neoplastic human breast tissue: identification of interleukin-8 as a potential regulatory factor in breast tumours. Int J Cancer 72:937–941
75. Miller LJ, Kurtzman SH, Wang Y et al (1998) Expression of interleukin-8 receptors on tumor cells and vascular endothelial cells in human breast cancer tissue. Anticancer Res 18:77–81
76. Strieter RM, Kunkel SL, Elner VM et al (1992) Interleukin-8. A corneal factor that induces neovascularization. Am J Pathol 141:1279–1284
77. Koch AE, Polverini PJ, Kunkel SL et al (1992) Interleukin-8 as a macrophage-derived mediator of angiogenesis. Science 258:1798–1801
78. Hu DE, Hori Y, Fan TP (1993) Interleukin-8 stimulates angiogenesis in rats. Inflammation 17:135–143
79. Li A, Dubey S, Varney ML et al (2003) IL-8 directly enhanced endothelial cell survival, proliferation, and matrix metalloproteinases production and regulated angiogenesis. J Immunol 170:3369–3376
80. Kunz M, Hartmann A, Flory E et al (1999) Anoxia-induced up-regulation of interleukin-8 in human malignant melanoma. A potential mechanism for high tumor aggressiveness. Am J Pathol 155:753–763
81. www.rndsystems.com/products/human-cxcl8-il-8-quantikine-elisa-kit_d8000c. In Edition
82. Lyon DE, McCain NL, Walter J, Schubert C (2008) Cytokine comparisons between women with breast cancer and women with a negative breast biopsy. Nurs Res 57:51–58
83. Ahmed OI, Adel AM, Diab DR, Gobran NS (2006) Prognostic value of serum level of interleukin-6 and interleukin-8 in metastatic breast cancer patients. Egypt J Immunol 13:61–68
84. Fuksiewicz M, Kaminska J, Kotowicz B et al (2006) Serum cytokine levels and the expression of estrogen and progesterone receptors in breast cancer patients. Clin Chem Lab Med 44:1092–1097
85. Kozlowski L, Zakrzewska I, Tokajuk P, Wojtukiewicz MZ (2003) Concentration of interleukin-6 (IL-6), interleukin-8 (IL-8) and interleukin-10 (IL-10) in blood serum of breast cancer patients. Rocz Akad Med Bialymst 48:82–84
86. Zakrzewska I, Omyla J (2005) [The value of plasma interleukin-6 and interleukin-8 in monitoring of patients with breast cancer]. Pol Merkur Lekarski 18:424–426
87. Hamed EA, Zakhary MM, Maximous DW (2012) Apoptosis, angiogenesis, inflammation, and oxidative stress: basic interactions in patients with early and metastatic breast cancer. J Cancer Res Clin Oncol 138:999–1009
88. Pusztai L, Mendoza TR, Reuben JM et al (2004) Changes in plasma levels of inflammatory cytokines in response to paclitaxel chemotherapy. Cytokine 25:94–102
89. Derin D, Soydinc HO, Guney N et al (2007) Serum IL-8 and IL-12 levels in breast cancer. Med Oncol 24:163–168
90. Wesche J, Haglund K, Haugsten EM (2011) Fibroblast growth factors and their receptors in cancer. Biochem J 437:199–213
91. Taraboletti G, Rusnati M, Ragona L, Colombo G (2010) Targeting tumor angiogenesis with TSP-1-based compounds: rational design of antiangiogenic mimetics of endogenous inhibitors. Oncotarget 1:662–673

92. Folkman J, Shing Y (1992) Angiogenesis. J Biol Chem 267:10931–10934
93. Powers CJ, McLeskey SW, Wellstein A (2000) Fibroblast growth factors, their receptors and signaling. Endocr Relat Cancer 7:165–197
94. Presta M, Dell'Era P, Mitola S et al (2005) Fibroblast growth factor/fibroblast growth factor receptor system in angiogenesis. Cytokine Growth Factor Rev 16:159–178
95. Xian W, Pappas L, Pandya D et al (2009) Fibroblast growth factor receptor 1-transformed mammary epithelial cells are dependent on RSK activity for growth and survival. Cancer Res 69:2244–2251
96. Xian W, Schwertfeger KL, Vargo-Gogola T, Rosen JM (2005) Pleiotropic effects of FGFR1 on cell proliferation, survival, and migration in a 3D mammary epithelial cell model. J Cell Biol 171:663–673
97. Yoshimura N, Sano H, Hashiramoto A et al (1998) The expression and localization of fibroblast growth factor-1 (FGF-1) and FGF receptor-1 (FGFR-1) in human breast cancer. Clin Immunol Immunopathol 89:28–34
98. Penault-Llorca F, Bertucci F, Adelaide J et al (1995) Expression of FGF and FGF receptor genes in human breast cancer. Int J Cancer 61:170–176
99. Neve RM, Chin K, Fridlyand J et al (2006) A collection of breast cancer cell lines for the study of functionally distinct cancer subtypes. Cancer Cell 10:515–527
100. Slavin J (1995) Fibroblast growth factors: at the heart of angiogenesis. Cell Biol Int 19:431–444
101. Folkman J, Merler E, Abernathy C, Williams G (1971) Isolation of a tumor factor responsible for angiogenesis. J Exp Med 133:275–288
102. Gospodarowicz D (1974) Localisation of a fibroblast growth factor and its effect alone and with hydrocortisone on 3T3 cell growth. Nature 249:123–127
103. Przybylski M (2009) A review of the current research on the role of bFGF and VEGF in angiogenesis. J Wound Care 18:516–519
104. Pepper MS, Ferrara N, Orci L, Montesano R (1992) Potent synergism between vascular endothelial growth factor and basic fibroblast growth factor in the induction of angiogenesis in vitro. Biochem Biophys Res Commun 189:824–831
105. Turner N, Lambros MB, Horlings HM et al (2010) Integrative molecular profiling of triple negative breast cancers identifies amplicon drivers and potential therapeutic targets. Oncogene 29:2013–2023
106. Giulianelli S, Cerliani JP, Lamb CA et al (2008) Carcinoma-associated fibroblasts activate progesterone receptors and induce hormone independent mammary tumor growth: a role for the FGF-2/FGFR-2 axis. Int J Cancer 123:2518–2531
107. Relf M, LeJeune S, Scott PA et al (1997) Expression of the angiogenic factors vascular endothelial cell growth factor, acidic and basic fibroblast growth factor, tumor growth factor beta-1, platelet-derived endothelial cell growth factor, placenta growth factor, and pleiotrophin in human primary breast cancer and its relation to angiogenesis. Cancer Res 57:963–969
108. Anandappa SY, Winstanley JH, Leinster S et al (1994) Comparative expression of fibroblast growth factor mRNAs in benign and malignant breast disease. Br J Cancer 69:772–776
109. Smith K, Fox SB, Whitehouse R et al (1999) Upregulation of basic fibroblast growth factor in breast carcinoma and its relationship to vascular density, oestrogen receptor, epidermal growth factor receptor and survival. Ann Oncol 10:707–713
110. Dabrosin C (2005) Positive correlation between estradiol and vascular endothelial growth factor but not fibroblast growth factor-2 in normal human breast tissue in vivo. Clin Cancer Res 11:8036–8041
111. Hewala TI, Abd El-Moneim NA, Ebied SA et al (2010) Diagnostic and prognostic value of serum nitric oxide, tumor necrosis factor-alpha, basic fibroblast growth factor and copper as angiogenic markers in premenopausal breast cancer patients: a case-control study. Br J Biomed Sci 67:167–176
112. Sliutz G, Tempfer C, Obermair A et al (1995) Serum evaluation of basic FGF in breast cancer patients. Anticancer Res 15:2675–2677

113. Kornacker M, Roth A, Christensen O et al (2008) Quantification of vascular endothelial growth factor, interleukin-8, and basic fibroblast growth factor in plasma of cancer patients and healthy volunteers—comparison of ELISA and microsphere-based multiplexed immunoassay. Clin Chem Lab Med 46:1256–1264
114. Larsson A, Skoldenberg E, Ericson H (2002) Serum and plasma levels of FGF-2 and VEGF in healthy blood donors. Angiogenesis 5:107–110
115. Fuhrmann-Benzakein E, Ma MN, Rubbia-Brandt L et al (2000) Elevated levels of angiogenic cytokines in the plasma of cancer patients. Int J Cancer 85:40–45
116. www.rndsystems.com/products/human-fgf-basic-quantikine-elisa-kit_dfb50. In Edition
117. Kim RH, Takabe K, Milstien S, Spiegel S (1791) Export and functions of sphingosine-1-phosphate. Biochim Biophys Acta 2009:692–696
118. Anelli V, Gault CR, Snider AJ, Obeid LM (2010) Role of sphingosine kinase-1 in paracrine/transcellular angiogenesis and lymphangiogenesis in vitro. FASEB J 24:2727–2738
119. Pyne S, Pyne NJ (2000) Sphingosine 1-phosphate signalling in mammalian cells. Biochem J 349:385–402
120. Nagahashi M, Ramachandran S, Kim EY et al (2012) Sphingosine-1-phosphate produced by sphingosine kinase 1 promotes breast cancer progression by stimulating angiogenesis and lymphangiogenesis. Cancer Res 72:726–735
121. Aoyagi T, Nagahashi M, Yamada A, Takabe K (2012) The role of sphingosine-1-phosphate in breast cancer tumor-induced lymphangiogenesis. Lymphat Res Biol 10:97–106
122. Cuvillier O, Ader I, Bouquerel P et al (2010) Activation of sphingosine kinase-1 in cancer: implications for therapeutic targeting. Curr Mol Pharmacol 3:53–65
123. Nava VE, Hobson JP, Murthy S et al (2002) Sphingosine kinase type 1 promotes estrogen-dependent tumorigenesis of breast cancer MCF-7 cells. Exp Cell Res 281:115–127
124. Takuwa N, Du W, Kaneko E et al (2011) Tumor-suppressive sphingosine-1-phosphate receptor-2 counteracting tumor-promoting sphingosine-1-phosphate receptor-1 and sphingosine kinase 1—Jekyll Hidden behind Hyde. Am J Cancer Res 1:460–481
125. Ader I, Malavaud B, Cuvillier O (2009) When the sphingosine kinase 1/sphingosine 1-phosphate pathway meets hypoxia signaling: new targets for cancer therapy. Cancer Res 69:3723–3726
126. Ruckhaberle E, Rody A, Engels K et al (2008) Microarray analysis of altered sphingolipid metabolism reveals prognostic significance of sphingosine kinase 1 in breast cancer. Breast Cancer Res Treat 112:41–52
127. Atkin GK, Chopada A (2006) Tumour angiogenesis: the relevance to surgeons. Ann R Coll Surg Engl 88:525–529
128. Bansal GS, Yiangou C, Coope RC et al (1995) Expression of fibroblast growth factor 1 is lower in breast cancer than in the normal human breast. Br J Cancer 72:1420–1426
129. Jaakkola S, Salmikangas P, Nylund S et al (1993) Amplification of fgfr4 gene in human breast and gynecological cancers. Int J Cancer 54:378–382
130. La Rosa S, Sessa F, Colombo L et al (2001) Expression of acidic fibroblast growth factor (aFGF) and fibroblast growth factor receptor 4 (FGFR4) in breast fibroadenomas. J Clin Pathol 54:37–41
131. Mohammed RA, Green A, El-Shikh S et al (2007) Prognostic significance of vascular endothelial cell growth factors -A, -C and -D in breast cancer and their relationship with angio- and lymphangiogenesis. Br J Cancer 96:1092–1100
132. Zhao YC, Ni XJ, Li Y et al (2012) Peritumoral lymphangiogenesis induced by vascular endothelial growth factor C and D promotes lymph node metastasis in breast cancer patients. World J Surg Oncol 10:165
133. Li X, Dang X, Sun X (2012) Expression of survivin and VEGF-C in breast cancer tissue and its relation to lymphatic metastasis. Eur J Gynaecol Oncol 33:178–182
134. Nakamura Y, Yasuoka H, Tsujimoto M et al (2003) Clinicopathological significance of vascular endothelial growth factor-C in breast carcinoma with long-term follow-up. Mod Pathol 16:309–314
135. Wang J, Guo Y, Wang B et al (2012) Lymphatic microvessel density and vascular endothelial growth factor-C and -D as prognostic factors in breast cancer: a systematic review and meta-analysis of the literature. Mol Biol Rep 39:11153–11165

136. Normanno N, De Luca A, Bianco C et al (2006) Epidermal growth factor receptor (EGFR) signaling in cancer. Gene 366:2–16
137. Hardy KM, Booth BW, Hendrix MJ et al (2010) ErbB/EGF signaling and EMT in mammary development and breast cancer. J Mammary Gland Biol Neoplasia 15:191–199
138. Foley J, Nickerson NK, Nam S et al (2010) EGFR signaling in breast cancer: bad to the bone. Semin Cell Dev Biol 21:951–960
139. Tabernero J (2007) The role of VEGF and EGFR inhibition: implications for combining anti-VEGF and anti-EGFR agents. Mol Cancer Res 5:203–220
140. Sun J (2010) Matrix metalloproteinases and tissue inhibitor of metalloproteinases are essential for the inflammatory response in cancer cells. J Signal Transduct 2010:985132
141. Qi JH, Ebrahem Q, Moore N et al (2003) A novel function for tissue inhibitor of metalloproteinases-3 (TIMP3): inhibition of angiogenesis by blockage of VEGF binding to VEGF receptor-2. Nat Med 9:407–415
142. Jiang X, Huang X, Li J et al (2000) [Relationship between tissue inhibitors of metalloproteinase and metastasis and prognosis in breast cancer]. Zhonghua Wai Ke Za Zhi 38:291–293, 219
143. Peterson NB, Beeghly-Fadiel A, Gao YT et al (2009) Polymorphisms in tissue inhibitors of metalloproteinases-2 and -3 and breast cancer susceptibility and survival. Int J Cancer 125:844–850
144. Lopez-Dee Z, Pidcock K, Gutierrez LS (2011) Thrombospondin-1: multiple paths to inflammation. Mediat Inflamm 2011:296069
145. Kyriakides TR, Maclauchlan S (2009) The role of thrombospondins in wound healing, ischemia, and the foreign body reaction. J Cell Commun Signal 3:215–225
146. Zhang X, Lawler J (2007) Thrombospondin-based antiangiogenic therapy. Microvasc Res 74:90–99
147. Clezardin P, Frappart L, Clerget M et al (1993) Expression of thrombospondin (TSP1) and its receptors (CD36 and CD51) in normal, hyperplastic, and neoplastic human breast. Cancer Res 53:1421–1430
148. Bertin N, Clezardin P, Kubiak R, Frappart L (1997) Thrombospondin-1 and -2 messenger RNA expression in normal, benign, and neoplastic human breast tissues: correlation with prognostic factors, tumor angiogenesis, and fibroblastic desmoplasia. Cancer Res 57:396–399
149. Abreu-Velez AM, Howard MS (2012) Collagen IV in normal skin and in pathological processes. N Am J Med Sci 4:1–8
150. Jiang CP, Wu BH, Chen SP et al (2013) High COL4A3 expression correlates with poor prognosis after cisplatin plus gemcitabine chemotherapy in non-small cell lung cancer. Tumour Biol 34:415–420
151. Nie XC, Wang JP, Zhu W et al (2013) COL4A3 expression correlates with pathogenesis, pathologic behaviors, and prognosis of gastric carcinomas. Hum Pathol 44:77–86
152. Apte RN, Dotan S, Elkabets M et al (2006) The involvement of IL-1 in tumorigenesis, tumor invasiveness, metastasis and tumor-host interactions. Cancer Metastasis Rev 25:387–408
153. Guo S, Gonzalez-Perez RR (2011) Notch, IL-1 and leptin crosstalk outcome (NILCO) is critical for leptin-induced proliferation, migration and VEGF/VEGFR-2 expression in breast cancer. PLoS One 6:e21467
154. Ren JG, Jie C, Talbot C (2005) How PEDF prevents angiogenesis: a hypothesized pathway. Med Hypotheses 64:74–78
155. Rundqvist H, Johnson RS (2013) Tumour oxygenation: implications for breast cancer prognosis. J Intern Med 274:105–112
156. Fukuhara S, Sako K, Noda K et al (2010) Angiopoietin-1/Tie2 receptor signaling in vascular quiescence and angiogenesis. Histol Histopathol 25:387–396
157. Tait CR, Jones PF (2004) Angiopoietins in tumours: the angiogenic switch. J Pathol 204:1–10
158. Woodfin A, Voisin MB, Nourshargh S (2007) PECAM-1: a multi-functional molecule in inflammation and vascular biology. Arterioscler Thromb Vasc Biol 27:2514–2523

Chapter 4
Perioperative Biologic Perturbation and Cancer Surgery: Targeting the Adrenergic-Inflammatory Response and Microcirculatory Dysregulation

Jonathan Hiller, Robert Schier, and Bernhard Riedel

Abstract Many of the physiological responses that comprise the surgical stress response are known to promote cancer-signaling pathways. Tissue resection and exposure to the pharmaco-physiological stressors of anesthesia required for surgery activate local and systemic inflammatory cytokines, up-regulate cyclooxygenase with increased prostaglandin production, and increase adrenergic activity. The activation of neuro-hormonal pathways is increasingly linked with cancer propagation. Retrospective evidence suggests that the use of anesthetic techniques and adjuncts that modulate these pathways and commonly available to practicing anesthesiologists may benefit patients scheduled for cancer surgery. Minimising the inflammatory response, preventing perioperative immunosuppression, and optimizing fluid delivery may have oncological benefits (improved disease free survival, reduced postoperative complications with timely delivery of adjuvant therapies) that extend beyond enhanced postoperative recovery. This review will consider key components of local and systemic inflammatory response, relevant immune cell mediators, perioperative endothelial dysfunction, and relevant perioperative therapies specific to the care of the patient receiving cancer surgery.

Keywords Perioperative • Cancer • Anesthesia • Surgery • Stress

---

J. Hiller, MBBS (Hons.), GCEpi, FANZCA (✉)
Department of Anaesthesia, Perioperative and Pain Medicine, Peter MacCallum Cancer Centre, Melbourne, VIC, Australia

University of Melbourne, Parkville, VIC, Australia

Monash University, Clayton, VIC, Australia
e-mail: jonathan.hiller@petermac.org

R. Schier, M.D., Ph.D.
Department of Anaesthesiology and Intensive Care Medicine, University Hospital of Cologne, Cologne, Germany

B. Riedel, MBChB, FCA, FANZCA, PhD
Department of Anaesthesia, Perioperative and Pain Medicine, Peter MacCallum Cancer Centre, Melbourne, VIC, Australia

University of Melbourne, Parkville, VIC, Australia

M.W. Retsky, R. Demicheli (eds.), *Perioperative Inflammation as Triggering Origin of Metastasis Development*, DOI 10.1007/978-3-319-57943-6_4

4.1 Introduction

Over the last decade focus has increasingly been placed on the role of anesthesiologists as perioperative physicians. This is, in part, due to the recognition that surgery results in a substantial physiological impact. More specifically, the role of the perioperative physician in improving long-term cancer outcomes is gaining increasing attention, as uncomplicated recovery from surgery is vital to ensuring an uninterrupted cancer journey that may include adjuvant therapy. Similarly, anaesthetic techniques and perioperative adjuncts may impact cancer-signaling pathways and thus impact cancer recurrence and survival. It is therefore essential that optimal management of the perioperative period in cancer patients considers preoperative optimization of modifiable risk factors and careful management of non-modifiable risk factors to ensure optimal recovery. This focus on the perioperative journey has led to improvements in risk stratification of patients, preoperative optimization (prehabilitation) programs, careful selection of anesthetic technique and perioperative adjuvants, enhanced recovery goals, and strategies to avoid 'failure-to-rescue' when complications do occur.

The surgical stress response involves physiological processes that are teleological remnants of our ancestral need to survive trauma, injury, and infection. This primordial axis, however, may be disadvantageous in the context of appropriate inflammatory response and resolution following the stress of cancer resection surgery in, most frequently, the elderly. The biological perturbation of surgical stress is underpinned by activation of the adrenergic-inflammatory pathway and associated immunosuppression: systemic release of catecholamines, local release of inflammatory mediators (interleukins, cytokines, prostaglandins) culminating in the activation of leukocytes, platelets and the endothelium. Platelet and neutrophil activation also triggers neutrophil extracellular trap (NET) formation within the sinusoids (measuring single cell diameter) of end organs such as the liver and lungs, with extracellular DNA strands that trap bacteria and parasites. While teleologically advantageous, unfortunately these NETs also trap circulating tumor cells that are known to be released into the circulation during cancer surgery [1]. Additionally, inflammatory mediators cleave the endothelial glycocalyx to facilitate an increase in capillary permeability and trans-capillary migration of leukocytes into the interstitial space, to facilitate removal of bacteria within the interstitial space. Prostaglandins mediate lymphodilation by signaling to lymphatic endothelial cells; and adrenergic signaling, via sympathetic activation, increases lymphatic contractility. As a consequence, lymphatic flow through the lymph nodes and lymphatic ducts of the parallel circulatory systems increase several fold under conditions of stress. While this is intended to mediate an immune response to infectious agents, it may unfortunately be the mechanism whereby minimal residual disease (MRD, cancer cells within the surgical field) enters the lymphatic system with regional dissemination of cancer following surgery or radiotherapy.

The perioperative period is further characterized by changes in T-lymphocyte, natural killer (NK) cell and monocyte function—resulting in temporary immunosuppression. The changes occur through the adrenergic-inflammatory effects of surgical stress, but also through the exposure to anesthetic agents, hypothermia, and blood transfusion. Endothelial dysfunction, a hallmark of many comorbid disease states, is triggered and/or exacerbated during the postoperative inflammatory period predisposing to tissue edema with increased risk of hypoperfusion and subsequent postoperative complications such as wound infection. Such complications lead to a protracted recovery period, delaying the delivery of adjuvant cancer therapies, and subsequently reducing long-term cancer survival.

Awareness of these perioperative factors has led to increasing emphasis on a 'cancer anesthetic' specifically focused on offsetting the perioperative stress response: avoiding adrenergic, inflammatory and immunosuppressive pathway activation during surgery. Fortunately, a number of anesthetic agents and perioperative adjuncts are available to help achieve this hitherto unrecognised role of improving outcomes following cancer surgery.

4.2 Importance of the Perioperative Period to Cancer Outcomes

The cornerstone of solid organ cancer treatment remains surgical excision. Unfortunately, for many patients, cancer progression (local recurrence or metastatic disease) following surgery is a frequent occurrence carrying significant mortality risk, for which a number of postulates have been proposed. First, despite optimal surgical techniques and apparent 'clear margins', MRD remains and progresses at the resection site. Secondly, mature isolated tumor cells remain in the interstitium following surgery and are transported using innate wound resolution (lymphatic) pathways [2, 3] leading to the clinical scenarios such as carcinoma-in-transit, regional lymph node recurrence, peritoneal carcinomatosis, and port site recurrence. Thirdly, perioperative iatrogenic displacement of blood-borne circulating tumor cells occurs [4, 5] leading to dissemination and seeding of epithelial mesenchymal transition-like or progenitor cancer cells [6–13], with potential entrapment in the sinusoids of the liver and lungs [1]. A number of studies have indicated a disadvantageous prognostic significance of circulating tumor cell release [9, 14, 15]. Lastly, immunoediting theory [16] suggests that pre-potential cancer cells (micrometastatic disease) held in 'equilibrium' in distant organs through active immunosurveillance, are postulated to, through a brief period of perioperative immunosuppression of endogenous innate immunity, 'escape' to form de novo malignancies [17, 18]. Removal of a primary tumor has been shown to increase growth rates of such distant micrometastatic disease [19, 20].

A number of animal studies have demonstrated that intervening in a simulated perioperative setting to offset inflammation and immune impairment have resulted in improved cancer outcomes [21–24]. This supports the theoretical framework that biological perturbation during the perioperative period, through systemic and local pro-cancerous processes, places a patient at an increased risk of cancer recurrence. As such, by limiting perioperative adrenergic-inflammatory activity, immunosuppression, and increased lymphatic flow through focused implementation of commonly used anesthetic techniques and adjuvants (favoring anti-adrenergic, anti-inflammatory, anti-angiogenic, anti-lymphangiogenic techniques) perioperative clinicians may provide additional benefit to plausibly limit cancer recurrence following surgery. Numerous randomised clinical trials are being conducted to translate these findings.

4.3 Perioperative Adrenergic-Inflammatory Processes

The first 48–72 h following a surgical procedure, hereafter the 'perioperative period', is characterized as a period during which physiological stress and pharmacologic agents modulate physiological derangements.

4.3.1 Surgical Stress Response

Patients presenting for cancer resection surgery present a unique challenge for anesthesiologists. Additional to the age-associated, co-morbid diseases of the commonly older patient, cancer itself imposes a physiological strain on patients through their disease (anemia, malnutrition), paraneoplastic syndromes, and psychological stress of a cancer diagnosis. Patients may be further exposed to the debilitating "double hit" [25] effect of combined neoadjuvant chemo-radiotherapy. This translates to a baseline level of impaired functional capacity, chronic inflammation, and immune deficiency even before approaching surgery. Patients' abilities to respond to surgical stress are further compromised by the pre-existing state of malnourishment, deconditioning, and immunosuppression [26, 27]. Perioperatively, patients are then further exposed to psychological, physiological and immunological stress [28–31]. Historically, this has been referred to as the 'surgical stress response' that arises as a consequence of not only surgical excision, but also exposure to numerous perioperative events (Table 4.1). The stress response is characterized by impaired homeostasis of the neuroendocrine (hypothalamic-adrenocorticoid up-regulation), sympathetic nervous system, inflammation (cytokine and prostaglandin release), metabolism (hyperglycemia, protein breakdown), and host innate immune (natural killer cell and T-helper cell impairment) systems.

Table 4.1 'Surgical stress response' that arises as a consequence of surgical excision and exposure to numerous perioperative events

Pharmacological • Opioids • Corticosteroid agents • Anesthetic agents	**Physiological** • Hyperglycemia • Blood product transfusion • Hyperoxia and hypoxia • Hypothermia • Muscle breakdown and ketosis • Infection • Pathogen exposure
Psychological • Pain • Anxiety and fear	**Surgical** • Surgical excision and tissue trauma • Tumor cell release

4.3.2 Local Inflammation

Skin incision inevitably results in tissue inflammation and lymphatic dilation, and an innate response that promotes wound healing [32]. Tissue healing is dependent on a localized inflammatory response characterized by vasodilation, local release of growth factors, angiogenesis and dilation of lymphatic channels. These mediators that co-ordinate the process of wound healing are also directly linked with the inflammatory processes of the tumor microenvironment [33]. The release of local angiogenic growth factors and inhibition of angiostatin and endostatin secretion may facilitate local tumor cell escape to develop malignancy [34, 35].

As acute inflammatory mediators in tissue, prostaglandins and vascular endothelial growth factors (VEGF) facilitate angiogenic and lymphangiogenic processes [36]. Lymphatic dilation is a key component of cellular repair [37, 38]. However, locally released prostaglandins and VEGF are also key components of cancer invasion [39, 40], and high VEGF expression is associated with accelerated cancer progression and more aggressive disease [41–44]. These cytokines are up-regulated in response to surgical trauma [45]. Given their role in cancer pathways, in the presence of residual disease, exaggerated up-regulation of prostaglandins and VEGF is hence postulated to be disadvantageous [46–49].

Leukocyte invasion of healing tissue is an appropriate component of wound healing that includes the recruitment of blood-borne monocytes [50]. Of note, peri-incisional wound inflammation shifts macrophages to the M2 sub-type, which is associated with an immunosuppressed tumor microenvironment and cancer progression [51]. M2 macrophages up-regulate stromal cyclooxygenase (COX), matrix metalloproteinase (MMP) and VEGF expression—all mediators of cancer progression [52].

4.3.3 Immune Cells Relevant to Perioperative Period

In brief, perioperative immune suppression can be considered by examining the pathophysiological changes occurring in three distinct leukocyte cell types.

4.3.3.1 Macrophages

As components of host innate immunity cells, phagocytic macrophages are subclassified into classically activated (M1) and alternatively activated (M2) lineages [52].

- M1 macrophages have a key role in the localized stimulation of T-helper lymphocytes. M1 differentiated macrophages secrete cytotoxic superoxide anions and free radicals.
- M2 macrophages are classically induced by pro-inflammatory states. Conceivably, this teleological development was rooted in the need for lymphangiogenic processes and resolution of pathogen associated wound trauma. M2 macrophages are also increasingly considered as Tumor Associated Macrophages (TAMs) that promote a localized immunosuppressed environment facilitating tumor growth [53]. TAMs are integral to the process of lymphatic vessel formation and tumor invasion [48]. TAM presence is used as a prognostic marker of cancer outcome [54].

4.3.3.2 $CD4^{+}$–Th1 'Helper' Lymphocytes

T-helper lymphocytes will differentiate to sub-types (to Th1 or Th2) based on their exposure to a number of cytokines and interleukins (e.g. IL-2, IL-4, IL-10) [55].

- Progenitor T-lymphocytes differentiate to Th1 under the influence of IL-2. Th1 cells can be considered as anti-tumor effector cells and, with M1 macrophages, facilitate the activation of $CD8^{+}$ cytotoxic T-lymphocytes as well as natural killer (NK) cells [56]. Immunoediting theory and host immunosurveillance are strongly based on the role of Th1 lymphocytes to co-ordinate macrophage based antigen-presenting cells and enhance tumor surveillance [16].
- Also facilitating an immunosuppressed tumor microenvironment are Th2 lymphocytes that assist in tumor progression [57, 58]. Progenitor Th2 lymphocytes differentiate under the influence of IL-4 and IL-10, and favor non-cellular immunity to actively inhibit NK and cytotoxic T-lymphocytes. Th2 cells can be broadly considered to promote tumor growth and metastasis. Th2 cells dominate Th1 cells after severe injury such as surgical stress [59].

4.3.3.3 Natural Killer Cells

- Representing 8–16% of peripheral blood mononuclear cells, NK cells may be considered key anti-tumor effector cells and vital components of host immunosurveillance and tumor cell destruction [60, 61]. A hallmark of the perioperative period and response to surgical inflammation is the suppression of NK cells. Volatile anesthesia agents will also suppress NK cells [62]. Natural killer cells function synergistically to potentiate cytotoxic T-lymphocytes [63]. Poor cancer outcomes are associated in patients with poor NK cell function and cytotoxicity [64–66].

4.3.3.4 Neutrophils

- As the most abundant of the circulating leukocytes, neutrophils play a key role in the acute inflammatory response. The role of neutrophils in the cancer context is complex. In the tumor microenvironment, neutrophil secretion of VEGF and matrix metalloproteinases facilitate cancer invasion, and immature neutrophils (myeloid-derived suppressor cells) promote localized immunosuppression.
- Neutrophil activation and subsequent expulsion of DNA (chromatin) is a key step in the formation of Neutrophil-Extracellular Traps (NETs). Teleologically advantageous in the trapping of pathogens following tissue trauma to decrease bacteremia, NET formation within the sinusoids of end organs such as the liver and lungs also traps circulating tumor cells released during surgery. This process may initiate micrometastasis and is associated with a reduction in disease free survival [1].
- A recent systematic review found a perioperative elevated neutrophil-lymphocyte ratio associated with a reduction in recurrence free survival following surgery for resection of solid tumor [67].

4.3.3.5 Platelets

- Platelets are vital in the first response to tissue injury initiating primary thrombosis and endothelial activation. Platelet activation is likely to be a co-factor in the formation of NETs [1].
- In controlling inflammatory processes in the tumor microenvironment, platelet release of pro-inflammatory hormones and cytokines can potentiate cancer progression [68].
- Two retrospective studies have found a perioperative elevated platelet-lymphocyte ratio associated with a reduction in recurrence free survival following surgery for resection of solid tumor [69, 70].

4.3.3.6 Perioperative, Clinical Significance of Immune Cells

Coincident with the inflammatory response to surgical stress are changes in patients' immune cell profile [17]. Broadly, the perioperative physiological and pharmacological stressors lead to impairment of the innate immune system and a shift from a patient's capacity to optimally recognize and destroy cancer cells. Surgical stress induces a shift of T-lymphocyte differentiation from a Th1 to Th2 dominance [71] together with direct inhibition of NK and cytotoxic T-lymphocyte proliferation [72]. This differential state is partly influenced by circulating cytokines and catecholamines [55, 60]. Interestingly, non-invasive surgical techniques, likely through a reduction in inflammatory burden, reduce perioperative immune suppression (and Th2 dominance) [71, 73]. The catecholamine surge associated with perioperative stress may reduce the Th1/Th2 lymphocyte ratio [74–76] and has been shown to further depress the impaired Th1 lymphocyte activity reported in cancer patients [73]. Sympathetic nervous system activity and circulating noradrenaline facilitates macrophages towards an M2 sub-type [77]. This polarization is partially mediated by beta-2 adrenergic receptors on the macrophage cell surface, and may account for the suggestion that non-selective beta-blockers have a protective effect against cancer progression [78–80].

NK cells and NK cell cytotoxicity is significantly depressed for 24–72 h following exposure to surgical stress [81, 82]. Specifically, suppression of NK cell number and activity has been reported following lung, breast, and colorectal surgery [83]. As vital anti-tumor effector cells, NK cells are normally active in the presence of Th1 cells and in response to IFN-gamma [84]. The reduction in perioperative NK cell activity may be due to the surgical stress response—specifically through increased circulating epinephrine and cortisol, or through a reduction in IFN-gamma [85, 86]. Overall, these perioperative changes promote an immunological state less competent to manage residual disease or circulating cancer cells and has been implicated in cancer recurrence and metastatic disease [87].

4.3.4 Inflammatory Mediators of the Surgical Stress Response

This stress response to surgery is characterized by up-regulation of a number of acute phase physiological pathways. With surgical incision, the hypothalamic-pituitary-adrenal axis is immediately activated and sympathetic up-regulation leads to suppressed cell mediated immunity [88]. Raised catecholamine levels are a feature of the perioperative period [89, 90], through activation of neural sympathetic outflow and adrenal medulla adrenaline and noradrenaline release [91]. The up-regulation of the sympathetic nervous system is likely to begin prior to surgical incision through anxiety, fear and hypothermia [92, 93]. Catecholamine levels remain elevated for at least 24 h following surgery [90].

In health, prostaglandins are vital to the maintenance of the cellular microenvironment: fluid permeability, endothelial maintenance, and lymphatic flow modification [36, 94]. Surgery and associated tissue trauma release prostaglandins locally and into the systemic circulation [45]. Cyclooxygenase (cox) exists in two isoforms—cox1 and (inducible) cox2. The latter enzyme's activity is greatly increased in the setting of active inflammation and is a focus for perioperative stress response strategies. Cox activity is difficult to measure due to the instability of its key product prostaglandin-E, though prostaglandins appear to be elevated for up to 48 h following minor surgery [45]. Cerebrospinal fluid prostaglandin E2 levels elevate in response to surgery [95]. Co-incident with the rise in prostaglandins following tissue trauma, inflammatory cytokines (IL-1, IL-6 and IL-8) remain elevated for up to 48 h [96–99].

Because of the implicit involvement of the sympathetic nervous system, prostaglandins and subsequent up-regulation of systemic cytokines, a focus of research has been the perioperative blockade of these pathways to modulate the surgical stress response and improve patients' outcomes.

4.3.5 Microcirculation Changes and Endothelial Dysfunction

Endothelial dysfunction results in impairment of the microcirculation with a loss of the endothelium's key physiological tendency toward vasodilation, fibrinolysis, and anti-aggregation. Perioperative inflammatory response results in the endothelium undergoing a change in its phenotype from a baseline quiescent state to an activated, or pathological dysfunctional state characterized by loss of the glycol-polysaccharide 'glycocalyx' layer. The set point of the endothelium reflects the balance between the underlying chronic health of the endothelium, acute exacerbating triggers such as inflammation and oxidative stress, and the 'regenerative' ability of the bone marrow that releases endothelial progenitor cells into the peripheral circulation [100, 101].

To maintain physiological microcirculation, the bioavailability of key mediators such as nitric oxide is crucial, otherwise endothelial dysfunction will result in vasoconstriction, pro-inflammatory, and pro-thrombotic changes. In a perioperative setting, microcirculatory changes as described above serve as an appropriate adaptive physiologic response to acute stressors like surgical trauma. Furthermore, elderly patients presenting for cancer surgery often have underlying vascular disease based on comorbid risk factors such as diabetes mellitus, hypertension, hyperlipidemia, and obesity that result in clinically unapparent but underlying endothelial dysfunction [102].

The pro-inflammatory and pro-oxidant milieu resulting from surgical trauma further injures the endothelium and is ubiquitous in the perioperative period [103–105]. Plausibly, the loss of glycocalyx, increased extravasation, and subsequent tissue edema is disadvantageous in cancer surgery, given the presence of circulating tumor cells and residual tumor cells in the interstitium whose removal is dependent on lymphatic processes.

A temporal link exists between acute systemic inflammatory load and acute deterioration in endothelial function. In human volunteers, a pro-inflammatory cytokine challenge resulted in a transient loss of endothelial vasodilator function, recovery taking up to seven days [106]. Interestingly, this process is reversible. Studies indicating that removal of the inflammatory source (a 6 month aggressive treatment for chronic periodontitis) [107] or though anti-inflammatory strategies (hydrocortisone or high dose aspirin) [106, 108] improve endothelial vasodilator function. Hu et al. found patients receiving a laparotomy, when compared with less invasive laparoscopic surgery, had greater and more prolonged deterioration in endothelial dysfunction for up to seven postoperative days [105]. A deterioration in endothelial-dependent vasodilation occurs in the first 24–48 h following surgical treatment [107], which reflects an important clinical correlation: the peak incidence of postoperative myocardial infarction occurs at 48 h following surgery, when flow stagnation and increased thrombogenicity manifest [109].

Patients undergoing major cancer surgery are at substantial risk for postoperative morbidity, with 30–60% of patients developing complications [110, 111]. The risk of postoperative complications may relate to perioperative endothelial dysfunction: impaired vascular homeostasis and reduced tissue (organ) perfusion. Research has hence focused on both the measurement of endothelial-dependent vascular function and the prevention of its dysregulation in order to minimize the risk for perioperative cardiovascular complications [112]. Measurement tools include characterization of endothelial vasodilatory function (e.g. assess vascular function through endothelial dependent vasodilation), quantification of vascular damage (e.g. measurement of endothelial, thrombogenic and inflammatory biomarkers) and levels of denuded circulating endothelial cells or endothelial microparticles. In addition, analyzing the endothelial regenerative capacity via endothelial progenitor cell (EPC), a key stem cell line for endothelial repair, has been a recent focus of clinical research [113]. In patients with metabolic syndrome, EPC levels decrease following surgery—a potential correlate with the postoperative morbidity seen in these patients [102]. To prevent endothelial damage mobilization, proliferation, survival and homing of EPCs is important, and microcirculatory impairment is an early pathogenic event in end-organ damage (cardiomyopathy, nephropathy, retinopathy, and neuropathy) [102].

It appears the fundamental determinant for endothelial dysfunction is activation of inflammatory pathways (such as the surgical stress response). The same processes, exacerbated specifically by neutrophil-platelet activation, lead to subsequent NET formation [1]. As such, maintaining endothelial integrity to prevent complications related to surgery or circulating tumor cell entrapment by NETs may be an important strategy in the perioperative care of the cancer patient. This is especially important when one considers that surgical morbidity results in significant prolonged hospital stay, with a substantial delay in return to intended oncologic therapy (RIOT). Reduced RIOT has been attributed to surgical complications and shown to increase risk for poor oncologic outcome in breast, liver, and pancreatic cancer surgery [114, 115].

4.4 Modifying Inflammatory Response and Preventing Endothelial Dysfunction

4.4.1 Appropriate Fluid Delivery

Given the susceptibility of the endothelial glycocalyx to inflammatory insult, with consequent increased permeability and lymphatic flow, it is crucial that anesthetic techniques for cancer surgery incorporate a strong anti-inflammatory strategy. Further consideration should also be given to judicious goal-directed fluid therapy as fluid overload may result in beta natriuretic peptide release which, in turn, cleaves the endothelial glycocalyx [116].

A plausible link with increased lymphatic flow and residual cancer cells impacting on cancer recurrence through residual cells in lymph nodes has been described [117].

Prevention of tissue edema through optimal, goal directed fluid delivery would likely reduce lymphatic flow and is also known to reduce postoperative complications [118]. The extent to which optimal perioperative fluid delivery and lymphatic flow reduction impacts upon a timely return to intended oncologic (adjuvant) therapy (i.e. RIOT) or long-term oncological outcomes requires further study within the setting of adequately powered prospective studies.

4.4.2 Regional Anesthesia

Epidurals have been extensively investigated as a means of reducing perioperative opioid requirements following intra-cavity surgery [119]. Additional benefits from the use of epidural anesthesia have been the reduction in neural sympathetic outflow and circulating catecholamines, and subsequent reduction in the perioperative stress response. Neuraxial analgesia have been shown to reduce cytokine assessed inflammatory response through cancer surgery [99], preserve endothelial function [120], and possibly reduce lymphatic flow [121].

Epidural analgesia inhibits neural sympathetic activity and the catecholamine rise of surgical incision both in animal models [122] and in patients receiving major surgery [89, 90]. Preventing the adrenaline surge maintains lymphocyte numbers, activity and the Th1/Th2 ratio to preserve cell-mediated immunity [91, 123]. This may occur through the preservation of Th1 cell number, and maintenance of interferon (IFN)-gamma levels [123, 124] crucial to adaptive immune defense and anti-tumorigenic cell-mediated immunity [91, 96, 125–128]. Regional anesthesia reduces other markers of the surgical stress response such as elevated cortisol and hyperglycemia [97, 129]. As a strategy to improve clinical outcomes, epidural analgesia's reduction in the surgical stress response has been shown to improve post-operative morbidity in surgical sub-populations [91, 119, 130].

Specific to cancer surgery, retrospective studies have found an association between perioperative epidural analgesia and improvements in long-term cancer recurrence [131–133]. A mooted explanation for this is the reduced catecholamine levels and β-adrenergic activity following neuraxial analgesia [90, 134]. Numerous studies are currently recruiting patients to prospective trials examining the influence of perioperative analgesia with a primary endpoint of cancer recurrence and survival (NCT01318161, NCT00684229, NCT02801409).

4.4.3 Beta-Blockers

An alternate means of minimising the sympathetic nervous system component of the surgical stress response is through the use of beta-blocker medication. In animal models, limiting the stress response of surgery through beta-blockade has led to improved cancer outcomes.

When modelling the surgical stress response in animals, prevention of β-adrenergic activation through the use of beta-blockers increased in NK cell number and activity with resultant improvements in cancer outcomes [21, 22]. The peak period of immunosuppression occurs 24 h following incision, partially induced by unregulated sympathetic hyperactivity [135]. Also during this time frame is a reduction in NK cell cytotoxicity, Th1 and B cell decline and a rise in IL-10. The use of peri-incision selective β(1)-blockade prevents immunosuppression, presumably through reduction in sympathetic nervous system activity [136].

There are few published trials demonstrating the utility of beta-blockers to offset the immunosuppressive component of the surgical stress response. Small trials have shown that beta-blockers preserve NK cell cytotoxicity [85, 86, 96]. One study prospectively examined the effect of placebo or perioperative atenolol (a non-selective beta-blocker) in patients receiving abdominal surgery [137]. While no difference in adrenaline or noradrenaline levels were observed, β-blockade modified the stress and inflammatory response as indicated by faster recovery from anesthesia, reduced pain, and reduced opioid requirement.

Traditionally, trials examining perioperative beta-blockade have focused on its role in preventing post-operative cardiovascular events such as myocardial infarction and stroke. Investigators hypothesize that improvements seen through the use of beta-blockers would be mediated through limiting of the surgical stress response [138, 139]. The largest of these trials is the 8351 patient 'POISE' study which found that perioperative administration of the non-selective beta-blocker metoprolol led to a reduction in post-operative myocardial infarction (176 [4.2%] vs. 239 [5.7%] patients; 0.73, 0.60–0.89; $p = 0.002$) [140]. However, this occurred at the cost of excess deaths in the metoprolol group compared with the placebo group (129 [3.1%] vs. 97 [2.3%] patients; 1.33, 1.03–1.74; $p = 0.0317$) due to an increased rate of post-operative hypotension and stroke. While the increased risk of stroke may be specific to metoprolol rather than to all beta-blockers, caution must be used in their perioperative administration [141].

A number of retrospective studies have found an association between non-selective beta-blocker use and improved cancer outcomes [142, 143]. These studies have arisen in the setting of patients simultaneously treated with beta-blocker anti-hypertensive medication coincidentally with their cancer diagnosis.

The use of non-selective beta-blockers has appeal due to increased mechanistic evidence of β-adrenergic signaling in tumor progression, macrophage recruitment and metastasis in animal models. The perioperative period is dominated by a period of intense catecholamine activity. Modification of β-adrenergic activity and reduction in surgical stress through beta-blocker use may improve patients' cancer outcomes through regulation of the pathogenic behavior of residual disease and preservation of host immune responses. No study to date has considered the role of perioperatively commenced beta-blockers and improvement in patients' cancer outcomes.

4.4.4 Non-steroidal Anti-inflammatory Agents (NSAID)

Due to the increased tissue expression of cyclooxygenase and prostaglandin production in the perioperative period, the use of selective (cox2) NSAID agents is an appealing strategy to minimize the surgical inflammatory response. Surgical stress response can be partially suppressed through NSAID administration. In non-cancer surgery, a rise in systemic and wound prostaglandin levels was partially inhibited through the use of NSAIDs [45, 144]. However, in cancer surgery a single dose of diclofenac during surgery was unable to suppress post-operative PGE2 rise [31]. Following cardiac surgery, NSAIDs have been shown to suppress the inflammation (IL-6, IL-8) and potentiate anti-inflammatory cytokines (IL-10) [145]. A number of trials have demonstrated that, either through a reduction in surgical stress response or opioid related side effects, patients receiving perioperative NSAIDs have improved pain control and improved clinical outcomes [146–148].

The role of NSAIDs in minimising stress response has been demonstrated in a number of animal models where attempts to model the 'perioperative' period in animals has arisen through an interest in off-setting the inflammatory and immunological changes associated with surgery that are cancer promoting [21, 22, 149, 150]. Perioperative NK cell suppression induced through sham laparotomy is prevented through the use of single or multiple doses of NSAID agents [151]; in multiple murine studies such interventions have been shown to reduce cancer growth [21, 150, 152]. In animals, cox2 specific agents (etodolac) have been shown to be particularly efficacious in preventing melanoma [22] and lung cancer growth in both the surgical [153] and non-surgical setting [154–157].

The successful demonstration of NSAIDs' improvement in tumor progression in animal models is probably a consequence of the vital role prostaglandins have in cancer progression. At the cancer cell-stroma interface, tumor cells utilize prostaglandins to achieve growth and metastasis via newly-formed lymphatic channels and blood vessels [158–162]. The perioperative up-regulation of prostaglandins and VEGF, and consequent facilitation of lymphatic and vascular channel dilation, provides an ideal conduit for iatrogenic tumor cell dissemination in the post-surgical period. NSAIDs have been shown to have an integral role in reversing prostaglandin-mediated lymphangiogenesis and lymphatic dilation that ultimately lead to reduced tumor dissemination and metastasis [47, 87, 163, 164].

Investigators have questioned whether NSAID administration in the perioperative period of cancer surgery may impact on patients' long-term cancer outcomes. It has been observed that in humans, tumors with high cox expression by breast [165], lung [166] and cervical [167] cancers are associated with poor prognosis. These findings, combined with animal evidence led to a number of trials prospectively analysing whether NSAIDs might impact cancer outcomes. Selective cox2 inhibitors prevent colon cancer progression from adenomas [168, 169]. Cox2 inhibitor 'chemoprophylaxis' in ex-smokers at high risk of cancer development resulted in reduced lung cancer biomarkers with subsequent clinical benefit [170, 171]. Cohort studies support a beneficial role of cox2 inhibitors in patients with lung cancer [172]. Subsequent trials of cox2 inhibitors added to chemotherapy regimens in advanced lung cancer have not consistently shown survival benefit [173–177]. Hence, the role for cox2 inhibitors in the prevention of cancer appears to be in early chemoprophylaxis against cancer development rather than cox2 inhibition in established disease [178]. These observations have led investigators to research the benefit of administering NSAIDs during the period of cancer surgery—a pro-inflammatory, immunosuppressed period of low volume disease.

A number of retrospective studies have found an association between perioperatively administered NSAIDs and cancer outcomes following breast cancer surgery [179–182]. NSAIDS appear to impact on the first peak of the bimodal recurrence pattern observed in breast cancer patients following surgery [183]. Prospective randomized studies of 2 week preoperative courses of the cox2 inhibitor celecoxib found improvements in the tumor microenvironment (increased tumor apoptosis, VEGF suppression, reduced lymphangiogenesis) in bladder [184], prostate [185], and oesophageal [186] cancers. There is a paucity of evidence regarding long-term outcomes following the randomized intervention of a perioperative NSAID. The largest study to date is the follow-up of a 1500 patient randomized trial of aspirin in patients receiving gastroesophagectomy; the investigators found a 10% reduction (51% aspirin, 41% placebo) in 5-year survival from the use of perioperative aspirin [187].

As such, NSAIDs (in particular cox2 inhibitors) have a role in reducing pain and the stress response to surgery, have clear anti-cancer properties, and in animal 'perioperative' models of cancer prevent overt tumor development. Preliminary evidence of specific anti-cancer benefit from NSAIDs use in the perioperative period is plausible, given the conditions of low volume disease and a pro-inflammatory state.

4.4.5 *Total Intravenous Anesthesia (TIVA)*

A number of preclinical in vitro and in vivo studies indicate differing effects of anesthesia agents on both inflammatory pathways and cancer cells. In the majority of cases, general anesthesia is administered via techniques of intravenous or inhalational (volatile) agents. Anesthesia agent-specific effects have already been identified with regard to postoperative outcomes; TIVA, using propofol, is used for the prevention of post operative nausea and vomiting in high risk patients [188].

In murine studies, propofol has been identified as a prostaglandin E suppressant through inhibition of cox in both murine studies [189, 190] and human monocytes [191]. Clinically, propofol appears to have protective influence on endothelial inflammatory mediator release by reducing IL-1, IL-6 and IL-8 when compared with sevoflurane (volatile) based anesthesia [192]. These findings have been confirmed in studies examining serial plasma levels of cytokines following open cholecystectomy [193].

The role of propofol as the choice anesthesia agent specific for cancer surgery has been mooted due to its properties as a cox inhibitor [194]. Furthermore, in murine studies, propofol appears to act as an immune enhancer and has been shown to have anti-tumor properties [195]. A large 11,345 patient retrospective study recently published found an association between volatile anesthesia, compared with TIVA, and reduced survival after propensity matching: hazard ratio 1.59 (95% Confidence Interval 1.30–1.95) [196]. The apparent benefit for patients that appeared in the 12 months following surgery indicates that TIVA may have a role in modifying the perioperative stress response and medium-term morbidity. Alternatively, the benefit may lie in avoidance of volatiles, which may be tumor promoting by activating biological pathways (e.g. HIF-1 alpha) that could be tumorigenic. The impact of TIVA on cancer recurrence rates was not examined.

4.4.6 Lidocaine

The use of systemic lidocaine has been studied extensively in the perioperative setting for its role in improving short-term patient outcomes and inhibition of the surgical stress response. Lidocaine acts through blockade of the voltage-gated sodium channel in the neuronal cell membrane. It is postulated that it is through a systemic reduction in neuronal signaling that profound analgesic benefits are achieved for patients in the post-operative period—in particular following abdominal surgery in which neuraxial analgesia is not implemented [197]. Compared with opioid based analgesia, the addition of systemic lidocaine therapy reduces inflammation (IL-6, IL-8), markers of immune function (complement activation, CD11b) following laparotomy that led to a reduction in opioid consumption and improvements in clinical outcomes including patients' earlier discharge from hospital [198]. Furthermore, lidocaine clearly suppressed pro-inflammatory behavior (IL1, IL6 secretion) of peripheral blood mononuclear cells in the peri-surgical setting [199]. Improvements in non-oncologic clinical outcomes from perioperative lidocaine use have been confirmed in other trials of colon resection surgery [200, 201].

Additionally, a number of studies have demonstrated key anti-proliferative properties of local anesthetics, in particular lidocaine. In a number of cancer cell lines, lidocaine promotes cancer cell apoptosis [202, 203] and anti-proliferation of mesenchymal stem cells [204]. In the clinical setting, epidural lidocaine is associated with a reduction in cancer recurrence rates following radical prostatectomy surgery [131]. It is difficult to extrapolate whether lidocaine's benefit (if any) is observed due to systemic exposure of the drug, associated reduction in inflammatory response, or to a reduction in opioid and anesthesia requirements [205].

4.5 Conclusion

The expansion of our understanding of the pathophysiological processes involved in cancer progression, and the awareness that many of these processes are temporarily activated through the perioperative period, has led researchers and anesthesiologists to view the provision of care at this time to be tailored specifically for the patient receiving cancer resection surgery.

Furthermore, retrospective evidence suggests that specific anesthetic approaches and adjuvants may beneficially impact not only recovery time, but also facilitate more rapid RIOT, potentially increasing disease free survival. A 'cancer anesthetic' appears to be increasingly defined as one that focuses on anti-adrenergic and anti-inflammatory strategies that reduce cytokine production and prevent endothelial dysfunction: intravenous anesthesia, goal directed fluid therapy, cox2 inhibitors, neuraxial anesthesia and potentially perioperative beta-blockade. A number of prospective trials are currently recruiting patients; the results of these studies will more effectively guide practice.

References

1. Tohme S et al (2016) Neutrophil extracellular traps promote the development and progression of liver metastases after surgical stress. Cancer Res 76(6):1367–1380
2. Camara O et al (2006) Seeding of epithelial cells into circulation during surgery for breast cancer: the fate of malignant and benign mobilized cells. World J Surg Oncol 4:67
3. Tvedskov TF et al (2012) Iatrogenic displacement of tumor cells to the sentinel node after surgical excision in primary breast cancer. Breast Cancer Res Treat 131(1):223–229
4. Akiyoshi S et al (2013) Laparoscopic surgery minimizes the surgical manipulation of isolated tumor cells leading to decreased metastasis compared to open surgery for colorectal cancer. Surg Today 43(1):20–25
5. Eguchi H et al (2009) Presence of minute cancer cell dissemination in peritoneal lavage fluid detected by reverse transcription PCR is an independent prognostic factor in patients with resectable pancreatic cancer. Surgery 146(5):888–895
6. Ge MJ et al (2006) Observation of circulating tumour cells in patients with non-small cell lung cancer by real-time fluorescent quantitative reverse transcriptase-polymerase chain reaction in perioperative period. J Cancer Res Clin Oncol 132(4):248–256
7. Katoh H et al (2009) Prognostic significance of peritoneal tumour cells identified at surgery for colorectal cancer. Br J Surg 96(7):769–777
8. Li J et al (2005) [Detection of blood dissemination during the operation of lung cancer and its significance]. Zhonghua wai ke za zhi [Chin J Surg] 43(2):76–79
9. Rolle A et al (2005) Increase in number of circulating disseminated epithelial cells after surgery for non-small cell lung cancer monitored by MAINTRAC(R) is a predictor for relapse: a preliminary report. World J Surg Oncol 3(1):18
10. Sawabata N et al (2007) Circulating tumor cells in peripheral blood caused by surgical manipulation of non-small-cell lung cancer: pilot study using an immunocytology method. Gen Thorac Cardiovasc Surg 55(5):189–192
11. Temesi R et al (2012) Impact of positive intraabdominal lavage cytology on the long-term prognosis of colorectal cancer patients. World J Surg 36(11):2714–2721
12. Tsakok T et al (2012) Washout after lobectomy: is water more effective than normal saline in preventing local recurrence? Interact Cardiovasc Thorac Surg 14(2):200–204
13. Weitz J, Herfarth C (2001) Surgical strategies and minimal residual disease detection. Semin Surg Oncol 20(4):329–333
14. Ma X-L et al (2012) Meta-analysis of circulating tumor cells as a prognostic marker in lung cancer. Asian Pac J Cancer Prev 13(4):1137–1144

15. Yamashita JI et al (2000) Detection of circulating tumor cells in patients with non-small cell lung cancer undergoing lobectomy by video-assisted thoracic surgery: a potential hazard for intraoperative hematogenous tumor cell dissemination. J Thorac Cardiovasc Surg 119(5):899–905
16. Dunn GP, Old LJ, Schreiber RD (2004) The immunobiology of cancer immunosurveillance and immunoediting. Immunity 21(2):137–148
17. Kurosawa S, Kato M (2008) Anesthetics, immune cells, and immune responses. J Anesth 22(3):263–277
18. Retsky M et al (2013) Reduction of breast cancer relapses with perioperative non-steroidal anti-inflammatory drugs: new findings and a review. Curr Med Chem 20(33):4163–4176
19. Fisher B, Gunduz N, Saffer EA (1983) Influence of the interval between primary tumor removal and chemotherapy on kinetics and growth of metastases. Cancer Res 43(4):1488–1492
20. Gunduz N, Fisher B, Saffer EA (1979) Effect of surgical removal on the growth and kinetics of residual tumor. Cancer Res 39(10):3861–3865
21. Benish M et al (2008) Perioperative use of beta-blockers and COX-2 inhibitors may improve immune competence and reduce the risk of tumor metastasis. Ann Surg Oncol 15(7):2042–2052
22. Glasner A et al (2010) Improving survival rates in two models of spontaneous postoperative metastasis in mice by combined administration of a beta-adrenergic antagonist and a cyclooxygenase-2 inhibitor. J Immunol 184(5):2449–2457
23. Goldfarb Y et al (2012) Fish oil attenuates surgery-induced immunosuppression, limits post-operative metastatic dissemination and increases long-term recurrence-free survival in rodents inoculated with cancer cells. Clin Nutr 31(3):396–404
24. Wada H et al (2007) Combined spinal and general anesthesia attenuates liver metastasis by preserving TH1/TH2 cytokine balance. Anesthesiology 106(3):499–506
25. Jones LW et al (2009) Exercise intolerance in cancer and the role of exercise therapy to reverse dysfunction. Lancet Oncol 10(6):598–605
26. Fearon KC et al (2013) Patient optimization for gastrointestinal cancer surgery. Br J Surg 100(1):15–27
27. Marik PE, Zaloga GP (2010) Immunonutrition in high-risk surgical patients: a systematic review and analysis of the literature. JPEN J Parenter Enteral Nutr 34(4):378–386
28. Colvin LA, Fallon MT, Buggy DJ (2012) Cancer biology, analgesics, and anaesthetics: is there a link? Br J Anaesth 109(2):140–143
29. Heaney A, Buggy DJ (2012) Can anaesthetic and analgesic techniques affect cancer recurrence or metastasis? Br J Anaesth 109(Suppl 1):i17–i28
30. Kavanagh T, Buggy DJ (2012) Can anaesthetic technique effect postoperative outcome? Curr Opin Anaesthesiol 25(2):185–198
31. O'Riain SC et al (2005) Inhibition of the stress response to breast cancer surgery by regional anesthesia and analgesia does not affect vascular endothelial growth factor and prostaglandin E2. Anesth Analg 100(1):244–249
32. Huggenberger R et al (2011) An important role of lymphatic vessel activation in limiting acute inflammation. Blood 117(17):4667–4678
33. Heinrich EL et al (2012) The inflammatory tumor microenvironment, epithelial mesenchymal transition and lung carcinogenesis. Cancer Microenviron 5(1):5–18
34. O'Reilly MS et al (1994) Angiostatin: a novel angiogenesis inhibitor that mediates the suppression of metastases by a Lewis lung carcinoma. Cell 79(2):315–328
35. O'Reilly MS et al (1997) Endostatin: an endogenous inhibitor of angiogenesis and tumor growth. Cell 88(2):277–285
36. Kalish BT et al (2013) The growing role of eicosanoids in tissue regeneration, repair, and wound healing. Prostaglandins Other Lipid Mediat 104–105:130–138
37. Greco KV et al (2006) Lymphatic regeneration across an incisional wound: inhibition by dexamethasone and aspirin, and acceleration by a micronized purified flavonoid fraction. Eur J Pharmacol 551(1–3):131–142
38. Narayan K, Cliff WJ (1981) In vivo morphology and ultrastructure of thyroid autografts in rabbit ear chambers. Q J Exp Physiol 66(3):237–252

39. Ferrandina G et al (2002) Increased cyclooxygenase-2 expression is associated with chemotherapy resistance and poor survival in cervical cancer patients. J Clin Oncol 20(4):973–981
40. Zhang R et al (2009) [Expression of P53, COX2 and CD44V6 in early-stage squamous carcinoma of cervix with lymph vascular space invasion positive and negative and its relationship with prognosis]. Zhonghua Yi Xue Za Zhi 89(47):3341–3345
41. Gou H-F et al (2011) Expressions of COX-2 and VEGF-C in gastric cancer: correlations with lymphangiogenesis and prognostic implications. J Exp Clin Cancer Res 30:14
42. Hashimoto I et al (2001) Vascular endothelial growth factor-C expression and its relationship to pelvic lymph node status in invasive cervical cancer. Br J Cancer 85(1):93–97
43. Kopfstein L et al (2007) Distinct roles of vascular endothelial growth factor-D in lymphangiogenesis and metastasis. Am J Pathol 170(4):1348–1361
44. Lutgendorf SK et al (2009) Depression, social support, and beta-adrenergic transcription control in human ovarian cancer. Brain Behav Immun 23(2):176–183
45. Zhao H et al (2011) Comparison of different loading dose of celecoxib on postoperative anti-inflammation and analgesia in patients undergoing endoscopic nasal surgery-200 mg is equivalent to 400 mg. Pain Med 12(8):1267–1275
46. Alessandri G et al (1987) Influence of gangliosides on primary and metastatic neoplastic growth in human and murine cells. Cancer Res 47(16):4243–4247
47. Karnezis T, Shayan R, Caesar C et al (2012) VEGF-D promotes tumor metastasis by regulating prostaglandins produced by the collecting lymphatic endothelium. Cancer Cell 21(2):181–195
48. Schoppmann SF et al (2002) Tumor-associated macrophages express lymphatic endothelial growth factors and are related to peritumoral lymphangiogenesis. Am J Pathol 161(3):947–956
49. Stacker SA, Achen MG (2008) From anti-angiogenesis to anti-lymphangiogenesis: emerging trends in cancer therapy. Lymphat Res Biol 6(3–4):165–172
50. Viswanathan K, Dhabhar FS (2005) Stress-induced enhancement of leukocyte trafficking into sites of surgery or immune activation. Proc Natl Acad Sci U S A 102(16):5808–5813
51. Harvey NL, Gordon EJ (2012) Deciphering the roles of macrophages in developmental and inflammation stimulated lymphangiogenesis. Vasc cell 4(1):15
52. Hao N-B et al (2012) Macrophages in tumor microenvironments and the progression of tumors. Clin Dev Immunol 2012:948098
53. Solinas G et al (2009) Tumor-associated macrophages (TAM) as major players of the cancer-related inflammation. J Leukoc Biol 86(5):1065–1073
54. Medrek C et al (2012) The presence of tumor associated macrophages in tumor stroma as a prognostic marker for breast cancer patients. BMC Cancer 12:306
55. Kurosawa S (2012) Anesthesia in patients with cancer disorders. Curr Opin Anaesthesiol 25(3):376–384
56. Powrie F, Coffman RL (1993) Cytokine regulation of T-cell function: potential for therapeutic intervention. Immunol Today 14(6):270–274
57. Joyce JA, Pollard JW (2009) Microenvironmental regulation of metastasis. Nat Rev Cancer 9(4):239–252
58. Quail DF, Joyce JA (2013) Microenvironmental regulation of tumor progression and metastasis. Nat Med 19(11):1423–1437
59. Mack VE et al (1996) Dominance of T-helper 2-type cytokines after severe injury. Arch Surg 131(12):1303–1308. Discussion 1308–9
60. Kurosawa S et al (1993) Early appearance and activation of natural killer cells in tumor-infiltrating lymphoid cells during tumor development. Eur J Immunol 23(5):1029–1033
61. Kurosawa S et al (1995) Early-appearing tumour-infiltrating natural killer cells play a crucial role in the generation of anti-tumour T lymphocytes. Immunology 85(2):338–346
62. Huitink JM et al (2010) Volatile anesthetics modulate gene expression in breast and brain tumor cells. Anesth Analg 111(6):1411–1415
63. Kos FJ, Engleman EG (1996) Immune regulation: a critical link between NK cells and CTLs. Immunol Today 17(4):174–176

64. Fujisawa T, Yamaguchi Y (1997) Autologous tumor killing activity as a prognostic factor in primary resected nonsmall cell carcinoma of the lung. Cancer 79(3):474–481
65. Koda K et al (1997) Preoperative natural killer cell activity: correlation with distant metastases in curatively research colorectal carcinomas. Int Surg 82(2):190–193
66. Takeuchi H et al (2001) Prognostic significance of natural killer cell activity in patients with gastric carcinoma: a multivariate analysis. Am J Gastroenterol 96(2):574–578
67. Paramanathan A, Saxena A, Morris DL (2014) A systematic review and meta-analysis on the impact of pre-operative neutrophil lymphocyte ratio on long term outcomes after curative intent resection of solid tumours. Surg Oncol 23(1):31–39
68. Sharma D et al (2014) Platelets in tumor progression: a host factor that offers multiple potential targets in the treatment of cancer. J Cell Physiol 229(8):1005–1015
69. Goh BKP et al (2016) Blood neutrophil-to-lymphocyte and platelet-to-lymphocyte ratios are independent prognostic factors for surgically resected gastrointestinal stromal tumors. Surgery 159(4):1146–1156
70. Que Y et al (2015) Preoperative platelet-lymphocyte ratio is superior to neutrophil-lymphocyte ratio as a prognostic factor for soft-tissue sarcoma. BMC Cancer 15:648
71. Evans C et al (2009) Impact of surgery on immunologic function: comparison between minimally invasive techniques and conventional laparotomy for surgical resection of colorectal tumors. Am J Surg 197(2):238–245
72. Kuroda E, Yamashita U (2003) Mechanisms of enhanced macrophage-mediated prostaglandin E2 production and its suppressive role in Th1 activation in Th2-dominant BALB/c mice. J Immunol 170(2):757–764
73. Ishikawa M et al (2009) Perioperative immune responses in cancer patients undergoing digestive surgeries. World J Surg Oncol 7:7
74. Elenkov IJ, Chrousos GP (2002) Stress hormones, proinflammatory and antiinflammatory cytokines, and autoimmunity. Ann N Y Acad Sci 966:290–303
75. Greenfeld K et al (2007) Immune suppression while awaiting surgery and following it: dissociations between plasma cytokine levels, their induced production, and NK cell cytotoxicity. Brain Behav Immun 21(4):503–513
76. Vallejo R et al (2003) Perioperative immunosuppression in cancer patients. J Environ Pathol Toxicol Oncol 22(2):139–146
77. Grailer JJ et al (2014) Induction of M2 regulatory macrophages through the β2-adrenergic receptor with protection during endotoxemia and acute lung injury. J Innate Immun 6(5):607–618
78. Horowitz M et al (2015) Exploiting the critical perioperative period to improve long-term cancer outcomes. Nat Rev Clin Oncol 12:213–226
79. Sloan EK et al (2010) The sympathetic nervous system induces a metastatic switch in primary breast cancer. Cancer Res 70(18):7042–7052
80. Watkins JL et al (2015) Clinical impact of selective and nonselective beta-blockers on survival in patients with ovarian cancer. Cancer 121(19):3444–3451
81. Cata JP et al (2013) Effects of surgery, general anesthesia, and perioperative epidural analgesia on the immune function of patients with non-small cell lung cancer. J Clin Anesth 25(4):255–262
82. Nosotti M et al (2011) Leukocyte subsets dynamics following open pulmonary lobectomy for lung cancer: a prospective, observational study. Interact Cardiovasc Thorac Surg 13(3):262–266
83. Ramirez MF et al (2015) Innate immune function after breast, lung, and colorectal cancer surgery. J Surg Res 194(1):185–193
84. Gajewski TF, Schreiber H, Fu Y-X (2013) Innate and adaptive immune cells in the tumor microenvironment. Nat Immunol 14(10):1014–1022
85. Madden KS, Sanders VM, Felten DL (1995) Catecholamine influences and sympathetic neural modulation of immune responsiveness. Annu Rev Pharmacol Toxicol 35:417–448
86. Robertson MJ, Ritz J (1990) Biology and clinical relevance of human natural killer cells. Blood 76(12):2421–2438

87. Mantovani A, Sica A (2010) Macrophages, innate immunity and cancer: balance, tolerance, and diversity. Curr Opin Immunol 22(2):231–237
88. Shakhar G, Ben-Eliyahu S (2003) Potential prophylactic measures against postoperative immunosuppression: could they reduce recurrence rates in oncological patients? Ann Surg Oncol 10(8):972–992
89. Moore CM et al (1994) Effects of extradural anaesthesia on interleukin-6 and acute phase response to surgery. Br J Anaesth 72(3):272–279
90. Moore CM et al (1995) Hormonal effects of thoracic extradural analgesia for cardiac surgery. Br J Anaesth 75(4):387–393
91. Ahlers O et al (2008) Intraoperative thoracic epidural anaesthesia attenuates stress-induced immunosuppression in patients undergoing major abdominal surgery. Br J Anaesth 101(6):781–787
92. Khadke VV, Khadke SV, Khare A (2012) Oral propranolol—efficacy and comparison of two doses for peri-operative anxiolysis. J Indian Med Assoc 110(7):457–460
93. Mavridou P et al (2013) Patient's anxiety and fear of anesthesia: effect of gender, age, education, and previous experience of anesthesia. A survey of 400 patients. J Anesth 27(1):104–108
94. Salvemini D, Kim SF, Mollace V (2013) Reciprocal regulation of the nitric oxide and cyclooxygenase pathway in pathophysiology: relevance and clinical implications. Am J Physiol Regul Integr Comp Physiol 304(7):R473–R487
95. Buvanendran A et al (2006) Upregulation of prostaglandin E2 and interleukins in the central nervous system and peripheral tissue during and after surgery in humans. Anesthesiology 104(3):403–410
96. Dong H, Zhang Y, Xi H (2012) The effects of epidural anaesthesia and analgesia on natural killer cell cytotoxicity and cytokine response in patients with epithelial ovarian cancer undergoing radical resection. J Int Med Res 40(5):1822–1829
97. Fant F et al (2013) Thoracic epidural analgesia inhibits the neuro-hormonal but not the acute inflammatory stress response after radical retropubic prostatectomy. Br J Anaesth 110(5):747–757
98. Frick VO et al (2012) Thoracotomy procedures effect cytokine levels after thoracoabdominal esophagectomy. Oncol Rep 27(1):258–264
99. Moselli NM et al (2011) Intraoperative epidural analgesia prevents the early proinflammatory response to surgical trauma. Results from a prospective randomized clinical trial of intraoperative epidural versus general analgesia. Ann Surg Oncol 18(10):2722–2731
100. Asahara T et al (1997) Isolation of putative progenitor endothelial cells for angiogenesis. Science 275(5302):964–967
101. Hill JM et al (2003) Circulating endothelial progenitor cells, vascular function, and cardiovascular risk. N Engl J Med 348(7):593–600
102. Avogaro A et al (2011) Endothelial dysfunction in diabetes: the role of reparatory mechanisms. Diabetes Care 34(Suppl 2):S285–S290
103. Chello M et al (2005) Effects of atorvastatin on arterial endothelial function in coronary bypass surgery. Eur J Cardiothorac Surg 28(6):805–810
104. Clapp BR et al (2004) Inflammation-induced endothelial dysfunction involves reduced nitric oxide bioavailability and increased oxidant stress. Cardiovasc Res 64(1):172–178
105. Hu YJ et al (2013) Impact of non-cardiovascular surgery on reactive hyperaemia and arterial endothelial function. Clin Exp Pharmacol Physiol 40(7):466–472
106. Bhagat K, Vallance P (1997) Inflammatory cytokines impair endothelium-dependent dilatation in human veins in vivo. Circulation 96(9):3042–3047
107. Tonetti MS et al (2007) Treatment of periodontitis and endothelial function. N Engl J Med 356(9):911–920
108. Farb MG et al (2014) Cyclooxygenase inhibition improves endothelial vasomotor dysfunction of visceral adipose arterioles in human obesity. Obesity 22(2):349–355
109. Biccard BM, Rodseth RN (2010) The pathophysiology of peri-operative myocardial infarction. Anaesthesia 65(7):733–741

110. Duque JL et al (1997) Early complications in surgical treatment of lung cancer: a prospective, multicenter study. Grupo Cooperativo de Carcinoma Broncogénico de la Sociedad Española de Neumología y Cirugía Torácica. Ann Thorac Surg 63(4):944–950
111. Licker M et al (2002) Risk factors for early mortality and major complications following pneumonectomy for non-small cell carcinoma of the lung. Chest 121(6):1890–1897
112. Deanfield JE, Halcox JP, Rabelink TJ (2007) Endothelial function and dysfunction: testing and clinical relevance. Circulation 115(10):1285–1295
113. Gokce N (2011) Clinical assessment of endothelial function: ready for prime time? Circ Cardiovasc Imaging 4(4):348–350
114. Aloia TA et al (2014) Return to intended oncologic treatment (RIOT): a novel metric for evaluating the quality of oncosurgical therapy for malignancy. J Surg Oncol 110(2):107–114
115. Gagliato Dde M et al (2014) Clinical impact of delaying initiation of adjuvant chemotherapy in patients with breast cancer. J Clin Oncol 32(8):735–744
116. Marik PE, Lemson J (2014) Fluid responsiveness: an evolution of our understanding. Br J Anaesth 112(4):617–620
117. Gottschalk A et al (2012) Can regional anaesthesia for lymph-node dissection improve the prognosis in malignant melanoma? Br J Anaesth 109(2):253–259
118. Pearse RM et al (2014) Effect of a perioperative, cardiac output-guided hemodynamic therapy algorithm on outcomes following major gastrointestinal surgery: a randomized clinical trial and systematic review. JAMA 311(21):2181–2190
119. Rigg JRA et al (2002) Epidural anaesthesia and analgesia and outcome of major surgery: a randomised trial. Lancet 359(9314):1276–1282
120. Lauer S et al (2009) Thoracic epidural anesthesia time-dependently modulates pulmonary endothelial dysfunction in septic rats. Critical Care 13(4):R109
121. Hiller JG, et al (2016) Neuraxial Anesthesia Reduces Lymphatic Flow: Proof-of-Concept in First In-Human Study. Anesth Analg 123:1325–7
122. Enigk F et al (2014) Thoracic epidural anesthesia decreases endotoxin-induced endothelial injury. BMC Anesthesiol 14:23
123. Zhou D et al (2012) Effects of anesthetic methods on preserving anti-tumor T-helper polarization following hepatectomy. World J Gastroenterol 18(24):3089–3098
124. Nowarski R et al (2013) Innate immune cells in inflammation and cancer. Cancer Immunol Res 1(2):77–84
125. Kawasaki T et al (2007) Effects of epidural anaesthesia on surgical stress-induced immunosuppression during upper abdominal surgery. Br J Anaesth 98(2):196–203
126. Rao VSR et al (2006) Potential prognostic and therapeutic roles for cytokines in breast cancer (Review). Oncol Rep 15(1):179–185
127. Xu YJ et al (2014) Effect of thoracic epidural anaesthesia on serum vascular endothelial growth factor C and cytokines in patients undergoing anaesthesia and surgery for colon cancer. Br J Anaesth 113 Suppl 1:i49–55
128. Yokoyama M et al (2005) The effects of continuous epidural anesthesia and analgesia on stress response and immune function in patients undergoing radical esophagectomy. Anesth Analg 101(5):1521–1527
129. Volk T et al (2003) Stress induced IL-10 does not seem to be essential for early monocyte deactivation following cardiac surgery. Cytokine 24(6):237–243
130. Tønnesen E, Wahlgreen C (1988) Influence of extradural and general anaesthesia on natural killer cell activity and lymphocyte subpopulations in patients undergoing hysterectomy. Br J Anaesth 60(5):500–507
131. Biki B et al (2008) Anesthetic technique for radical prostatectomy surgery affects cancer recurrence: a retrospective analysis. Anesthesiology 109(2):180–187
132. de Oliveira GSJ et al (2011) Intraoperative neuraxial anesthesia but not postoperative neuraxial analgesia is associated with increased relapse-free survival in ovarian cancer patients after primary cytoreductive surgery. Reg Anesth Pain Med 36(3):271–277

133. Hiller J et al (2010) A retrospective observational study examining the admission arterial to end-tidal carbon dioxide gradient in intubated major trauma patients. Anaesth Intensive Care 38(2):302–306
134. Riedel BJ, Wright IG (1997) Epidural anesthesia in coronary artery bypass grafting surgery. Curr Opin Cardiol 12(6):515–521
135. Nelson CJ, Lysle DT (1998) Severity, time, and beta-adrenergic receptor involvement in surgery-induced immune alterations. J Surg Res 80(2):115–122
136. Woiciechowsky C et al (1998) Sympathetic activation triggers systemic interleukin-10 release in immunodepression induced by brain injury. Nat Med 4(7):808–813
137. Zaugg M et al (1999) Beneficial effects from beta-adrenergic blockade in elderly patients undergoing noncardiac surgery. Anesthesiology 91(6):1674–1686
138. Blessberger H et al (2014) Perioperative beta-blockers for preventing surgery-related mortality and morbidity. Cochrane Database Syst Rev 9:CD004476
139. Mostafaie K, Bedenis R, Harrington D (2015) Beta-adrenergic blockers for perioperative cardiac risk reduction in people undergoing vascular surgery. Cochrane Database Syst Rev 1:CD006342
140. POISE Study Group et al (2008) Effects of extended-release metoprolol succinate in patients undergoing non-cardiac surgery (POISE trial): a randomised controlled trial. Lancet 371(9627):1839–1847
141. Ashes C et al (2013) Selective β1-antagonism with bisoprolol is associated with fewer postoperative strokes than atenolol or metoprolol: a single-center cohort study of 44,092 consecutive patients. Anesthesiology 119(4):777–787
142. Melhem-Bertrandt A et al (2011) Beta-blocker use is associated with improved relapse-free survival in patients with triple-negative breast cancer. J Clin Oncol 29(19):2645–2652
143. Powe DG et al (2010) Beta-blocker drug therapy reduces secondary cancer formation in breast cancer and improves cancer specific survival. Oncotarget 1(7):628–638
144. Zhu Y et al (2014) Effect of perioperative parecoxib on postoperative pain and local inflammation factors PGE2 and IL-6 for total knee arthroplasty: a randomized, double-blind, placebo-controlled study. Eur J Orthop Surg Traumatol 24(3):395–401
145. Wu Q et al (2013) The efficacy of parecoxib on systemic inflammatory response associated with cardiopulmonary bypass during cardiac surgery. Br J Clin Pharmacol 75(3):769–778
146. Ng A, Smith G, Davidson AC (2003) Analgesic effects of parecoxib following total abdominal hysterectomy. Br J Anaesth 90(6):746–749
147. Riest G et al (2008) Preventive effects of perioperative parecoxib on post-discectomy pain. Br J Anaesth 100(2):256–262
148. Wattchow DA et al (2009) Clinical trial: the impact of cyclooxygenase inhibitors on gastrointestinal recovery after major surgery—a randomized double blind controlled trial of celecoxib or diclofenac vs. placebo. Aliment Pharmacol Ther 30(10):987–998
149. Bar-Yosef S et al (2001) Attenuation of the tumor-promoting effect of surgery by spinal blockade in rats. Anesthesiology 94(6):1066–1073
150. Melamed R et al (2005) Marginating pulmonary-NK activity and resistance to experimental tumor metastasis: suppression by surgery and the prophylactic use of a beta-adrenergic antagonist and a prostaglandin synthesis inhibitor. Brain Behav Immun 19(2):114–126
151. Yakar I et al (2003) Prostaglandin e(2) suppresses NK activity in vivo and promotes postoperative tumor metastasis in rats. Ann Surg Oncol 10(4):469–479
152. Backhus LM et al (2006) Perioperative cyclooxygenase 2 inhibition to reduce tumor cell adhesion and metastatic potential of circulating tumor cells in non-small cell lung cancer. J Thorac Cardiovasc Surg 132(2):297–303
153. Goldfarb Y et al (2011) Improving postoperative immune status and resistance to cancer metastasis: a combined perioperative approach of immunostimulation and prevention of excessive surgical stress responses. Ann Surg 253(4):798–810
154. Diperna CA et al (2003) Cyclooxygenase-2 inhibition decreases primary and metastatic tumor burden in a murine model of orthotopic lung adenocarcinoma. J Thorac Cardiovasc Surg 126(4):1129–1133

155. Qadri SSA et al (2005) Surgically induced accelerated local and distant tumor growth is significantly attenuated by selective COX-2 inhibition. Ann Thorac Surg 79(3):990–995. Discussion 990–5
156. Tanaka T et al (2005) Treatment of lung cancer using clinically relevant oral doses of the cyclooxygenase-2 inhibitor rofecoxib: potential value as adjuvant therapy after surgery. Ann Surg 241(1):168–178
157. Zhang M et al (2011) Inhibitory effect of celecoxib in lung carcinoma by regulation of cyclooxygenase-2/cytosolic phospholipase A_2 and peroxisome proliferator-activated receptor gamma. Mol Cell Biochem 355(1–2):233–240
158. Iwata C et al (2007) Inhibition of cyclooxygenase-2 suppresses lymph node metastasis via reduction of lymphangiogenesis. Cancer Res 67(21):10181–10189
159. Ruan D, So S-P (2014) Prostaglandin E2 produced by inducible COX-2 and mPGES-1 promoting cancer cell proliferation in vitro and in vivo. Life Sci 116(1):43–50
160. Timoshenko AV et al (2006) COX-2-mediated stimulation of the lymphangiogenic factor VEGF-C in human breast cancer. Br J Cancer 94(8):1154–1163
161. Ungefroren H et al (2011) Interaction of tumor cells with the microenvironment. Cell Commun Signal 9:18
162. Xin X et al (2012) Targeting COX-2 and EP4 to control tumor growth, angiogenesis, lymphangiogenesis and metastasis to the lungs and lymph nodes in a breast cancer model. Lab Invest 92(8):1115–1128
163. Karnezis T, Shayan R, Fox S et al (2012) The connection between lymphangiogenic signalling and prostaglandin biology: a missing link in the metastatic pathway. Oncotarget 3(8):893–906
164. Roche-Nagle G et al (2004) Antimetastatic activity of a cyclooxygenase-2 inhibitor. Br J Cancer 91(2):359–365
165. Costa C et al (2002) Cyclo-oxygenase 2 expression is associated with angiogenesis and lymph node metastasis in human breast cancer. J Clin Pathol 55(6):429–434
166. Khuri FR et al (2001) Cyclooxygenase-2 overexpression is a marker of poor prognosis in stage I non-small cell lung cancer. Clin Cancer Res 7(4):861–867
167. Liu H et al (2011) COX-2 expression is correlated with VEGF-C, lymphangiogenesis and lymph node metastasis in human cervical cancer. Microvasc Res 82(2):131–140
168. Bertagnolli MM et al (2009) Five-year efficacy and safety analysis of the Adenoma Prevention with Celecoxib Trial. Cancer Prev Res 2(4):310–321
169. Steinbach G et al (2000) The effect of celecoxib, a cyclooxygenase-2 inhibitor, in familial adenomatous polyposis. N Engl J Med 342(26):1946–1952
170. Mao JT et al (2006) Celecoxib decreases Ki-67 proliferative index in active smokers. Clin Cancer Res 12(1):314–320
171. Mao JT et al (2011) Lung cancer chemoprevention with celecoxib in former smokers. Cancer Prev Res 4(7):984–993
172. Slatore CG et al (2009) Association of nonsteroidal anti-inflammatory drugs with lung cancer: results from a large cohort study. Cancer Epidemiol Biomarkers Prev 18(4):1203–1207
173. Altorki NK et al (2003) Celecoxib, a selective cyclo-oxygenase-2 inhibitor, enhances the response to preoperative paclitaxel and carboplatin in early-stage non-small-cell lung cancer. J Clin Oncol 21(14):2645–2650
174. Edelman MJ et al (2008) Eicosanoid modulation in advanced lung cancer: cyclooxygenase-2 expression is a positive predictive factor for celecoxib + chemotherapy—Cancer and Leukemia Group B Trial 30203. J Clin Oncol 26(6):848–855
175. Groen HJM et al (2011) Randomized, placebo-controlled phase III study of docetaxel plus carboplatin with celecoxib and cyclooxygenase-2 expression as a biomarker for patients with advanced non-small-cell lung cancer: the NVALT-4 study. J Clin Oncol 29(32):4320–4326
176. Koch A et al (2011) Effect of celecoxib on survival in patients with advanced non-small cell lung cancer: a double blind randomised clinical phase III trial (CYCLUS study) by the Swedish Lung Cancer Study Group. Eur J Cancer 47(10):1546–1555

177. Mutter R et al (2009) A phase II study of celecoxib in combination with paclitaxel, carboplatin, and radiotherapy for patients with inoperable stage IIIA/B non-small cell lung cancer. Clin Cancer Res 15(6):2158–2165
178. Khuri FR (2011) The dawn of a revolution in personalized lung cancer prevention. Cancer Prev Res 4(7):949–953
179. Forget P et al (2010) Do intraoperative analgesics influence breast cancer recurrence after mastectomy? A retrospective analysis. Anesth Analg 110(6):1630–1635
180. Forget P et al (2014) Intraoperative use of ketorolac or diclofenac is associated with improved disease-free survival and overall survival in conservative breast cancer surgery. Br J Anaesth 113(Suppl 1):i82–i87
181. Retsky M, Demicheli R et al (2012) Promising development from translational or perhaps anti-translational research in breast cancer. Clin Transl Med 1(1):17
182. Retsky M, Rogers R et al (2012) NSAID analgesic ketorolac used perioperatively may suppress early breast cancer relapse: particular relevance to triple negative subgroup. Breast Cancer Res Treat 134(2):881–888
183. Demicheli R et al (2008) Recurrence dynamics does not depend on the recurrence site. Breast Cancer Res 10(5):R83
184. Dhawan D et al (2010) Effects of short-term celecoxib treatment in patients with invasive transitional cell carcinoma of the urinary bladder. Mol Cancer Ther 9(5):1371–1377
185. Sooriakumaran P et al (2009) A randomized controlled trial investigating the effects of celecoxib in patients with localized prostate cancer. Anticancer Res 29(5):1483–1488
186. Liu J-F et al (2008) The effects of a COX-2 inhibitor meloxicam on squamous cell carcinoma of the esophagus in vivo. Int J Cancer 122(7):1639–1644
187. Liu J-F et al (2009) A preliminary study on the postoperative survival of patients given aspirin after resection for squamous cell carcinoma of the esophagus or adenocarcinoma of the cardia. Ann Surg Oncol 16(5):1397–1402
188. Gan TJ et al (2003) Consensus guidelines for managing postoperative nausea and vomiting. Anesth Analg 97(1):62–71
189. Inada T, Hirota K, Shingu K (2015) Intravenous anesthetic propofol suppresses prostaglandin E2 and cysteinyl leukotriene production and reduces edema formation in arachidonic acid-induced ear inflammation. J Immunotoxicol 12(3):261–265
190. Inada T, Kubo K, Ueshima H et al (2011) Intravenous anesthetic propofol suppresses prostaglandin E2 production in murine dendritic cells. J Immunotoxicol 8(4):359–366
191. Kambara T et al (2009) Propofol suppresses prostaglandin E(2) production in human peripheral monocytes. Immunopharmacol Immunotoxicol 31(1):117–126
192. Wakabayashi S et al (2014) Effects of anesthesia with sevoflurane and propofol on the cytokine/chemokine production at the airway epithelium during esophagectomy. Int J Mol Med 34(1):137–144
193. Ke JJ et al (2008) A comparison of the effect of total intravenous anaesthesia with propofol and remifentanil and inhalational anaesthesia with isoflurane on the release of pro- and anti-inflammatory cytokines in patients undergoing open cholecystectomy. Anaesth Intensive Care 36(1):74–78
194. Inada T, Kubo K, Shingu K (2011) Possible link between cyclooxygenase-inhibiting and antitumor properties of propofol. J Anesth 25(4):569–575
195. Kushida A, Inada T, Shingu K (2007) Enhancement of antitumor immunity after propofol treatment in mice. Immunopharmacol Immunotoxicol 29(3–4):477–486
196. Wigmore TJ, Mohammed K, Jhanji S (2016) Long-term survival for patients undergoing volatile versus IV anesthesia for cancer surgery: a retrospective analysis. Anesthesiology 124(1):69–79
197. Brinkrolf P, Hahnenkamp K (2014) Systemic lidocaine in surgical procedures: effects beyond sodium channel blockade. Curr Opin Anaesthesiol 27(4):420–425
198. Herroeder S et al (2007) Systemic lidocaine shortens length of hospital stay after colorectal surgery: a double-blinded, randomized, placebo-controlled trial. Ann Surg 246(2):192–200

199. Yardeni IZ et al (2009) The effect of perioperative intravenous lidocaine on postoperative pain and immune function. Anesth Analg 109(5):1464–1469
200. Swenson BR et al (2010) Intravenous lidocaine is as effective as epidural bupivacaine in reducing ileus duration, hospital stay, and pain after open colon resection: a randomized clinical trial. Reg Anesth Pain Med 35(4):370–376
201. Wongyingsinn M et al (2011) Intravenous lidocaine versus thoracic epidural analgesia: a randomized controlled trial in patients undergoing laparoscopic colorectal surgery using an enhanced recovery program. Reg Anesth Pain Med 36(3):241–248
202. Chang Y-C et al (2014) Local anesthetics induce apoptosis in human breast tumor cells. Anesth Analg 118(1):116–124
203. Piegeler T et al (2012) Antimetastatic potential of amide-linked local anesthetics: inhibition of lung adenocarcinoma cell migration and inflammatory Src signaling independent of sodium channel blockade. Anesthesiology 117(3):548–559
204. Lucchinetti E et al (2012) Antiproliferative effects of local anesthetics on mesenchymal stem cells: potential implications for tumor spreading and wound healing. Anesthesiology 116(4):841–856
205. Fraser SP, Foo I, Djamgoz MBA (2014) Local anaesthetic use in cancer surgery and disease recurrence: role of voltage-gated sodium channels? Br J Anaesth 113(6):899–902

Chapter 5
Circulating Tumor Cells as Predictive Marker in Metastatic Disease

Mazen A. Juratli, Dmitry A. Nedosekin, Mustafa Sarimollaoglu, Eric R. Siegel, Ekaterina I. Galanzha, and Vladimir P. Zharov

Abstract Numerous studies have demonstrated that circulating tumor cell (CTC) number in peripheral blood correlates with therapy efficiency in various tumors, and can serve as a prognostic marker of metastasis development. Recent clinical data support many oncologists' opinion that some medical procedures may provoke metastasis by triggering increased tumor cell shedding into circulation, but no systematic study has been performed. The development of an *in vivo* flow cytometry method for real-time CTC quantification can provide insights on CTC release dynamics during different medical interventions and possibly long and short term outcome predictions.

Noninvasive enumeration of CTCs is the most direct way to confirm the central hypothesis that tumor manipulations during medical interventions can promote liberation of CTC into the bloodstream. Incisional biopsy and complete tumor resection in melanoma-bearing mice were conducted and the CTC rate was monitored before, during, and for a short-term after the procedures. Incisional biopsy significantly increased CTC counts (up to 60-fold), whereas complete tumor resection significantly decreased CTC counts. Long-term *in vivo* monitoring of CTC triggered by punch biopsy and complete tumor resection was performed on breast cancer- bearing mice. After punch biopsy, the number of CTC increased. In contrast, complete tumor resection significantly decreased the CTC count. New techniques were proposed for labeling newly released CTCs in order to identify them among previously circulating cells.

M.A. Juratli (✉)
Department of General and Visceral Surgery, Goethe-University Hospital of Frankfurt, Frankfurt am Main, Germany

Winthrop P. Rockefeller Cancer Institute, Arkansas Nanomedicine Center, University of Arkansas for Medical Sciences (UAMS), 4301 West Markham, Little Rock, AR 72205, USA
e-mail: Mazen.Juratli@kgu.de

D.A. Nedosekin • M. Sarimollaoglu • E.R. Siegel • E.I. Galanzha • V.P. Zharov
Winthrop P. Rockefeller Cancer Institute, Arkansas Nanomedicine Center, University of Arkansas for Medical Sciences (UAMS), 4301 West Markham, Little Rock, AR 72205, USA
e-mail: DNedosekin@uams.edu; MSarimollaoglu@uams.edu; SiegelEricR@uams.edu; EGalanzha@uams.edu; ZharovVladimirP@uams.edu

M.W. Retsky, R. Demicheli (eds.), *Perioperative Inflammation as Triggering Origin of Metastasis Development*, DOI 10.1007/978-3-319-57943-6_5

These findings have broad clinical implications to reduce viable CTCs release during diagnostics and treatments by real-time monitoring of CTC dynamics followed by well-timed treatment to reduce CTCs in the blood.

Keywords Circulating tumor cell • Melanoma • Breast cancer • Surgery • Biopsy • *In vivo* flow cytometry

5.1 Circulating Tumor Cells (CTCs)

Up to 90% of cancer deaths are related to metastasis in distant organs due to the hematogenous and lymphatics dissemination of circulating tumor cells (CTCs) shed from the primary tumor [1–5]. Despite major effort, challenges remain in treating advanced stages of disease in patients in whom distant metastases develop [1–3]. It would be extremely helpful to have an ultrasensitive blood cancer test (liquid biopsy) for early stages of metastatic diseases, when well-timed therapy is more effective. CTCs at early disease stages are present in the bloodstream in extremely low concentrations: ≤10 CTC/mL. The invasion of tumor cells in the circulation may occur very early in tumor development, thus emphasizing the potential importance of sensitive detection of CTCs and circulating tumor microemboli (CTM).

5.2 Cancer Treatment and CTC Release

A growing body of clinical data suggests that medical diagnostic and therapeutic procedures such as surgery, chemotherapy and radiation therapy may trigger tumor cell shedding into the circulation and thus increase the risk of metastasis. However, data on CTC release due to medical interventions such as tumor palpation, biopsy, or surgery is controversial [6–10]. Some previous studies have shown an increase in CTC number using *in vitro* methods after surgical tumor resection [9], while others observed a decrease in CTC count after surgery or metastases resection [10, 11]. Wind et al. [12] reported significantly fewer CTC during laparoscopic surgery compared to open surgery in patients with colon cancer during tumor resection. The major drawback of these studies is that CTC enumeration is performed several hours after tumor resection, and likely could miss the transient increase in CTC number during or immediately after surgery because of the short CTC lifetime (0.5–4 h depending on CTC metastatic activity) [13–16]. Moreover, the effective difference between surgical invasiveness of cancer such as incisional biopsy and excisional biopsy in term of CTC release into the blood stream is suggested to play an important role in tumor diagnosis and treatment. Incisional biopsy could result in increased risk of metastasis by increasing the CTC count [8, 17]. This effect was observed both using an *ex vivo* model and after the biopsy.

Real-time *in vivo* fluorescence imaging was used to reveal an increase in CTC count in lymphatic vessels after applying 25 or 250 g of pressure for 10 s on the tumor, but no dynamics studies were performed and no correlation with metastasis progression has been established [18]. Unfortunately, this and most other previous studies have not reported crucial tumor manipulation details (e.g. palpation, compression, or partial resection) or lack a comprehensive comparison of the outcomes for different manipulations.

5.3 Principles of *In Vivo* Flow Cytometry with Photoacoustic and Fluorescence Detection Techniques

In vivo flow cytometry (FC), which was invented in 2004, can quantitatively monitor circulating cells *in vivo*, both noninvasively and dynamically [19–28]. Pigmented and fluorescent cells can be detected *in vivo* using dual-contrast photoacoustic (PA) fluorescence flow cytometry (PAFFC) [22]. The method uses laser irradiation of peripheral blood vessels to induce acoustic waves (PA effect) from pigmented cells (e.g., melanoma with intrinsic melanin as PA contrast agent) or fluorescence from cells containing fluorescent proteins (e.g. green fluorescent protein, GFP) in blood flow. The transient increase in blood PA background caused by the presence of a pigmented cell is detected by an ultrasound transducer attached to the skin. The photomultiplier tube detects transient increase in fluorescence from vessels [29–31]. The PA background is associated with the absorption of randomly distributed red blood cells (RBCs) in the irradiated volume, whereas the fluorescence background is related to the autofluorescence from blood and plasma components. In fluorescence flow cytometry (FFC), a cell emits fluorescence photons under continuous wave (CW) laser excitation, whereas PA flow cytometry (PAFC) uses nanosecond pulse lasers to generate PA signals (Fig. 5.1).

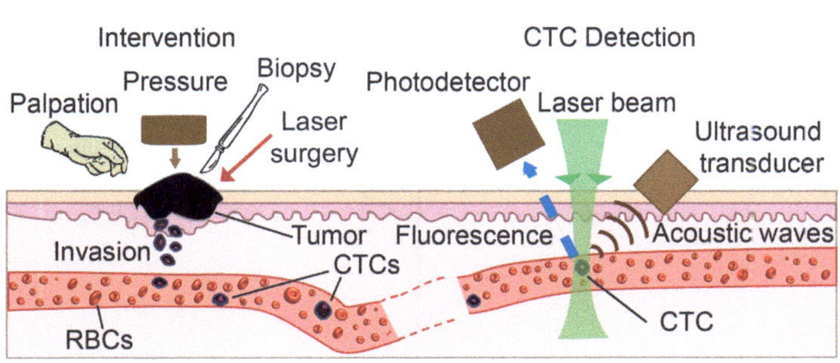

Fig. 5.1 Principle of *in vivo* flow cytometry using PA and fluorescence methods for real-time monitoring of melanoma and breast CTCs directly in the bloodstream during palpation, pressure, biopsy, and surgery. (Reproduced from Juratli et al. [22, 25])

5.4 Relationship Between Cancer Treatment and CTC Release

Using tumor-bearing mouse models, the CTC dynamic was studied during cancer treatment and afterwards. Melanoma and breast cancer cell lines inoculated in nude mice were used. The effect of biopsy and surgery on CTC dynamics was studied.

5.4.1 CTC Dynamics, and Tumor Growth in Tumor-Bearing Mice Without Interventions (Control)

Breast cancer tumor-bearing mice (n = 6) were used as control group to identify the normal rate for CTC release by the tumor. CTCs were detected by FFC and using their intrinsic fluorescence contrast (GFP expression). The average CTC count varied between 0.5 and 2 cells/min during the first 8 weeks of tumor growth, and peaked at the third and fifth weeks (Fig. 5.2). Fluctuating CTC count did not strongly correlate with tumor size in our orthotropic tumor-bearing mouse model [23].

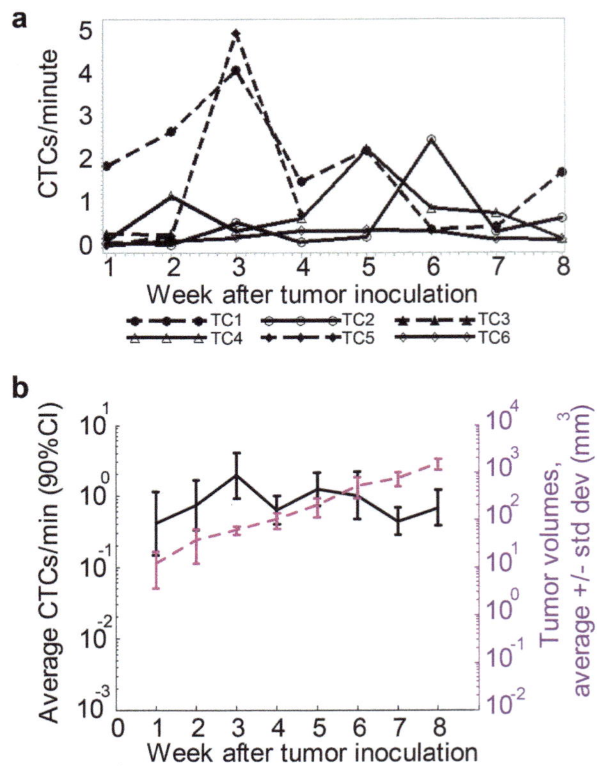

Fig. 5.2 (**a**) Profile plot of CTC detection rates (in CTCs/minute) measured weekly from six different mice inoculated with breast cancer cells (MDA-MB-LUC2-GFP) during the 8 weeks after tumor inoculation, (**b**) profile plot of the average number of CTC signals per minute and average tumor volume during the same 8 weeks. Values and error bars represent the averages and SDs of CTC counts from n = 6 mice. (Reproduced from Juratli et al. [23])

5.4.2 *Tumor Biopsy-Related CTC Release*

Two kinds of biopsy using two different tumor-bearing mouse models were conducted to study the effect of biopsy on CTC dynamics. Incisional biopsy in a melanoma-bearing mouse model and punch biopsy in a breast cancer-bearing mouse model were performed.

5.4.2.1 Incisional Biopsy in Melanoma-Bearing Mouse Model

Five Melanoma-bearing mice were tested using *in vivo* PAFC, relying on the intrinsic melanin in CTCs. Mice were monitored continuously for 60 min before, 15 min during, and 260 min after incisional biopsy. The baseline CTC detection rate was 1.3 cells/10 min before biopsy began. During the 15-min biopsy period, CTC rate soared to 75.1 cells/10 min, a 58-fold increase compared to baseline ($P < 0.0001$). During the first hour after the biopsy concluded, CTC rate remained high at 44.3 cells/10 min, which was 34-fold higher than the baseline ($P < 0.0001$). It decreased thereafter, but remained significantly elevated at sixfold above baseline ($P = 0.049$) during the second hour after biopsy, and at threefold above baseline ($P = 0.007$) afterwards (Fig. 5.3a–c) [22].

In two instances, we performed a second incisional biopsy 1 h after the first one. We also detected a total of 200 CTCs during the first 10 min after the second biopsy. This number was less than the first time, where we observed a total of 380 CTCs during the same period (Fig. 5.3d) [22].

5.4.2.2 Punch Biopsy in Breast Cancer-Bearing Mouse Model

A punch biopsy was conducted in six mice bearing MDA-231-MB-GFP breast cancer tumor 2 weeks after tumor inoculation. A 2.0 mm biopsy punch with a plunger system (BPP-20F 2.0 mm w/plunger, Miltex, Inc.) was used for biopsy. Cells expressing GFP were detected using FFC.

During the 8 weeks of monitoring, CTC detection rate varied from 0.2 to 1.6 cells/min (Fig. 5.4a, b). In comparison to control group (Sect. 5.4.1), average CTC rate after the biopsy was steadier (Fig. 5.4a, b). Tumor volume increased continuously throughout the experiment (Fig. 5.4b–e). The punch biopsy performed at the second week after tumor inoculation did not affect the tumor volume in five of the total of six mice. The tumor volume increased continuously during the 8 weeks after tumor inoculation. However, the punch biopsy immediately caused a significant increase in the number of CTCs at week 2. The baseline average CTC rate during 1 h before the biopsy (0.64 cells/min) was elevated to 1.17 cells/min for the 2 h after biopsy ended ($P = 0.021$; Fig. 5.4d) [23].

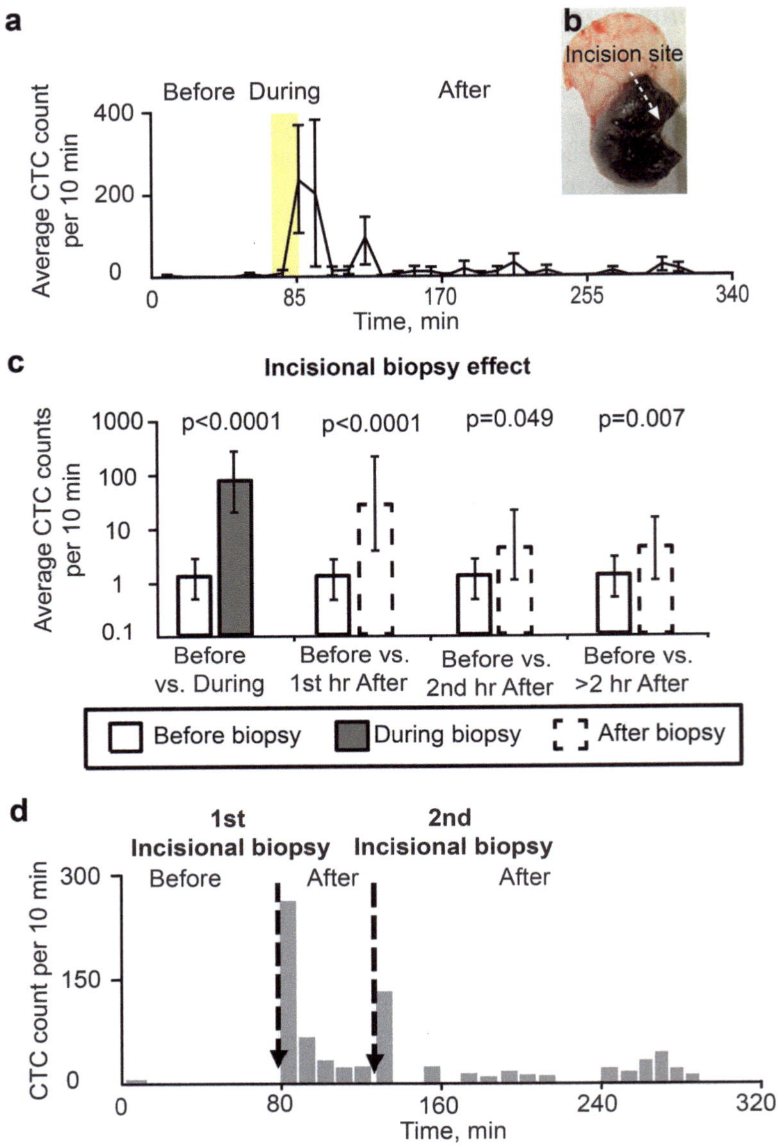

Fig. 5.3 (**a**) Histogram of average CTC counts per 10-min window for 70 min before, 15 min during (*yellow region*) and 260 min after incisional biopsy. Values and error bars represent the averages and SDs of CTC counts from n = 5 mice during each 10-min bin, (**b**) tumor after incisional biopsy, (**c**) CTC detection rates in counts per 10 min before vs. during biopsy, and before vs. after biopsy. Values (error bars) represent the estimates (90% confidence intervals) determined from mixed-models Poisson-regression analysis, (**d**) example of histogram of CTCs release before, and after two different incisional biopsies in the same mouse (B16F10-GFP) (duration of each incisional biopsy: approx. ~1 min). (Reproduced from Juratli et al. [22, 25])

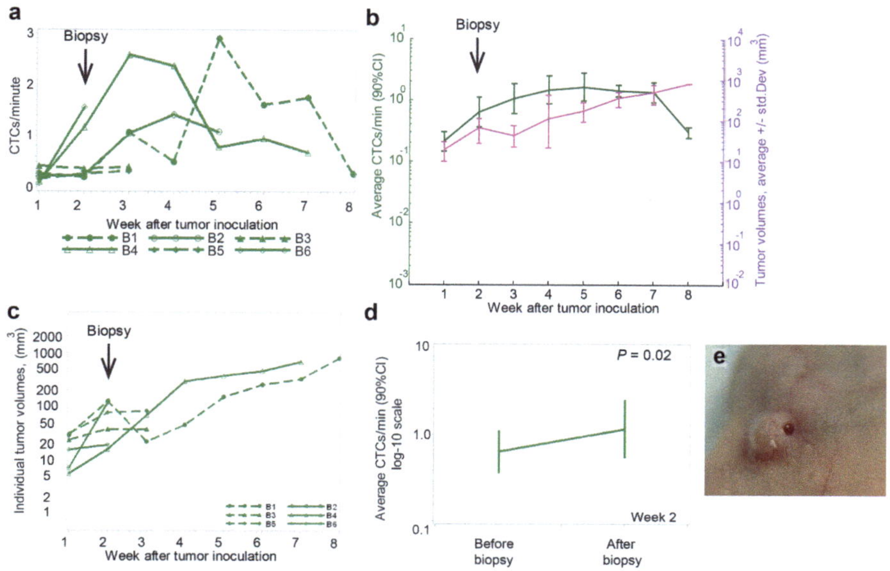

Fig. 5.4 (**a**) Profile plot of CTC detection rate number of CTCs per minute measured weekly from six mice inoculated with breast cancer cells (MDA-MB-LUC2-GFP) during the 8 weeks after tumor inoculation. Punch biopsy was performed at week 2 after tumor inoculation, (**b**) profile plot over time of the average number of CTC signals per minute and average of the tumor volume during the same 8 weeks. Values and error bars represent the averages and SDs of CTC counts from n = 6 mice. The average CTC rate per 8 weeks was calculated for five mice at week 3, three mice at week 5 and two mice at week 7, (**c**) individual tumor volumes from six mice. Punch biopsy was performed at week 2 after tumor inoculation, (**d**) profile plot of the average number of CTC signals per minute from 60 min before to 120 min after the punch biopsy, showing a 1.82-fold increase in the CTC-detection rate ($P = 0.02$), (**e**) image of the tumor after a punch biopsy. (Reproduced from Juratli et al. [23])

5.4.3 *Tumor Surgery-Related CTC Release*

To study the effect of surgery on CTC dynamics, complete tumor resection was conducted in melanoma-bearing mouse model and in breast cancer-bearing mouse model.

5.4.3.1 Complete Tumor Resection in Melanoma-Bearing Mouse Model

Seven mice with melanoma tumors on their right ears underwent tumor resection. PAFC was performed to enumerate CTCs in a blood vessel of the left ear, before and after the tumor resection. During the 50 min of baseline recording prior to tumor resection, a total of 35 CTCs were detected among the 7 mice (an average of 1 CTC/10 min). In contrast, no increase in CTC rate was observed during

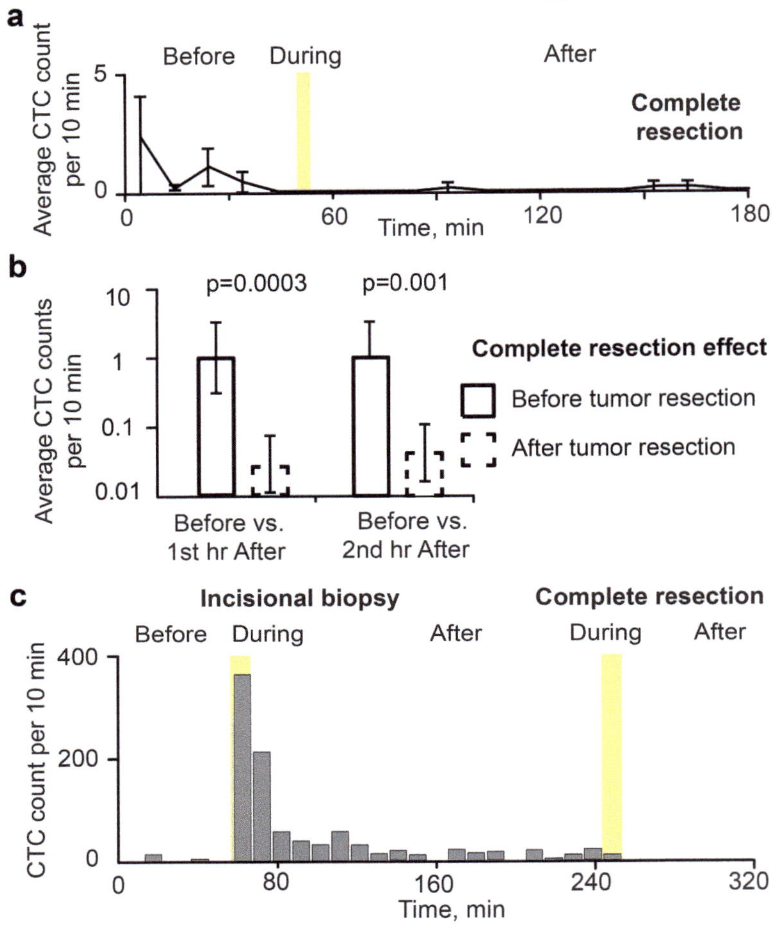

Fig. 5.5 (**a**) Histogram of average CTC signal number per 10 min from before, 5 min during (*yellow region*) and after complete tumor resection. Values and error bars represent the averages and SDs of CTC counts from n = 7 mice during each 10-min bin, (**b**) CTC detection rates in counts per 10 min before vs. the first hour and second hour after surgery. During complete resection, no CTCs were detected. Values (error bars) represent the estimates (90% confidence intervals) determined from mixed-models Poisson-regression analysis, (**c**) Example of histogram of CTCs release before, and after incisional biopsy (duration of incisional biopsy: approx. 10 min), and tumor complete resection with tumor manipulation (duration of complete tumor resection: approx. 10 min) (B16F10-GFP). (Reproduced from Juratli et al. [22, 25])

surgery, and only one CTC was detected during the first hour after resection (0.023 CTCs/10 min; $P = 0.0002$), and only two CTCs were detected during the second hour after resection (0.047 CTCs/10 min; $P = 0.0005$) among the seven mice. Two to three hours after tumor resection, no CTCs were detected in any mouse (Fig. 5.5a, b) [22].

5.4.3.2 Incisional Biopsy Followed by Complete Tumor Resection in Melanoma-Bearing Mouse Model

In two cases, a complete tumor resection was conducted 2 h after the incisional biopsy. The tumor (B16F10-GFP) was squeezed with a surgical instrument during resection. Twenty CTCs were observed during 10 min of resection time and no CTCs were detected up to 1 h after the complete resection was completed (Fig. 5.5c) [22].

5.4.3.3 Complete Tumor Resection in Breast Cancer-Bearing Mouse Model

On a group of six mice, tumor resection was conducted 2 weeks after inoculation of MDA-MB-231 breast cancer cells in the mammary gland. In five of them, tumor-free margins were achieved and there was no residual tumor left, which was confirmed by histology exams performed on the resected tumors.

A dramatic decrease in the number of CTCs was observed compared to the control group (Sect. 5.4.1); from 0.1 CTCs/min at second week to ~0.01 CTCs/min at weeks three-to-eight (Fig. 5.6a, b). However, CTC recurrence in small numbers was detected during the 5 weeks following surgery (Fig. 5.6a, b).

No tumor visibly re-grew in any of the mice during the 6 weeks after tumor resection (Fig. 5.6b). A short-term effect of complete tumor resection was also profound. While a total of 28 CTCs were detected during 1 h before resection (0.08 CTCs/min, $n = 6$), no CTCs were observed during and for 2 h after the resection ($P = 0.03$) (Fig. 5.6d) [23].

In one of the mice (S5), histology exam of the resected tumor revealed a positive tumor margin (Fig. 5.5a). The CTC rate for this mouse was the highest in the group for 6 weeks after the surgery, and the maximum CTC rate was observed 2 weeks after the surgery [23].

5.4.4 Novel Techniques for Identification of Released CTC

The quantification of CTC release triggered by manipulation is complicated by the presence of CTCs that were shed from tumor sometime before the manipulation. This requires the use of complex statistical methods to confirm the release of CTCs as the result of manipulations. Novel tools for labeling tumor cells bring a promise of simple identification of newly released CTCs among already circulating ones. Both photoswitchable fluorescent proteins (e.g. Dendra2 [32, 33]) as contrast agents for fluorescence flow cytometry and photoswitchable nanoparticles (NPs) for PA detection have been proposed to identify manipulation-released CTCs [32, 34].

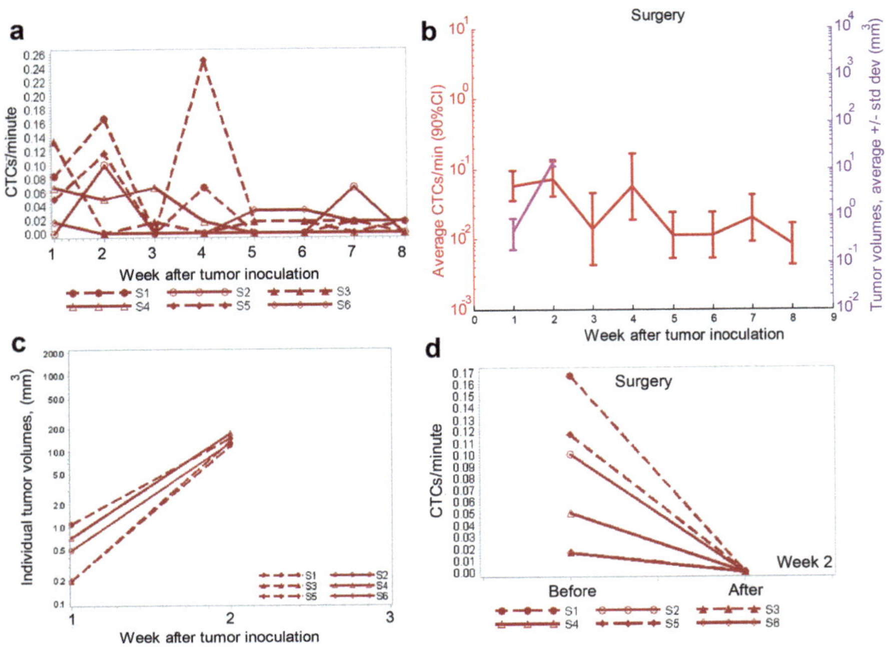

Fig. 5.6 (**a**) Profile plot of CTC detection rates (in CTCs/minute) measured weekly from six mice inoculated with breast cancer cells (MDA-MB-LUC2-GFP). Surgery was conducted at Week 2 after tumor inoculation, (**b**) profile plot of the average number of CTC signals per minute and average tumor volume during 8 weeks from n = 5 mice after excluding the mouse which received partial tumor resection. Values and error bars represent the averages and SDs of CTC counts from n = 5 mice, (**c**) individual tumor volumes from six mice. Surgery was performed at week 2 after tumor inoculation, (**d**) profile plot of the average number of CTC signals per minute from 60 min before and 120 min after the surgery. (Reproduced from Juratli et al. [23])

5.4.4.1 Photoswitchable Fluorescent Proteins

Photoswitchable fluorescent protein Dendra2 normally fluoresces in green, however, it can be irreversibly switched into red color using 405 nm laser [35]. A photoswitchable fluorescence cytometry (PFC) for noninvasive enumeration of red and green cells, as well as switching of primary tumor cells and of individual CTCs in blood flow was developed [34]. The principles of CTCs identification using photoswitchable proteins were demonstrated using a mouse ear model of metastatic carcinoma (MTLn3 adenocarcinoma cells expressing Dendra2 protein). Thin ear structures and isolated tumor location allow successful photoswitching of all the primary tumor cells, and noninvasive fluorescence imaging to control switching efficacy laser. Dual color (green and red) monitoring of CTCs released from the primary tumor has indicated that only green cells are released from the primary tumor, and possibly, from already established metastases. However, after the primary tumor was completely converted into "red" state (i.e. Dendra2 protein in all the primary tumor cells was switched to red color), it was able to detect both green

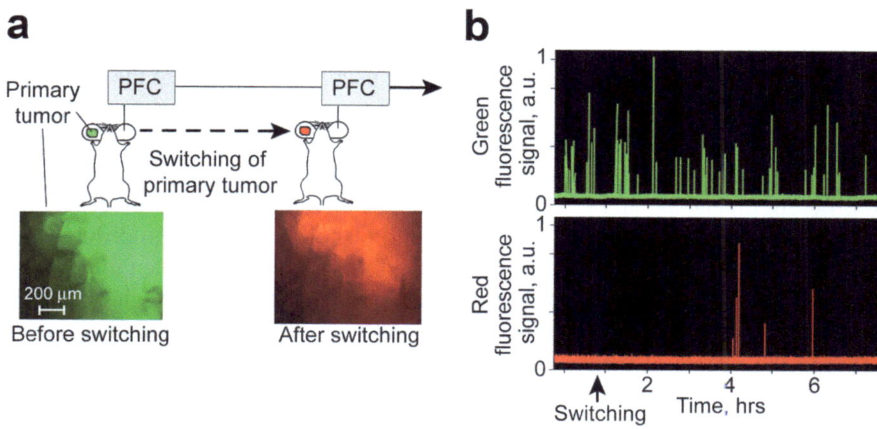

Fig. 5.7 (**a**) Concept of switching the primary tumor cells from *green* to *red* state; (**b**) dual color detection of circulating cells in peripheral blood flow (56 μm diameter ear vein) after photoswitching of the primary tumor. *Green signals* correspond to non-switched CTCs shed into flow before switching of the primary tumor, *red signals* correspond to photoswitched cells released after conversion. (Reproduced from Nedosekin et al. [34])

(old CTCs) and red (recently released CTCs) in circulation. Without manipulation, first red CTCs were detected ~180 min after switching indicating that it was spontaneous shedding [25]. Moreover, high irregularity in the dynamics of new CTCs release was observed. The same model can be extended to study release of CTCs from metastases (non-switched metastases will keep producing green CTCs), given that primary tumor may shed only red cells and all the old green CTCs will eventually leave the circulation (Fig. 5.7) [34].

5.5 Discussion and Conclusion

The major cause of cancer-associated mortality is tumor metastasis. CTCs which during successful dissemination invade the surrounding primary tumor tissue, intravasate into blood, lymph and cerebrospinal fluid and could form metastases [36, 37]. Therefore, one of the most promising approaches to prevent metastatic disease is the early detection of CTCs and to avoid interventions which could lead to an increase in CTC rate.

This work was designed with the overall goal to determine the dynamic fluctuation of CTCs during medical interventions using breast cancer and melanoma-bearing mouse models. The PAFC and FFC allowed us to monitor the CTC dynamics noninvasively and in real-time in physiologically and clinically relevant conditions. The well-established murine xenograft mouse model was used in these studies. This model has several advantages to determine CTC dynamics during tumor growth and medical interventions because of (1) the use of actual human tumor tissue; (2)

results could be obtained during the few weeks from tumor inoculation; (3) the organ environment in which the tumor growth could be reproduced [38]. However, the immunological deficit is a disadvantage for using this model. For the first time, it was possible to monitor the same mouse frequently up to 8 weeks after tumor inoculation and to study the change in CTC rate during tumor biopsy and surgery.

This work aimed to determine the short term of the CTC dynamic fluctuation due to different diagnostic and treatment procedures. Here experimental evidence that incisional biopsy increased the CTC rate up to 60-fold during the procedures in a melanoma-bearing mouse model was presented. In contrast, complete tumor resection led to decrease of CTC rate and in some cases to disappearance shortly afterwards. One of the most interesting findings in this work could be the discrepancy between the effects of incisional biopsy versus excisional biopsy on CTC count. This analysis is very timely and relevant, as tumor manipulation is a key point of interest for the practicing surgeon. To study the CTC dynamics for long-term after procedures, breast cancer-bearing mice were used. In this study, marked increase in CTC rate was determined during the punch biopsy. In the melanoma-bearing mouse model, however, a higher level of CTC rate was monitored shortly afterwards. Different outcome was observed after complete tumor resection by disappearance of the CTCs. However, in some cases low level of CTC re-elevation during 6 weeks after the procedure was observed in the breast cancer-bearing mice.

The results of this work provide further support that tumor manipulation, by offering greater opportunity for tumor cell invasion into the circulation, could result in shedding of malignant cells into the circulatory system and possibly in turn will affect the prognosis by increasing the risk of metastasis [39]. However, these data must be interpreted with caution because of the immunological deficit of the tumor bearing-mouse models used and because of the CTCs, which are rare and not all may be clinically relevant in the human body [37]. Thus, further research is needed to examine CTC dynamic in human *in vivo* during tumor growth and medical interventions.

References

1. Galanzha EI, Zharov VP (2013) Circulating tumor cell detection and capture by photoacoustic flow cytometry in vivo and ex vivo. Cancers (Basel) 5:1691–1738
2. Pantel K, Brakenhoff RH, Brandt B (2008) Detection, clinical relevance and specific biological properties of disseminating tumour cells. Nat Rev Cancer 8:329–340
3. Kaiser J (2010) Medicine. Cancer's circulation problem. Science 327:1072–1074
4. Yu M, Bardia A, Wittner BS, Stott SL, Smas ME et al (2013) Circulating breast tumor cells exhibit dynamic changes in epithelial and mesenchymal composition. Science 339:580–584
5. Yu M, Stott S, Toner M, Maheswaran S, Haber DA (2011) Circulating tumor cells: approaches to isolation and characterization. J Cell Biol 192:373–382
6. Weitz J, Kienle P, Lacroix J, Willeke F, Benner A et al (1998) Dissemination of tumor cells in patients undergoing surgery for colorectal cancer. Clin Cancer Res 4:343–348
7. Louha M, Nicolet J, Zylberberg H, Sabile A, Vons C et al (1999) Liver resection and needle liver biopsy cause hematogenous dissemination of liver cells. Hepatology 29:879–882

8. Loughran CF, Keeling CR (2011) Seeding of tumour cells following breast biopsy: a literature review. Br J Radiol 84:869–874
9. Katharina P (2011) Tumor cell seeding during surgery-possible contribution to metastasis formations. Cancers (Basel) 3:2540–2553
10. Patel H, Le Marer N, Wharton RQ, Khan ZA, Araia R et al (2002) Clearance of circulating tumor cells after excision of primary colorectal cancer. Ann Surg 235:226–231
11. Fan ZC, Yan J, Liu GD, Tan XY, Weng XF et al (2012) Real-time monitoring of rare circulating hepatocellular carcinoma cells in an orthotopic model by in vivo flow cytometry assesses resection on metastasis. Cancer Res 72:2683–2691
12. Wind J, Tuynman JB, Tibbe AG, Swennenhuis JF, Richel DJ et al (2009) Circulating tumour cells during laparoscopic and open surgery for primary colonic cancer in portal and peripheral blood. Eur J Surg Oncol 35:942–950
13. He W, Wang H, Hartmann LC, Cheng JX, Low PS (2007) In vivo quantitation of rare circulating tumor cells by multiphoton intravital flow cytometry. Proc Natl Acad Sci U S A 104:11760–11765
14. Riethdorf S, Fritsche H, Muller V, Rau T, Schindlbeck C et al (2007) Detection of circulating tumor cells in peripheral blood of patients with metastatic breast cancer: a validation study of the CellSearch system. Clin Cancer Res 13:920–928
15. Bednarz-Knoll N, Alix-Panabieres C, Pantel K (2011) Clinical relevance and biology of circulating tumor cells. Breast Cancer Res 13:228
16. Wei X, Sipkins DA, Pitsillides CM, Novak J, Georgakoudi I et al (2005) Real-time detection of circulating apoptotic cells by in vivo flow cytometry. Mol Imaging 4:415–416
17. Kusukawa J, Suefuji Y, Ryu F, Noguchi R, Iwamoto O et al (2000) Dissemination of cancer cells into circulation occurs by incisional biopsy of oral squamous cell carcinoma. J Oral Pathol Med 29:303–307
18. Hayashi K, Jiang P, Yamauchi K, Yamamoto N, Tsuchiya H et al (2007) Real-time imaging of tumor-cell shedding and trafficking in lymphatic channels. Cancer Res 67:8223–8228
19. Novak J, Georgakoudi I, Wei X, Prossin A, Lin CP (2004) In vivo flow cytometer for real- time detection and quantification of circulating cells. Opt Lett 29:77–79
20. Georgakoudi I, Solban N, Novak J, Rice WL, Wei X et al (2004) In vivo flow cytometry: a new method for enumerating circulating cancer cells. Cancer Res 64:5044–5047
21. Nedosekin DA, Sarimollaoglu M, Galanzha EI, Sawant R, Torchilin VP et al (2013) Synergy of photoacoustic and fluorescence flow cytometry of circulating cells with negative and positive contrasts. J Biophotonics 6:425–434
22. Juratli MA, Sarimollaoglu M, Siegel ER, Nedosekin DA, Galanzha EI et al (2014) Real-time monitoring of circulating tumor cell release during tumor manipulation using in vivo photoacoustic and fluorescent flow cytometry. Head Neck 36:1207–1215
23. Juratli MA, Siegel ER, Nedosekin DA, Sarimollaoglu M, Jamshidi-Parsian A et al (2015) In vivo long-term monitoring of circulating tumor cells fluctuation during medical interventions. PLoS One 10:e0137613
24. Zharov VP, Galanzha EI, Tuchin VV (2005) Integrated photothermal flow cytometry in vivo. J Biomed Opt 10:051502
25. Juratli MA, Sarimollaoglu M, Nedosekin DA, Melerzanov AV, Zharov VP et al (2014) Dynamic fluctuation of circulating tumor cells during cancer progression. Cancers (Basel) 6:128–142
26. Menyaev YA, Nedosekin DA, Sarimollaoglu M, Juratli MA, Galanzha EI et al (2013) Optical clearing in photoacoustic flow cytometry. Biomed Opt Express 4:3030–3041
27. Sarimollaoglu M, Nedosekin DA, Menyaev YA, Juratli MA, Zharov VP (2014) Nonlinear photoacoustic signal amplification from single targets in absorption background. Photoacoustics 2:1–11
28. Nedosekin DA, Juratli MA, Sarimollaoglu M, Moore CL, Rusch NJ et al (2013) Photoacoustic and photothermal detection of circulating tumor cells, bacteria and nanoparticles in cerebrospinal fluid in vivo and ex vivo. J Biophotonics 6:523–533

29. Galanzha EI, Kim JW, Zharov VP (2009) Nanotechnology-based molecular photoacoustic and photothermal flow cytometry platform for in-vivo detection and killing of circulating cancer stem cells. J Biophotonics 2:725–735
30. Galanzha EI, Shashkov EV, Spring PM, Suen JY, Zharov VP (2009) In vivo, noninvasive, label-free detection and eradication of circulating metastatic melanoma cells using two- color photoacoustic flow cytometry with a diode laser. Cancer Res 69:7926–7934
31. Galanzha EI, Zharov VP (2012) Photoacoustic flow cytometry. Methods 57:280–296
32. Galanzha EI, Nedosekin DA, Sarimollaoglu M, Orza AI, Biris AS et al (2015) Photoacoustic and photothermal cytometry using photoswitchable proteins and nanoparticles with ultrasharp resonances. J Biophotonics 8:81–93
33. Yao J, Kaberniuk AA, Li L, Shcherbakova DM, Zhang R et al (2016) Multiscale photoacoustic tomography using reversibly switchable bacterial phytochrome as a near-infrared photochromic probe. Nat Methods 13:67–73
34. Nedosekin DA, Verkhusha VV, Melerzanov AV, Zharov VP, Galanzha EI (2014) In vivo photoswitchable flow cytometry for direct tracking of single circulating tumor cells. Chem Biol 21:792–801
35. Kedrin D, Gligorijevic B, Wyckoff J, Verkhusha VV, Condeelis J et al (2008) Intravital imaging of metastatic behavior through a mammary imaging window. Nat Methods 5:1019–1021
36. Pantel K, Alix-Panabieres C (2012) Detection methods of circulating tumor cells. J Thorac Dis 4:446–447
37. Plaks V, Koopman CD, Werb Z (2013) Cancer. Circulating tumor cells. Science 341: 1186–1188.
38. Richmond A, Su Y (2008) Mouse xenograft models vs GEM models for human cancer therapeutics. Dis Model Mech 1:78–82
39. Davies MM, Mathur P, Carnochan P, Saini S, Allen-Mersh TG (2002) Effect of manipulation of primary tumour vascularity on metastasis in an adenocarcinoma model. Br J Cancer 86:123–129

Chapter 6
Randomized Clinical Trials on Breast Cancer in Nigeria and Other Developing Countries: Challenges and Constraints

Osaro Erhabor, Frank Udomah, Yakubu Abdulrahaman, Isaac Zama, Momodu Imoru, Teddy Charles Adias, Tosan Erhabor, Lori J., Amos Dangana, Bibiana Nonye Egenti, Christy Fredrick, Godswill Chikwendu Okara, Ikechukwu Iwueke, Olutayo Ifedayo Ajayi, and Emokpae Abiodun

Abstract Worldwide, breast cancer is the commonest cancer among women, and its incidence is rising exponentially particularly in developing countries. Compared with Caucasian women, women in developing countries experience a disproportionate burden of aggressive Triple Negative Breast Cancer for reasons that remain unknown and understudied. There is a high incidence of late stage presentation, low level of public awareness of the disease, suboptimal health infrastructure, lack of universal access to affordable interventions and poor prognosis.

A randomized controlled trial or randomized control trial (RCT) is a type of scientific (often medical) experiment, where the people being studied are allocated at random (by chance alone) to receive one of several clinical interventions. These

O. Erhabor (✉) • F. Udomah • Y. Abdulrahaman • I. Zama • M. Imoru
Faculty of Medical Laboratory Science, Department of Haematology and Blood Transfusion Science, Usmanu Danfodiyo University, Sokoto, Nigeria

Department of Human Physiology, University of Benin, Benin, Nigeria

Department of Medical Laboratory Science, University of Benin, Benin, Nigeria
e-mail: n_osaro@yahoo.com

T.C. Adias
Department of Microbiology, Federal University Otuoke, Otuoke, Bayelsa State, Nigeria

T. Erhabor
Medical Laboratory Science Council of Nigeria, Abuja, Nigeria

Lori J.
Department of Chemistry, Bingham University, Karu, Nigeria

A. Dangana
Department of Haematology, University of Abuja Teaching Hospital, Abuja, Nigeria

B.N. Egenti
Department of Community Medicine, College of Health Sciences, University of Abuja, Abuja, Nigeria

M.W. Retsky, R. Demicheli (eds.), *Perioperative Inflammation as Triggering Origin of Metastasis Development*, DOI 10.1007/978-3-319-57943-6_6

kinds of studies are vital in the development of new treatments and interventions for serious diseases like breast cancer, malaria, TB and HIV which are ravaging developing and often resource-poor countries. The need for more randomized clinical trials on breast cancer in developing countries cannot be overemphasized as it creates a unique opportunity to generate data and possibly develop affordable interventions that are responsive to the peculiar health challenges rather than relying on data from the West which may not be representative. Several limiting factors exist that can potentially affect the effectiveness of these trials. These challenges include; ethical challenges, bureaucracy in government, late stage of presentation, high prevalence of triple negative breast cancers, follow up challenges, cost-related challenges, sub optimal health infrastructure, poor implementation of clinical governance, suboptimal number of trained clinical trial personnel, poor laboratory capacity, informed consent-related issues, poor data management, suboptimal number of trained statisticians, challenge of poor awareness and stigma associated with breast cancer, logistics and accessibility issues concerning management of health products, education and communication-related challenges and cultural and religious issues. Objective approaches to these challenges are vital to the successful implementation of fit-for-purpose randomized clinical trial particularly on breast cancer in Nigeria and other developing countries.

Keywords Breast cancer • Triple negative • Clinical trials • Nigeria • Potential problems • Variable water quality and electricity • Opportunity

6.1 Introduction

A randomized controlled trial or randomized control trial (RCT) is a type of scientific research, where the people being studied are allocated at random (by chance alone) to receive one of several clinical interventions. [1]. They are used to test the efficacy or effectiveness of various types of medical intervention with the aim of obtaining evidence-based information about effectiveness, adverse effects and drug

C. Fredrick
Department of Pathology, College of Health Sciences, University of Abuja, Abuja, Nigeria

G.C. Okara
Dr. Hassan's Hospital and Diagnostic Centre, Abuja, Nigeria

I. Iwueke
Department of Pathology, Federal Neuro Psychiatric Hospital Kware, Kware, Sokoto State, Nigeria

O.I. Ajayi
Department of Human Physiology, University of Benin, Benin, Nigeria

E. Abiodun
Department of Medical Laboratory Science, University of Benin, Benin, Nigeria

reactions. The RCT is one of the simplest and most powerful tools in clinical research. In RCTs one of these interventions serve as a standard (control) upon which the comparison with the test is based. The control may be a standard practice, a placebo or no intervention at all. Individuals in a RCT are called participants or subjects. The aim of RCTs is a quantitative measure to compare the outcomes (subjects) and control after the subjects receive the interventions. In sum, RCTs are quantitative, comparative, controlled experiments in which the investigators study two or more interventions in a series of individuals who receive them in random order. Peculiarities with RCTs are that they are controlled experiments, have a clinical event as an outcome measure, done in a clinical setting, involve subjects suffering from a specific disease or health condition upon which the trial is based and participants are randomly assigned to different groups that compare different treatments.

Randomization allocates participants in a study to different groups without taking any similarities or differences between them into account. The implication is that each subject has equal chance of receiving each intervention. In a RCT, individuals with a similar disease or condition are randomly assigned (to prevent bias) to two or more groups to test the efficacy of a specific drug or treatment. One of the groups (subject or the experimental group) receives the treatment being investigated while the other (control or the comparison group) receives an alternative drug which is usually devoid of the active ingredient or treatment (placebo). Both groups (subjects and control group) are monitored (followed up) over a period of time to determine the efficacy and potential side effect of the drug or treatment. Differences between the subject and control groups are compared statistically to justify if the differences observed between the two groups are statistically significant or due to chance. The philosophy of random selection is to prevent bias. A key requirement is that after randomization, both groups are followed in exactly the same way and placed under the same conditions. The only differences between the two groups lie in the treatment or care they receive. This is the only way to justify that the differences observed in both the subjects and the control arm are due to the active ingredient present in the drug or treatment given to subject which the control group did not have. The most important advantage of randomization is that it reduces the chance of introducing bias, balancing both known and unknown prognostic factors, in the assignment of treatments. RCTs that contain the intervention group in which subjects receive the experimental drug or treatment while control groups receive standard treatment are termed placebo-controlled.

Carrying out RCT's on breast cancer in Nigeria and other developing countries can be quite challenging. Several limiting factors exist that can potentially affect the effectiveness of these trials. These challenges include; ethical challenges, bureaucracy in government, late stage of presentation, high prevalence of triple negative breast cancers, follow up challenges, cost-related challenges, sub optimal health infrastructure, poor implementation of clinical governance, suboptimal number of trained clinical trial personnel, poor laboratory capacity, informed consent-related issues, poor data management, suboptimal number of trained statisticians, challenge of poor awareness and stigma associated with breast cancer, logistics and accessibility issues concerning management of health products, education and communication-related challenges (majority have no formal education) and cultural and religious issues.

The sample size is often calculated using relevant formula to achieve maximized statistical power. Use of equal numbers of subjects and control participants can potentially maximize statistical power. It should however be noted that unequal groups sizes can be more powerful for some types of analyses particularly multiple comparisons of several doses of a particular treatment against a placebo control using Dennett's procedure. Dennett's test or procedure is a multiple comparison procedure developed by Canadian statistician Charles Dunnett to compare each of a multiple number of treatments (multiple comparisons or many-to-one comparisons) against a single control. Sometimes, sample size requirement can be based on the expectation by regulatory or funding agencies requiring that a minimum of subjects be given the trial treatment. Many potential subjects in Nigeria and other developing countries are potentially more likely to enroll in a trial if they have a higher likelihood of being given the trial medication or treatment particularly if the treatment is expensive and beyond their reach or if patients have tried other available options without effectiveness [2]. Every effort must be made to minimize selection bias. There is a high tendency for investigators in Nigeria and other developing countries to consciously or unconsciously preferentially enroll subjects to which they are potentially associated based on ethnic, religious or family sentiments into the treatment arms. This tendency is more pronounced when the trial treatment is expensive and beyond the reach of a majority of patients. For randomized trials to be effective in Nigeria and other developing countries, the principle of unpredictability must be a core requirement. It is vital that patient assignment be done by neutral investigators who have no prior information of the participants (blinded selection) [3]. The only way an RCT can be effective in Nigeria and other developing countries is for it to be blinded, ensuring the implementation of evidence-based best practices to prevent subjects, control participants, caregivers, investigators or outcome assessors from knowing which intervention was received.

However, there are some cases where it is practically impossible to achieve blinding and masking particularly if a RCT involves a treatment that requires active participation of the subjects or in a situation where subjects have to be offered a physical therapy or intervention. Unblinded or open RCTs particularly in developing countries tend to be biased toward beneficial effects only if the RCT's outcomes were subjective as opposed to objective [4–6]. In RCTs, particularly those in developing countries involving treatments for a debilitating disease, an unblinded investigator compared to a blinded investigator is more likely to enroll a patient he knows in the treatment arm particularly if he feels based on findings in previous trials that the potential benefits of treatments will outweigh treatment-associated side effects. An RCT in Nigeria and other developing countries needs to be pragmatic with requirements that subjects, controls, data managers and investigators are blinded to ensure the authenticity of data generated and the unbiased objective evaluation of trial outcomes.

6.2 Peculiarities with Developing Countries

Developing or third world also called less developed, resource poor, low-income or underdeveloped countries are those with underdeveloped industrial base and a generally low Human Development Index (HDI) and low GDP (Gross Domestic

Product), a monetary value of all the finished goods and services produced within a country's borders over a specific period of time often calculated on an annual basis [7]. There are several characteristics associated with developing or third world countries; citizens tend to have lower life expectancy, be less educated or educationally disadvantaged and have access to less money (income). On the other hand, a developed country is one in which many citizens enjoy a free and healthy life, high life expectancy, highly educated, high income, live in a safe environment, high Human Development Index and high Gross Domestic Product. Countries such as Japan in Asia, Canada and the United States in Northern America, Australia and New Zealand in Oceania, countries in Europe, and Israel are generally considered to be developed countries, regions or areas. Based on International Monetary Fund (IMF) classification, all countries of the former Soviet Union (USSR) countries in Central Asia (Kazakhstan, Uzbekistan, Kyrgyzstan, Tajikistan and Turkmenistan) and Mongolia are not included under either developed or developing regions, but rather are referred to as "countries in transition".

The World Bank classifies countries into four income groups based on the 2011 Gross National Income (GNI)—the total domestic and foreign output claimed by residents of a country, consisting of gross domestic product (GDP) plus factor incomes earned by foreign residents, minus income earned in the domestic economy by non-residents GNI per capita using the following ranges of income [8].

- Low income countries had GNI per capita of US$1026 or less.
- Lower middle income countries had GNI per capita between US$1026 and US$4036.
- Upper middle income countries had GNI per capita between US$4036 and US$12,476.
- High income countries had GNI per capita above US$12,476.

The development of a country is measured based on certain indices such as income per capita, GDP, life expectancy, the literacy level, health system, standard of living, level of industrialization, HDI and the extent to which the country meets her set Millennium Development Goals (MDGs) from a blueprint developed by all of the world's countries and leading development institutions in order to evaluate growth. There is a tendency for the health system and infrastructure in developing countries to be suboptimal. This challenge is a bane to carrying out an effective RCT in Nigeria and other developing countries. According to WHO, the lack of strong healthcare infrastructure in parts of the developing world is currently one of the biggest barriers to increasing essential healthcare access. Of the millennium development goals, the health-related goals are the least likely to be met. It is disappointing that despite the availability of drugs, vaccines and health-related tools, there seems a failure in stewardship by leaders in developing countries. There seems a disconnect in Nigeria and other developing countries between intention and the strength of global health systems to deliver them.

Developing countries tend to be associated with poverty, suboptimal health infrastructure, logistics—related challenges, endemic diseases and a low level of investment in health care systems. These factors have a negative effect on the ease of performing RCTs that will be beneficial to the teeming number of the populations that are raved by disease. In Nigeria and most developing countries, there are often challenges associated with the procurement and distribution systems that actually deliver interventions to those in need. Challenges such as poor transport infrastructure and communication and cultural differences often become barriers to successful implementation of health programmes like an RCT for breast cancer. There is an urgent need to strengthen health systems in Nigeria and other developing countries to include improved access, coverage, quality, efficiency, waste and bureaucracy-associated challenges to enable them effectively to manage the limited health budget. Health system strengthening is critical particularly in Nigeria and other developing countries in the face of increasing disease burden and the fastest growing population of young and the aged. It is essential that the backbone that supports effective health delivery is strengthened. Nigeria and other developing countries face daunting challenges. Heath systems in these countries are failing to improve the health status of individuals, families and communities; defend the citizens against diseases that potentially threatens their health; provide universal access to a continually improving quality of healthcare and protection of the citizens against the financial burden of ill-health; inability to provide equitable access to a people-centered care irrespective of whether they are resident in urban or rural communities and inability of the citizens to have a say in decisions affecting their health and the health system as well as how money budgeted for health is spent [9].

If Nigeria and other developing countries are to achieve the health-related aspect of their set Millennium Development Goals (MDGs), there is an urgent need to enhance the quality of health care through objective reforms that improve the capacity (human, material and infrastructural) including health facilities, qualified staff, essential medicines and financing. Essentially, there is need for developing countries to establish a centrally coordinated, regionally and community-based surveillance systems for detecting and reporting disease outbreak and health problems; establish appropriate health financing mechanisms including social health insurance (National Health Insurance Scheme), taxation, community financing and other options that promote universal access to quality health services nationwide. Other challenges associated with health systems in developing countries include: shortage of health workers and challenge of migration of healthcare workers from developing to developed countries (brain drain). The reasons for the high rate of migration from developing to developed countries are not far-fetched; lack of health strengthening, challenges of economic globalization, global inequalities and their effect on wage scales, poor quality of life in their host countries, poor labor rights, insecurity, poor access to opportunity for human capacity development, lack of innovation associated with lack of assistive technology to improve existing local and crude manufacturing capacity, poor implementation of appreciative intelligence and lack of access to cutting edge technology available in developed economies. These factors complicate the ability to carry out an RCT particularly on breast cancer in Nigeria and other developing countries.

6.3 Challenges Associated with Carrying Out Randomized Clinical Trials on Breast Cancer in Nigeria

Most chemotherapeutic regimens being used for the management of breast cancer patients in the developing countries have been tested in clinical trials in the developed world, and findings may not be generalizable to the developing world, where patient and tumor characteristics may differ markedly. This is an ethical issue of public health significance. There is growing advocacy and justification to carry out more clinical trials in developing countries to generate evidenced-based information that can facilitate the effective management of women with breast cancer in developing countries.

Breast cancer is a rapidly emerging disease in developing countries and affected women tend to be younger, poor and present with late stage disease [10]. There are several challenges associated with research governance on breast cancer in Nigeria and other developing countries compared to the developed economies [11, 12]. Ethical approval tends not be as well structured as it is in the West. Tracing patients and follow-up is often difficult. Record keeping and data retrieval have deficiencies. Lack of accurate supporting databases such as cancer registries, population census, and demography make interpretation of research information difficult. Also, the health infrastructures tend to be suboptimal [13] the people tend to be poor, health tends not to be universal, many patients present to hospital late because they cannot afford cost of diagnosis, surgery and follow-up monitoring. The only way clinical trials on breast cancer can realistically happen in Nigeria and other developing countries is if diagnosis, surgery and post-surgical management is done at a no-cost implication to the participants. If this is not guaranteed, the chance of losing patients to follow-up is high. It is a vital safeguard to implement research, trial or study that takes into consideration these challenges particularly at the planning stages rather than to encounter them midway through the study [14]. Research to develop new treatments for breast cancer, particularly in developing countries from natural or repurposed products is urgently needed and this can be done safely within established clinical trials with the right health research ethics and regulatory frameworks [15]. There are several challenges associated with carrying out effective randomized clinical trials on breast cancer in Nigeria and other developing countries; follow up challenges, cost challenges, late stage presentation, high prevalence of triple negative breast cancers, suboptimal health infrastructure, lack of governance, suboptimal number of trained clinical trial personnel, poor laboratory capacity, informed consent-related challenges, ethical challenges, poor data management, suboptimal number of trained statisticians, challenge of poor awareness and stigma associated with breast cancer, high patronage of traditional healers and spiritualists dealing with conflict of interest, poor trial design, logistics and accessibility issues associated with the management of health products, education and communication-related challenges, challenge associated with randomization, cultural and religious issues and bureaucracy in government [8, 16, 17]. There is need for funding agencies to step in to solve these issues by massively investing in clinical trials in breast cancer in developing countries. What is desperately needed is international collaborations between researchers from developed countries and those from developing economies in carrying out fit-for-purpose randomized clinical trials aimed at providing evidence-based, resource-stratified guidelines for the management and control of breast cancer [18]. Carrying out meaningful randomized clinical trials on breast cancer in Nigeria and other developing countries is the only way to develop evidence-based, economically feasible, religious and culturally appropriate data for the effective management of breast cancer in developing countries.

One of the ways Nigeria and other developing countries can effectively fight the war against breast cancer is by developing new and affordable treatments through established clinical trials. Surgery is the main modality of local treatment for breast cancer. Surgery and/or radiotherapy can control loco-regional disease in the majority of patients. However, more than 60% of patients will ultimately die due to distant recurrence of disease. Two types of systemic adjuvant therapy have been used increasingly over the last years to successfully reduce the rate of breast cancer recurrence and death. Adjuvant chemotherapy involves a combination of cytotoxic anticancer drugs and adjuvant hormone therapy which deprives cancer cells of the hormone oestrogen, which some breast cancer cells need to grow. These therapeutic modalities are complementary and are often used in combination. However hormone therapy is not effective in triple negative patients and chemotherapy is only partially effective. In older reports i.e., before the routine use of adjuvant therapy most relapses (50–80%) reside in an early peak 1–3 years post surgery, while the others are distributed rather broadly around the sixth postoperative year. The hazard rate of early recurrence is greater in high risk patients (the type commonly seen in Nigeria and other developing countries) identified with poor primary tumour characteristics (large size, high grade and lymph node involvement). The need for RCTs on the use of these and other remedies in developing countries cannot be over emphasized. Recently, a Belgian group reported data from a retrospective disease free survival study of 327 consecutive patients who were compared according to the perioperative inexpensive and affordable analgesics administered (sufentanil, clonidine, ketorolac and ketamine) [19]. Chemotherapy, radiotherapy and endocrine therapy were performed according to the international expert consensus (9th and 10th St-Gallen consensus). Follow-up in that initial report was average 27.3 months with range of 13–44 months. Perioperative administration of the Non-Steroidal Anti-Inflammatory Drug (NSAID) ketorolac was associated with significantly superior disease-free survival in the first few years after surgery. The updated analysis confirmed that the benefit appears in the 9–18 months' hazards and is of magnitude 4–6-fold, consistent with the early report. It has been proposed that primary surgery causes transient systemic inflammation that results 1–3 years later in the early relapses.

This finding is in keeping with a number of recent reports suggesting that surgery may be less successful in patients with a pre-existing elevation of some inflammatory scores, such as the neutrophil/lymphocyte ratio (NLR), the prognostic value of which was observed as well in mastectomy as in conservative breast cancer surgery [20–22]. Also, triple negative breast cancer (TNBC) patients have frequency of 12%

in US population, 25% among African Americans and even more in developing countries [22]. TNBC is looked upon by clinicians as a "bad tumour" with high recurrence rate in spite of adjuvant chemotherapy. This pessimistic viewpoint seems justified since in the USA, TNBC has 12% incidence but accounts for approximately 20% of mortality in breast cancer. Recurrence dynamics of TNBC patients displays a dominant early peak that looks remarkably similar to the no-ketorolac group in the study by Forget and colleagues [19]. The more agressive TNBC, prevalent more in developing countries, therefore, appears to be an ideal study group with which to test the benefit of perioperative ketorolac in a clinical trial. Intraoperative NSAID administration has been associated with a lower incidence of early detection of postoperative distant metastases. As a consequence, it could be assumed that the effect of ketorolac may be higher in the subgroup of breast cancer patients in Nigeria and other developing countries with the highest risk of early recurrence [19]. It may be worthwhile to test the possible beneficial effect of perioperative ketorolac (an inexpensive and affordable NSAID) in a clinical trial among breast cancer patients in Nigeria and other developing countries. It makes economic, public health and humanitarian sense for grant providers to fund a clinical trial on this inexpensive and readily available and affordable medication among patients in developing countries who may not be fortunate enough as their counterparts in the developed world to afford more expensive adjuvant and adjuvant hormone therapy. It would be very interesting to compare their effect.

6.4 Challenges Associated with Carrying Out Clinical Trials in Breast Cancer in Nigeria

Breast cancer is a rapidly emerging disease in Nigeria and other developing countries. Affected women tend to be young, poor and present with late stage disease. Five-year survival is 5–15% compared with over 60% in developed countries [10]. There are several challenges associated with research governance on breast cancer in Nigeria and other developing countries compared to the developed economies [11, 12]. Ethics approval tends not be as well structured as it is in the West. Tracing patients and follow-up is often difficult. Record keeping and data retrieval have deficiencies. There is lack of accurate, supporting databases such as cancer registries, population census, and demography that make interpretation of research information difficult. Also, the health infrastructure tends to be suboptimal [13], the people tend to be poor, health tends not to be universal, many patients present to hospital late because they cannot afford cost of diagnosis, surgery and follow-up monitoring. The only way clinical trials on breast cancer can realistically happen in these environments is for diagnosis, surgery and post surgically management to be done at a no-cost implication to the participants. If not, the chance of losing patients to follow-up is high. It is a vital safeguard to anticipate research, trial or study that takes into consideration these challenges in the planning stages rather than to encounter them midway through the study [11, 12]. Research to develop these new treatments and others, particularly from repurposed or natural products is what is urgently needed and this can be done safely within established clinical trials with the right health research ethics regulatory frameworks [23]. There are several challenges militating against the carrying out of objective and fit for purpose quality randomized clinical trials in Nigeria and other developing countries. The aim of this chapter is to critically investigate these challenges.

6.5 High Prevalence of Triple Negative Breast Cancers (TNBC)

Survival from breast cancer is still poor in many developing countries including Nigeria. Efforts at earlier diagnosis must be aggressively pursued in developing countries as it is in the West. Multi-centre trials are advocated in order to determine whether breast cancer pursues a more aggressive course among breast cancer patients in Nigeria and other developing countries [24, 25]. However, some of the most effective breast cancer treatments today target proteins on the surface of breast cancer cells, such as human epidermal growth factor receptor 2 (HER2), estrogen receptors and progesterone receptors. The growth of TNBC cells is not supported by high presence of HER2, progesterone or estrogen receptors, thus therapies targeting those receptors are not considered effective. TNBC is one of the most aggressive types of cancer. Women diagnosed with TNBC are four times more likely to have the cancer metastasize to other organs (such as brain, lungs, liver, and bone) within 5 years than patients with other types of breast cancer. In a study published in Clinical Cancer Research in 2007, researchers found that the median time to metastatic recurrences in TNBC patients was just 2.6 years, while the median time for patients with other breast cancer types was 5.0 years. In addition, the survival time from diagnosis of distance metastatic TNBC was just 9 months compared with 22 months for other breast cancer types [26]. The results of combination therapy trials in the developed world for TNBC are somewhat promising, although more effective treatments are still needed. There is need for trials of different combination therapies in Nigeria and other developing countries where there is a large pool of patients. Patients with TNBC tend to have worse clinical outcomes partly as a result of lacking a therapeutic target. For 30 years, accumulating evidence suggests that obese women have poorer prognoses than lean ones after breast cancer treatment [27, 28]. In an observational prospective study of about 350,000 US women, higher body mass index (BMI) was significantly associated with increasing risk of dying from breast cancer [29]. Overweight patients often have larger tumors at diagnosis [30]. Overweight also had a negative influence on overall survival (OS) especially in premenopausal patients. With immunohistochemistry (IHC), breast cancer is classified into four groups based on IHC profile of estrogen receptor (ER), progesterone receptor (PR), and human epidermal growth factor receptor 2 (HER2) expression, positive (+) or negative (−). The IHC classification correlates well with intrinsic gene expression microarray categorization. ER positive tumors may benefit from being treated with selective ER modulators and aromatase inhibitors, whereas patients with HER2 positive tumors have been shown to experience a significant survival advantage when treated with humanized monoclonal antibodies against HER2. The typical type of breast cancer in Nigeria and other developing countries is TNBC and is usually considered the worst early breast cancer diagnosis since there are no known targeted therapies and patients often relapse and die early. The prognosis is even worse for women in developing countries where diagnostic capacity is poor, patients are poor and quality healthcare is not universally available. Expression of estrogen receptors (ER) and progesterone receptors (PR) and Human Epidermal Growth Factor Receptor (HER2) in breast carcinomas identify patients that are more likely to respond to adjuvant therapy. Breast cancer is the most common cancer among women globally.

Triple negative breast cancers are common in Nigeria (29.2%) and affect young females most and could be contributory to the poorer prognosis of breast cancer in this environment. These findings underscore the urgent need for research and RCTs into the etiology and treatment of the aggressive molecular subtypes that disproportionately affect young women in Nigeria and other developing countries. A previous report among breast cancer subjects in Calabar, Nigeria indicated that ER and PR were immunohistochemically detected in 24.0% and 13.9%, respectively [22]. Similarly, a report discussing Nigeria women with breast cancer in Abia State, Nigeria indicated that the majority of cases were high grade (100% were grade III), triple-negative (65%), and occur in young women (mean age 47 years) [31]. Several studies have suggested that breast cancer in Black women is associated with aggressive features and poor survival. A previous report in Jos, Nigeria examined molecular markers along with clinical stage and pathological grade in breast cancer. Results indicated that there is predominance of high grade, invasive ductal carcinomas which are likely to be ER and PR negative but p53 positive. These features suggest a biologically aggressive form of breast cancer among women in Nigeria and other developing countries with the possibility of poor response to conventional hormonal therapy and chemotherapy [11, 12]. Similarly, a study reported that the prevalence of ER negative tumors in breast cancer patients is much higher in Black women than in White women in the US. The prevalence of ER negative tumors significantly varied from 22.0% (41/186) in Eastern-Africa-born to 32.9% (47/143) in Western-Africa-born Blacks. The prevalence was similar in Western-Africa-born and Jamaica-born Blacks, but significantly lower in Eastern-Africa-born Blacks. Notably, the ER negative prevalence in Eastern-Africa-born Blacks was comparable to the US-born Whites with breast cancer [32]. Also, a study involving 507 patients diagnosed with breast cancer in Nigeria and Senegal indicated that, compared with White Women, Black Women experience a disproportionate burden of aggressive breast cancer. Triple negativity for HER2, ER and PR markers was predominant, including basal-like (27%) and unclassified subtype (28%). Other subtypes were luminal A (27%), luminal B (2%), and HER2 positive/ER negative (15%) [33]. A study to determine the prevalence of estrogen and progesterone receptors positive results was conducted among histologically diagnosed breast cancer cases at the University of Benin Teaching Hospital, Benin City, Nigeria. The steroid hormone receptor positivity was 17%. Estrogen and Progesterone receptor positivity were 14.1% and 9.6% respectively.

Advances in breast cancer research have demonstrated differences between Blacks in developing countries compared to Caucasians regarding tumour behaviour, patient outcome and response to treatment. The tumour suppressor gene p53 has been speculated to be involved in tumour biology of triple negative and/or basal-like breast cancer and more commonly observed in Black than Caucasian women. Targeting the p53 pathways for therapeutic usage might improve the poor outcome observed in women in developing countries and there is an urgent need to have this tested by way of a RCT. A previous report investigated the protein expression of p53 in tissue samples from a series of 308 Nigerian women. Clinicopathological parameters, biomarkers of functional significance in Breast Cancer and patient outcome of tumours expressing p53 in Nigerian women were correlated with a UK grade matched series. A significantly large proportion of breast cancer from Nigerian women showed high p53 expression compared with UK women. In those tumours showing positive p53 in the Nigerian series, a significant proportion were premenopausal, diagnosed before 50 years of age larger in size, with evidence of metastasis in lymph nodes. In addition, p53 positive expression was also significantly correlated with negative expression of ER and PR, BRCA1, MDM2, p21 and E-cadherin and positively associated with P-cadherin, triple negative phenotype, basal cytokeratin (CK) 5/6 expression and basal phenotype compared with the UK series. Survival analyses seem to indicate that Nigerian women with breast cancer were significantly associated with poor breast cancer specific survival [34]. TNBC is common in Nigeria and other developing countries and affects young females and contributes to the poorer prognosis of breast cancer. A previous report in Lagos, Nigeria to determine ER/PR, HER2 expression and their association with histological prognostic markers in female breast carcinomas indicated that 18.7% of breast cancers had IHC (ER, PR and HER2) done. IHC pattern was as follows: ER/PR+, HER2− = 39.6%; ER/PR−, HER2− (triple negative) = 29.2%; ER/PR+, HER2+ = 18.8%; ER/PR−, HER2+ = 12.5%, corresponding to Luminal A, TN/basal-like, Luminal B and HER2 over expressed respectively. A British study also found that Black women presented at a younger age with a higher frequency of grade 3, ER-negative tumors and had poorer outcomes than Caucasian patients with breast cancer [35].

Compared with Caucasians, women in Nigeria and other developing countries experience a disproportionate burden of aggressive breast cancer for reasons that remain unknown and understudied by means of RCTs. TNBCs does not respond to many standard breast cancer treatments, but clinical trials in the developed world on combination therapies are showing promise. There is however an urgent need to replicate these trials in Nigeria and other developing countries where more aggressive forms of breast cancers are prevalent. Although breast cancer survival rates are improving on the whole for affected women in the West, those for women in developing countries particularly those diagnosed with the triple-negative form remain significantly lower. In large part, this is because the more modern and targeted treatments are not readily available nor affordable.

Advances in understanding tumor biology, particularly signalling pathways, have led to the development and approval of many novel agents and have changed the landscape of therapy for patients with metastatic breast cancer particularly in the West. These many novel agents unfortunately are not available to a vast majority of breast cancer sufferers in the developing world. This is an ethical issue of public health importance that the world will need to deal with. While significant progress has been made in treating certain types of breast cancer, triple-negative metastatic breast cancer unfortunately remains especially challenging [36]. For patients with metastatic breast cancer, expanding therapeutic options through clinical trial participation in developing countries is a crucial part of modern oncology practice. There is need to test new strategies by way of RCTs in developing countries to overcome endocrine and human epidermal growth factor 2-neu (HER2) resistance through novel receptors, harnessing the immune system and new ways of targeting angiogenesis.

6.6 Challenge Associated with Cultural and Religious Issues

Nigerian and many developing countries are culturally and religiously sensitive. Nigeria like many developing countries is a highly religious nation. Religious affiliations vary from Christianity to Muslim along with the numerous indigenous religions. Religion involves a specific set of beliefs and practices, usually within an organized group. Spiritual or religious beliefs and practices can have a significant effect on patients with breast cancer (when and whether to seek medical care and in coping with their disease). Spiritual or religious beliefs and practices can have a positive effect on mental attitude; improve well-being and quality of life of women with breast cancer. Religion and spirituality plays a prominent role in the social and cultural life of people in most developing countries. Most women in Nigeria and other developing countries identify with a variety of faith-based groups where their leaders have a considerable measure of influence, built on a combination of trust and culture. Religious leaders in developing countries can be empowered to provide potential access for health promotion, clinical trials, health education and improvement in utilization of health services. A previous report has shown that an active role in religion, reporting a lengthy duration of worship at the same place was beneficial [37]. Church, mosques and faith leaders could play a greater role in raising awareness on the potential benefits of early breast self-examination, early detection, enrolment in clinical trials, the need to continue to go for regular medical care and attention even when they believe they have been healed spiritually, and the need to seek medical attention early following breast cancer diagnosis. Religious leaders in Nigeria and other developing countries can potentially reach a significant number of people within a short period of time. Local participants can play an important role in the planning of trials to ensure that protocols are culturally and religiously sensitive and beneficial [38]. Trials should also target the specific medical needs of the country as perceived by the country.

There is a strong impact of religion on people in developing countries. Faith organisations may provide potential access for health promotion and interventions related to breast cancer. The religious affiliation can have a significant effect on enrolment and success of clinical trials in developing countries. In a study involving 2154 Nigerian breast cancer patients of all ages and socio-economic groups, 87% presented in Stages III or IV, and only 13% in Stages I or II. All the participants were questioned on their reasons for not attending hospital sooner. The most common reason for delay (963 patients, 44.7%) was fear of mastectomy. Other reasons given include preference for prayer houses or spiritual healing homes, a belief that the lesion was inflammatory, preference for native doctors or herbalists and economic reasons [39]. Spirituality and religiosity are significant factors responsible for delay in screening for breast cancer among African-American women [40]. The overall survival rate among breast cancer patients is low and patients with early breast cancer had better survival than those with advanced disease [41]. Similarly, all female breast cancer patients referred to one of the general surgery out-patient clinics of Lagos State University Teaching Hospital in Nigeria were interviewed to evaluate the effects of selected socio-demographic factors on late presentation and reasons why breast cancer patients delay reporting for treatment. Ignorance of the nature of illness, belief in spiritual healing, fear of mastectomy and belief in herbal treatment were the leading reasons for delay [42]. Other variables related to delays included factors such as advancing age, low socioeconomic status, fear of diagnosis, consequences of cancer treatments, shame and embarrassment, fear of stigmatization, misconceptions about the aetiology of breast cancer, family priorities, denial, and spirituality including faith-influenced delays [40]. *Most developing countries are* highly religious and culturally sensitive. There is increasing advocacy for implementation of appropriate, evidence-based nursing care which include spiritually-based interventions that acknowledge the significance of God [43]. Breast cancer sufferers in developing countries face significant physical, emotional and social changes and difficulties following primary breast cancer diagnosis. Culturally sensitive therapeutic groups and interventions should be established in developing countries to help women with breast cancer and their spouses and families understand and cope with the disease and its long- term health and quality of life implications [44, 45].

Experience from Thailand indicates that patient and system delays in breast cancer care are important weaknesses of disease control in developing countries. System delay in hospitals outside the university needs to be improved by a good referral system.

Financial barriers limit the ability of women, especially the poorest social economic status (SES) group, to utilize screening and treatment services for early diagnosis and treatment of breast cancer. Interventions that will improve financial risk protection for women with breast cancer or at risk of breast cancer in developing countries are needed to ensure equitable access to screening and treatment services [46]. Evidence from Kaduna, Nigeria on the reason for delayed treatment among symptomatic breast cancer women is related to the quality of medical care, local beliefs, ignorance of the disease, and lack of acceptance of orthodox treatment. It is becoming increasingly clear that for breast cancer prevention programs in Nigeria and other developing countries to succeed, breast cancer awareness and screening programs should involve spiritual leaders and institutions. Institutional bottlenecks, the dearth of knowledge among primary care physicians and improvement in referrals from alternative practitioners and prayer houses are vital [47].

6.7 Challenge Associated with Late Stage at Presentation

The stage at which breast cancer is diagnosed has a tremendous impact on the type of treatment, recovery, and survival. In most cases, the earlier the cancer is detected and treated, the higher the survival rate for the patient. Late presentation of patients at advanced stages when little or no benefit can be derived from any form of therapy is the hallmark of breast cancer in most developing countries. This makes developing countries potential sites for RCTs involving advanced stage breast cancers. The mean age at diagnosis of breast cancer in Nigeria was 42.7 years (SD 12.2, range 18–85 years). Patients less than 40 years of age accounted for 39.8% of the total number of patients with infiltrating breast carcinoma [48]. Breast cancer is now the commonest malignancy affecting women in Nigeria [49]. It is likely to become an important public health issue in coming years. Diagnostic and treatment delays in Nigeria and other developing countries seem to be responsible for the high prevalence of more advanced and higher grade (stage III and IV) breast cancer in Nigeria. Nigerian breast cancers are often high-grade, late-stage, high-proliferating and occur in a younger population than those of the Western countries [48]. In developing countries, the mean age at presentation of breast cancer is low compared to the developed world. A significant number of cases of breast cancer among women in developing countries are the more advanced stages III and IV. A previous report compared the histology and patterns of occurrence of breast cancers in Nigeria (n = 297) and Finland (n = 285). The mean age at presentation was 42.7 years in Nigeria versus 58.7 years in Finland. In both populations, there was an association between reproductive factors and the occurrence of breast cancer. In Nigeria, 53.2% of cases belonged to stages III and IV, versus 6.7% in Finland. In Finland, there were higher frequencies of lobular, tubular and mucinous types than in Nigeria [48]. Early detection through the use of mammography, high-quality surgery, and adjuvant therapies including chemotherapy and targeted therapies, such as hormonal therapy and, more recently the HER2-directed agent trastuzumab, can be credited for much of the recent improvement in outcome for women with breast cancer in the USA. Experience about breast cancer in developing countries shows that it follows a pattern similar to other parts of the developed world except that many present late in mainly multiparous pre-menopausal and low income patients [50, 51]. Late presentation has a number of implications. It is often associated with aggressive features, poor survival and a high chance of occurrence of presenting to emergency unit as an oncologic emergency. A previous report to evaluate the pattern of oncologic emergencies seen in adult cancer patients in Ahmadu Bello University Teaching

Hospital, Zaria, Nigeria indicated that tumour haemorrhage is the commonest oncologic emergency commonly seen in metastatic and locally advanced disease in Nigeria [52]. A previous study to describe the frequency, stages, histological patterns, staging and grading of BRCA in a local scenario of a tertiary hospital in southern Nigeria indicated that late presentation (Stages III and IV) constituted 76.2% of breast cancer [53]. This finding is similar to reports of other researchers [54] who reported 67% and 64% respectively. Similarly, Adesunkanmi et al. [55] observed that 74% of BRCA present in Stages III and IV. The reason for the late presentation in Nigeria and other developing countries is partly attributable to poverty and ignorance. A previous report has shown that women with breast cancer living in areas with limited access to healthcare services are more likely to have been diagnosed with late stage breast cancer. A retrospective study carried out to examine 5 year survival from breast cancer cases diagnosed between 2005 and May 2008 in Nigerian women revealed that the different staging of disease and treatment are independent predictors of disease outcome, whereas age of diagnosis and menopausal status although associated with low hazards are not significant. The study observed a 5 year breast cancer survival rate in Lagos, Nigeria of 24.1% [56]. Poor survival rates among breast cancer patients in developing countries are mainly attributed to late presentation and poor follow-up, hence early detection through breast cancer awareness programs, appropriate logistics and better management of patients through guidelines for the treatment of breast cancer need to be implemented to improve survival in developing countries.

6.8 Challenge of Conflict of Interest by Investigators

Conflict of interest (COI) can potentially distort interpretation of research data in biomedical publications and its non-disclosure can affect the trustworthiness of science communication One of the major requirements in carrying out an RCT is that of allocation concealment to prevent bias [57]. One of the challenges that RCTs may face in developing countries is maintaining impartiality. Practices that introduce selection bias and confounders (both of which should be minimized by randomization) are prevalent in most developing countries and can possibly distort the results of the study. Most Cochrane reviews of drug trials published in 2010 did not provide information on trial funding sources or trial author-industry financial ties or employment. One of the factors militating against RCTs particularly in developing countries is concern with conflicts of interest between researchers and drug manufacturers on one end and trial participants on the other [58]. Conflicts of interest as defined by the Institute of Medicine are a set of circumstances that create a risk that professional judgment or actions regarding a primary interest will be unduly influenced by a secondary interest or factor [59]. Secondary interests can include an individual's desire to benefit financially from professional actions, to favor family, friends and colleagues from the same ethnic group, religious affiliations, city, country, or institution. The resultant conflict may be commercial (financial), intellectual, academic (academic competition), ideological, personal or regional. These interests are prevalent in developing countries and can be a source of bias in RCTs. Conflicts of interest due to research funding and other financial relations can influence how trials are designed and carried out. Financial ties of the authors of the reviews, has been associated with conclusions more likely to favor a sponsor's drug compared with systematic reviews and meta-analyses not linked to industry [60]. It is a well-known fact that financial relationships between industry and scientific investigators/academic institutions are widespread and can negatively influence medical research findings in favour of industry [8]. This may even be worse particularly in developing countries where wages are low. The chances of compromises are potentially higher. Current guidelines recommend that study-funding and author-industry financial ties be disclosed in published research reports, including reports of systematic reviews and meta-analyses [61]. Disclosures of funding sources and conflicts of interests (COI) are important because of the risk of possible bias in the results/findings. Most company or industry-funded studies tend to favor the sponsors [8, 62]. Many researchers can have financial or personal relationships with individuals or organizations that can have an undue influence of their actions. There is a high tendency for industry to provide inducement as consultant fees, honoraria, patent royalty, grants, stock ownership, speaker fees, royalties and salary payments to researchers [63]. It is vital that authors in developing countries adhere to the guidance on COI from learned associations such as the International Committee of Medical Journal Editors (ICMJE) [64] and disclose personal and financial relationships that might bias their work, and to state in clear terms whether potential conflicts do or do not exist. One of the ways to ensure public accountability and minimize concerns with conflicts of interest among researchers in developing countries is to ensure strict, objective and independent ethical reviews of all clinical research protocols [65].

6.9 Ethical and Informed Consent-Related Challenge

Scientific research worldwide faces a broad range of concerns. The ethical aspect of carrying out scientific research is a major issue in developing countries. Randomized clinical trials in developing countries are traditionally bedevilled with several challenges; they are associated with less regulation, poor implementation of the principle of informed consent, poor governance and lack of transparency [66, 67]. Study participants in developing countries are more likely to desire and be attracted by financial compensation sometimes without any background knowledge of the concept and potential risk associated with the trial [66]. There is the tendency for Ethical Review Boards (ERBs) not to be as stringent as they should in ensuring that a research design ensures that risks to subjects are reasonable in relation to anticipated benefits. In such cases, participants in the research may incur undue risks, inconveniences, or discomforts.

Poverty can potentially influence participation in clinical trials in developing countries. The promise for financial gratification may be a reason why industry-funded trials may thrive more in developing countries. Involvement of developing countries in breast cancer–related randomized clinical trials can potentially provide opportunity for early access to interventions [68]. Subjects are more predisposed to participating in these trials because they are often able to access treatment and laboratory monitoring investigations and interventions that are often not feasible or even affordable within the health care delivery systems available in these countries [69]. There is however need for good governance and due diligence in carrying out RCTs in developing countries to ensure that unaffordability and hopelessness associated with late presentation to hospital and management challenge is not used as an opportunity to recruit patients in developing countries as guinea pigs into trials without following all the ethical milestones that ideally should be followed.

Developing countries are often at the receiving end. They are exposed to all the trial-related risks and adverse effects while their counterparts in the developed world reap the benefit of the trials. The risk of exploitation of subjects or host communities in the West is minimized, because research to improve health and quality of life of the people are funded by society. In these societies, researchers and research institutions are part of the larger community, the health infrastructure is optimal and access to healthcare often universal. Research in developing countries creates a greater risk of exploitation of trial participants and the larger communities since they end up bearing the long-term risks of research while most of the benefits are enjoyed by people in developed countries [70].

Obtaining adequate informed consent in breast-cancer clinical trials in developing countries can be challenging [71, 72]. Linguistic, cultural and social norms and taboos make the process of informed consent in developing countries complex. It is vital that informed consent be culturally, politically, and socially sensitive. In some communities, compensation for participation in research may be expected, whereas in others, it may be considered offensive. The appropriate form and level of compensation depends on the local economic and social context. Concerns about inducement are frequently expressed. However, high potential social value and a favourable risk-benefit ratio dispel these concerns [73]. Developing countries tend to prefer compensation and benefits for participants and host communities. Trying to create a balance between fair compensation and undue inducement may result in less compensation for participants and the impoverished communities. Collection and disclosure of information should be confidential and sensitive to the peculiarities of the community with regards to culture, religious beliefs and in the local language using culturally appropriate phrases and correspondences that the prospective participants understand. There may be need for collaborative partnership between the organizers of the RCTs and local community leaders and religious leaders particularly in religiously sensitive communities. In order to ensure that effective consent is obtained, there is need to involve the community and religious leaders in establishing recruitment procedures and incentives. It is also vital that consent, information retrieval and disclosure are done in a culturally, linguistically and confidentially appropriate manner. Participants must be made aware that they have freedom to refuse or withdraw from the trial without any sanction or penalty. Participants must have access to information on any treatment-related negative effects [74]. In most developing countries where many can neither read nor write, other appropriate alternative procedures can be used to document informed consent. Such procedure can include thumb printing, written documentation of verbal consent and tape recordings of verbal consent.

Participants in trials in developing countries must be made aware of their rights to participate or withdraw from research [75]. Since the ethical conduct of RCTs does not end when informed consent is obtained [65], it is vital that participants in breast cancer research in developing countries are kept duly informed particularly when new discoveries are made particularly those that relate to treatment-related risks that may arise during the RCTs. This is a way that investigators can build confidence of participants and local communities. It is vital that findings at the end of the trials are effectively communicated to participants and host communities. Having participated in the RCT, and being exposed to all the potential treatment-related adverse events, participants and host communities have a right to know what was found and the implications of the findings for public health, quality of life of participants and local healthcare policies. Ethical rules to protect participants in developing countries do not seem to be keeping pace with the increase in clinical trials. There is outcry that using impoverished populations for drug trials that is only beneficial to the developed world is a violation of the principle of ethical behaviour. Those planning, conducting and evaluating clinical trials on breast cancer in developing counties are ethically bound based on available guidance including the Helsinki Declaration (World Medical Association [76]), the Belmont Report, the Nuremberg Code [77] and the US "Common Rule" [75] to ensure that participants and communities benefit from the positive findings from the trial. This is the only way to ensure transparency, accountability and prevent exploitation.

6.10 Challenge of Suboptimal Number of Randomized Clinical Trials

Breast cancer is the most common cancer in women and the second largest cause of death from cancer in Nigeria and other developing world countries [78]. Evidence has shown that despite having lower breast cancer incidence rates in developing countries compared to the West, women in developing countries are more likely to be diagnosed with metastatic disease, have less access to live-saving breast cancer medication as well as other useful interventions and often have poorer prognosis [79]. Of the estimated 7.6 million cancer deaths, worldwide in 2007, 62% were in developing countries [80]. It is projected that there will be a 75% increase in cancer incidence in the developing world between the years 2000 and 2020. In order to prevent and manage this change in cancer incidence, significant organization and infrastructure is required to prevent, screen, treat and palliate cancer. As a result, the implications to health services delivery in developing countries are enormous. Health services research largely concerns itself with the factors influencing the need for health services, access to these services, quality and economic efficiency, in addition to the health outcomes of the individuals and populations involved [81]. There is also a disproportionately higher proportion of triple negative breast cancer—an aggressive form of the disease associated with poorer outcomes among women in developing economies compared to the west [82]. Developing countries face significant challenges in providing cost-effective and equitable screening for breast cancer. There are a number of factors contributing to this disparity between developing and developed economies in terms of breast cancer survival; risk factor awareness, cancer-related health education, beliefs, attitudes and behaviors, stigma, fear, access to healthcare services, access to screening, treatment and monitoring, taboo, fear of conventional treatment (mastectomy), mistrust of healthcare professionals, late stage presentation, religiosity, financial burden of healthcare and inaccessibility of services [83–87]. There are several drivers of advanced stage at diagnosis and low survival among women with breast cancer in developing countries; poor existing healthcare infrastructure, lack of early-detection programs, unaffordability, unavailability, inaccessibility and lack of adherence to treatment [88].

Although breast cancer incidence is lower in developing countries compared to that in the West, it is however rising rapidly because of longer life expectancy and dramatic changes in parity and lifestyle. The increasing burden of breast cancer in developing countries is exacerbated by late presentation and limited access to therapies, resulting in poorer outcomes [89]. Similarly, with limited budgets and an increasing incidence of breast cancer, governments in developing countries are facing difficult challenges on how to offer screening equitably and cost-effectively, and in particular, how to target limited resources to women at higher risk of developing breast cancer [90]. There is sufficient justification for more clinical trials on the development of readily available and affordable breast cancer treatment and interventions in developing countries.

6.11 Challenges Associated with Effective Follow-Up of Subjects

A significant number of people in developing countries live in remote areas without addresses and postcode as you have in the West. Access to telephone (landline and mobile) is still suboptimal in many developing countries. Communication with trial participants in rural communities can be challenging since many don't have access to means of communication like mobile phone. Many live in shanties without addresses and postcodes. Conducting clinical trials in developing countries often presents significant ethical, organizational, cultural and infrastructural challenges to researchers, pharmaceutical companies, sponsors and regulatory bodies. Globally, these regions are under-represented in research, yet this population stands to gain more from research as the burdens on the healthcare system are greater than those in developed resourceful countries. However, developing countries also offer an attractive setting for clinical trials because they often have larger treatment naive populations with higher incidence rates of disease and more advanced stages. These factors can present a reduction in costs and time required to recruit patients. So, balance needs to be found where research can be encouraged and supported in order to bring maximum public health benefits to these communities. The difficulties with such trials arise from problems with obtaining valid informed consent, ethical compensation mechanisms for extremely poor populations, poor health infrastructure and considerable socio-economic and cultural divides. There are several factors that can affect the carrying out of RCTs in developing countries including culture, religious, health infrastructure and socioeconomic status of the participants [91]. In most cases, access to the common means of effective follow up of participants (use of mobile phones and e-mails) may be non-existent. Most participants may not even have a fixed address with many living in slums and shanties. As a result of this challenge, many trial participants may be lost to follow-up. It is vital that attrition is taken into consideration in determining the sample sizes for trials in developing countries to compensate for participants who may be lost to follow-up [92, 93]. Lost to follow-up refers to participants who were actively participating in a trial but becomes unreachable at critical times when follow-up intervention or laboratory investigation is required. There is a high tendency for trial participants in developing countries to be lost to follow-up for a number of reasons; some may get better by taking the trial treatment or intervention and decide not to continue, others may suffer treatment-related side effect and may decide not to turn up at the point of follow-up. Some may have relocated from the study area or become ill or deceased. Some may not have transport fare to enable them to come to clinic for follow-up and many uneducated may find it difficult to remember scheduled follow-up dates [94]. Loss to follow up can introduce bias *and it can greatly affect the strength of the findings from the trial* because of incorrect estimation of the association between exposure and outcome. Also, there may be need to allocate extra resources to optimize recruitment efforts in developing countries. Another challenge associated with RCT in developing countries is the risk of trial abandonment because of problems with recruitment of participants. This challenge can sometimes disrupt the trial timetable and reduce the ability of the trial to detect treatment differences and treatment-related adverse events [95]. Recruitment challenges can be prevented by using appropriately trained recruitment staff that have good interpersonal skills and that are not ignorant of peculiarities of the community (cultural, religious, incentives, confidentiality and communication).

6.12 Financial Challenges and Accountability Associated with RCT in Developing Countries

Compared to developed countries, the cost of running a RCT is significantly less expensive in developing countries. There are several reasons for this, including lower wages, low overhead costs and less time is required to enroll participants [91, 96]. Participant compensation is very vital if trials are to succeed in developing countries even though it may seem unethical. Majority of people in developing countries do not have access to enough resources for transportation and sometimes feeding to facilitate regular follow up visits. Clinical trial responsibility for healthcare workers is often an additional workload. These workers need to be compensated for carrying additional clinical trial-related tasks beyond their normal roles and work schedules. A decent honorarium is vital for healthcare workers involved in RCT. Wages in most developing countries are low. Providing a decent honorarium for clinical trial staff can potentially improve their availability and productivity. These associated costs for trials can add up and make them prohibitively expensive. The cost implications of carrying out RCTs needs to be discussed by funders and institutions where research is to be conducted and ministries of health particularly because solutions could encourage more locally run research that benefits local public health goals. Delays due to financial and administrative hurdles can be sorted out by channeling funds directly to the point of expenditure. Inclusion of local investigators at the conception and design stages of a trial may help to reduce the likelihood of unforeseen expenditures. Financial audits can also help to safeguard accountability, but should not be an impediment to the research process.

6.13 Suboptimal Number of Trained Clinical Trial Personnel

In Nigeria and other developing countries, access to adequate human resources for RCTs is a major challenge. Getting an adequate number of staff that are knowledgeable on clinical trials (randomization, blinding) is often a huge problem. Also, while randomized clinical trials support structures (trained clinical trial personnel, data managers and statisticians) exist in the developed world, these structures are often non-existent in developing countries. Even when present they are often suboptimal. These support structures are often supposed to provide the required guidance ensuring that trials are legal, objective, dependable and compliant [97]. Capacity-building to carry out effective randomized clinical trials on breast cancer is vital if trials in Nigeria and other developing countries are to be effective and successful. There is an urgent need to develop internationally compliant clinical trial sites in Nigeria and other developing countries based on national research needs and the availability of competent or potentially trainable staff. These are ways to potentially improve the RCT culture and promote evidenced based best practices. These centers can become a hub for training other researchers and thereby improve capacity strengthening resulting in increased number of RCT compliant researchers who can promote the carrying out of high quality research in developing countries [98, 99]. Effective laboratory monitoring (trained laboratory scientists and required laboratory equipment) is vital to carrying out effective trials on breast cancer. Partnerships with laboratories in developed countries can help build laboratory capacity and promote investigator driven research [100]. There is need for effective networking between clinical trial operators in the West and those in developing countries to ensure sharing of best practices, mentorship and exchange of ideas [101].

6.14 Lack of Governance and Bureaucracy in Government

Post-trial access to care is often a challenge for most trial participants. Governments in developing countries continue to fail in their responsibility of providing universal access to treatment and laboratory investigations that can potentially improve the quality of lives of breast cancer patients as their counterparts in the West. As a result of this failure in stewardship by governments in developing countries, breast cancer-related mortality continues to be astronomically higher among women compared to the West. This is a humanitarian and ethical issue of public health importance that will need to be addressed. There are sometimes unnecessary administrative bottlenecks from government health departments that can potentially impede the ability of researchers to carry out breast cancer-related clinical trials in Nigeria and other developing countries. There tend to be too many hierarchically bottlenecks associated with getting approvals for purchases and expenditures. It is vital that these governance and organizational issues are dealt with before the trials begin to ensure that time frames are not distorted.

Accountability in medical research has become a focal requirement particularly in developing countries [102]. One of the major challenges associated with research governance in developing countries includes lack of responsiveness, sustainability and efficiency of health services where health systems are struggling to meet the growing challenges of disease burden in the midst of dwindling health budgets. Research governance is key to carrying out effective RCTs. The Research and Innovation committee of the European Commission published key principles on carrying out innovative scientific research. The six key principles include: engagement of all societal actors, gender equality, increased scientific knowledge and understanding in the population, free online access to results of publicly-funded research (publications and data), adherence to ethics to adequately respond to societal challenges and governance to ensure high quality results. "Responsible Research and Innovation" (RRI) is key to shaping governance as it affects scientific research. There are laid down codes of conduct with regard to carrying out effective medical research on human participants [76].

Governance is a set of processes that ensures effective stewardship in medical research. Governance ensures that medical research is carried out in continuous adherence with evidence-based best practices strictly following laid down code of conduct. Governance often involves all stakeholders including policy makers, researchers, industry and civil society groups and non-governmental agencies to protect the interest of the society.

Responsible Research Innovation has become a key element in carrying out medical research. Current European Commission research funding programme incorporates four Responsible Research Innovation dimensions: anticipation, reflexivity, inclusion and responsiveness. For medical research to be effective, policymakers are duty bound as good stewards to prevent harmful or unethical developments in research and innovation. It is the responsibility of policy makers to ensure Responsible Research and Innovation that integrates public engagement, gender equality, science education, open access and ethics [103].

From a research governance point of view, three major groups are very important: those with scientific and technological expertise (researchers), guided by legal expertise (ethico-legal expertise) and those included as part of public participation (subjects or advocacy groups). In most developing countries including Nigeria, Research governance is still a huge challenge and continues to be a bane to carrying out effective RCTs. There is an urgent need for the uptake of evidence-based best practices exemplified by the European RRI strategy for dealing with issues of good governance as it affects research and innovation as a way to building the confidence of the developed world on research initiatives in developing countries. From the funders point of view, research governance is critical to ensure the availability of public health and epidemiology research data in ways that are equitable, ethical and efficient [104, 105]. *If RCTs on breast cancer are to succeed in Nigeria and other developing countries,* trust-building, fairness, community involvement, independence and accountability of research governance mechanisms based on national and international framework are key [106].

6.15 Challenge of Poor Awareness and Stigma Associated with Breast Cancer

Breast cancer is the most common malignancy in women. Early diagnosis allows efficient treatment and increases survival. Stigma is a mental or physical mark that is characteristic of a defect or disease. Stigmas associated with breast cancer can present significant challenges to control the uptake of treatment and potential enrolment in trials. Breast cancer-related stigma can have a silencing effect on the sufferer. Breast cancer diagnosis has a significant social, economic and emotional effect particularly in developing countries. This is particularly due to unfounded cultural, religious myths, and taboos associated with the disease. There is need for a paradigm shift in the orientation of people in developing countries. There are several reasons why breast cancer patients in developing countries are stigmatized. Many people in developing countries still perceive breast cancer as contagious and fatal, many view the disease as a repercussion or punishment for sin and sexual immorality, breast cancer-related symptoms affect the breast, a part of the body that can cultivate stigma and fears about treatment (mastectomy) can also fuel stigma. Combating these stigmas, myths, taboos and overcoming silence is key to changing the mindset of the people. However, health belief models, people's health perceptions and attitudes influence the likelihood to present to health facility for treatment or to participate in RCTs.

Barriers to women undergoing breast cancer treatment include costs, risk for stigmatization, accessibility, low target population awareness and negative attitudes towards benefits of early breast cancer screening [107, 108]. Counselling can change interest in genetic testing only slightly and changing women's beliefs about the properties of testing might be one mechanism of doing so [109]. Cancer has the potential to provoke worries which should be assessed in order to adequately respond to patients' problems. Relatives have the emotional disposition and social potentials for playing informal care-giving roles; hence there is a need to strengthen institutional capabilities for community-based treatment of cancer. Cancer, particularly when it affects women and reproductive health, epitomizes the complexities and inequities of the epidemiological challenge faced by low- and middle-income countries [110].

Breast cancer-related stigma has far reaching implications; it can produce a silencing effect that can have a negative effect on breast cancer awareness. It can also negatively impact the patient's behavior. They are less likely to apply cancer-risk-reducing behaviors, seek available care and support including enrolment in RCTs. Culture of people in developing countries can fuel breast cancer related stigma and can have a significant effect on the outcome of health behaviors related to the prevention and control of the disease [111]. There is need to develop breast cancer prevention and control programs that take into consideration the cultural beliefs and values of the community. This can have a positive effect on the breast cancer-related stigma as well as psychological and behavioral outcomes following cancer diagnosis and treatment [112, 113].

Communication is key to decreasing breast cancer-related stigma in developing countries. There is need to invest in raising breast cancer-related awareness and education. There may be need to build breast-cancer education into the school curriculum. This may be a way to provide cancer education and potentially improve the cancer awareness among children and by extension the larger community. Religion is a belief in a supernatural power which governs the universe, and recognition of God as object of worship. In most developing countries, most people rely on their spirituality and faith when coping with illness which they believe have influence on positive outcomes [114]. Overall, we can say that spiritual care decreases aggressive end-of-life (EOL) care and improves quality of life [115, 116].

6.16 Logistics and Accessibility Issues Concerning Management of Health Products

Many in developing countries have benefited significantly from RCTs. The promise of future progress from ongoing RCTs is key to possible future access to more effective breast cancer treatment. Clinical trials supply chain management is key to successful RCTs. Ensuring that the right supply arrives in the right place, in the right quantity, in the right condition, at the right time and at the right cost effective price is key to the success of RCTs. Nigeria and other developing countries have logistic challenges with the management of health supplies. It is vital that the right clinical trial supply chain solution is put in place to prevent a stock out of vital trial supplies. For RCTs to be successful in Nigeria and other developing countries, it is vital that the correct study drug is available on time. For this to be achieved, the right logistics and inventory control professionals, processes, storage and transport facilities and adaptable technology must be in place. It is expedient that clinical trial supply chain management be implemented, is effective, efficient and compliant with the local regulations. It is vital to ensure that the manufacturing, packaging, cold chain/temperature management and inventory control management are guaranteed. Import/export and tax regulations in place in the country must be taken into consideration. If RCTs must succeed in Nigeria and other developing countries, clinical trial supply chain system to be implemented must ensure: prompt and regular delivery of clinical trial supplies, ancillary supplies including relevant medical devices, laboratory equipment and consumables. To ensure clinical trial materials arrive on time and in the right condition (just-in-time model), the storage and distribution is vital. Positioning the clinical trials materials closer to the patient can reduce lead times. There is also the need to implement the First In First Out (FIFO) model to prevent expiration of vital supplies. It is vital to prevent stock out as well as avoid waste by carrying out effective forecasting. Temperature management is vital when dealing with health products that require cold chain management. It is key that they are in place as a way of ensuring and verifying the conditions during transit.

6.17 Education, Communication, Poverty and Safety-Related Challenges

Developing countries face daunting challenges dealing with diseases such as HIV, malaria, TB, breast cancer and a host of other diseases for which RCTs, drugs and other interventions discovered in the West based on RCTs involving Caucasians may not be as effective among those in developing countries. It is vital to develop treatments that fit into the conditions in developing countries where there are regular power outages, poor access to clean portable water and suboptimal health infrastructure. Many people in developing countries tend to be uneducated. All these factors will need to be taken into consideration when planning RCTs in developing countries.

Although developing countries remain the most suitable settings to carry out RCTs because of cost effectiveness, a large pool of treatment naïve patients and findings from these RCTs can potentially address diseases of public health priority in these countries. Since many in developing countries are poorly educated and often lack health literacy, getting informed consent may be a huge challenge. Although consents and questionnaires are sometimes interviewer-administered, getting adequate informed consent may be problematic. In such situations, there is the potential risk for participants in RCTs to be exploited and for potentially risky studies to be forced down the throat of these participants. For these reasons, researchers conducting RCTs must be particularly sensitive to ethical concerns. Ethical review boards must ensure that the interest of participants is protected. It is vital that they insist that adequate consent is obtained. The capacity of ethical review boards (training, and resources) needs to be optimized to enable them to effectively carry out their statutory roles in protecting trial participants. There is increasing advocacy that if trial drug and interventions are found to be safe and effective, they should be made available at an affordable cost in the host country [117].

All RCTs in developing countries should offer participants a favourable risk-benefit ratio and ensure to a significant level that potential benefits outweigh the risks. Unlike in the developed world, where there is appropriate participant attitudes and behaviors with regards to RCTs [118], risk/benefit ratio assessment, unfounded misconceptions, wrong attitudes and beliefs about clinical trials, fear of painful processes and other adverse events are major concerns and determinants of parental consent in RCTs involving children in developing countries. Mistrust of healthcare professionals, trial burden, language barrier and fear of any trial-related complications are also common barriers to participation in clinical trials particularly in developing countries [119, 120]. Other factors identified as participation barriers in cancer-related RCTs in developing countries include participants' lack of transportation, lack of interest, job commitment, and medical problems [121]. Illiteracy, poverty, limited healthcare infrastructure, cultural and linguistic factors and limited number of qualified researchers and poor understanding of the nature of scientific research create room for possible exploitation. Improving communication with participants and building trust between researchers and trial participants is important for successful recruitment. There is the urgent need to develop an ethical framework for RCTs particularly on breast cancer in developing countries that minimize the possibilities of exploitation of the vulnerable population [65].

6.18 Advantages of Carrying Out Randomized Controlled Trials in Developing Countries

Nigeria and other developing low income countries disproportionately bear the rising global breast cancer burden [122]. There is an increasing need to carry out objective clinical research to address the disproportionate high breast cancer-related mortality seen among breast cancer patients in developing countries compared to the West. This is a moral issue of public health and humanitarian implication that needs to be tackled [123]. However, clinical trials are rapidly becoming increasingly globalized. Data between 1995 and 2005 indicate that Randomized Clinical Trial participation in sites outside of the United States more than doubled [66, 68]. A recent report indicates that 78% of clinical trials evaluating cancer therapies published between 2007 and 2011 were conducted in developed countries, while 22% of trials were conducted in developing countries [124]. However, many issues still need to be addressed particularly as they affects ethical concerns.

The advantages of proper randomization in breast cancer-related RCTs include: elimination of selection and treatment bias, it facilitates blinding (masking) of the identity of treatments a participant receives from participants, investigators and assessors and it justifies the use of the probability theory to prove that differences in outcome between the two groups are due to the treatment offered or that they may have occurred merely by chance. There are several advantages that centres in Nigeria and other developing countries can benefit by participating in RCTs; access to newer and expensive therapies that most patients would not be able to afford if they were asked to pay for them, access to other healthcare provisions that can potentially improve the quality of life and care during trials [69, 125], increased investment in human, infrastructure capital including equipment endowment and access to expensive reagents and intervention (mammogram, MRI scan, CT scan and radiotherapy) [125], improved global access and information exchange [68], access to professionals from collaborating centres in the developed world, collaboration—associated academic achievement and scholarly publication in scientific journals for researchers and financial status improvement from honorarium for researchers working in low income settings [69]. There is the urgent need to carry out objective RCTs in Nigeria and other developing countries focusing on critical aspects such as affordable and accessible low cost medication, early diagnosis, evidence-based primary prevention and early diagnosis through access to affordable and accessible screening. These initiatives can potentially improve the quality of care and by extension the QOL of patients in low income countries. The only real way to ensure improved outcomes among breast cancer patients in developing countries is to carry out quality and objective clinical trials and research. The need to continue to invest significantly in clinical trials geared towards improving access to appropriate and affordable breast cancer-related care relevant to local settings in Nigeria and other developing countries cannot be over emphasized. Furthermore, RCTs can be an opportunity for Health Care Workers to be paid a decent wage and to work based on standardised protocols. It is also an opportunity to improve the ailing medical and public health infrastructure. However most RCTs in developing countries place a negative ratio of benefits to burdens on the participants and the host communities since they bear the potential risks of research without any possible prospect of potentially benefiting from the findings of the researches.

6.19 Increasing Incidence of Breast Cancer among men in Developing Countries

Breast cancer in men is rare, accounting for <1% of all breast cancer cases [126] and <0.1% of cancer mortality in men [127–129]. It is almost 100 times less common among men than among women. The lifetime risk of a man getting breast cancer is about 1 in 1000. Although the epidemiologic literature regarding female breast cancer is extensive, there is paucity of data on the etiology of male breast cancer (MBC). Epidemiology of MBC shows similarities with female breast cancer. Genetically, factors associated with an increased risk of breast cancer in men include BRCA2 mutations, CHEK2, Klinefelter syndrome, AR gene mutations, CYP17 polymorphism, Cowden syndrome, and a positive family history. Other potential risk factors include: hormonal imbalances, obesity, testicular disorders (cryptorchidism, mumps orchitis, and orchiectomy) and radiation exposure. Suspected prostate cancer, gynecomastia, occupational exposures (electromagnetic fields, polycyclic aromatic hydrocarbons and high temperatures), dietary factors including meat and alcohol intake). About 4–40% of MBC has been attributed to inherited genetic mutations [130]. Commonly implicated genes include *BRCA2*, *AR* gene, cytochrome P45017 (*CYP17*), the XXY karyotype (Klinefelter syndrome), the *PTEN* tumor suppressor gene associated with Cowden syndrome, and the *CHEK2* gene.

A recent study revealed that having a history of breast cancer in a brother is associated with a higher risk of breast cancer than having an affected sister suggesting that MBC has a higher genetic basis than female breast cancer [131]. The Klinefelter syndrome, characterized by a 47-XXY karyotype, small testes, azospermia, and gynecomastia, has also been described as occurring in 3–7.5% of men with breast cancer [132]. Gynecomastia present in 6–38% of MBC patients has been described as a risk factor, although it is unclear whether gynecomastia is a risk factor for MBC or the risk factors for MBC are the same as those for gynecomastia [131]. The contributions of several other variables including smoking, alcohol consumption, and exposure to electromagnetic radiation remain uncertain [133].

In contrast to western countries, the incidence of MBC in sub-Saharan Africa ranges from 1.3 to 15% [134, 135]. In the UK, current estimates indicate around 300 cases annually. Incidence of male breast cancer has been increasing in developing countries. In a report from Zambia, 15% of breast cancer cases were male [136]. A retrospective study of all cases of male breast cancer managed in Jos University Teaching Hospital over a 17-year period indicated that out of a total of 302 cases of breast malignancies managed over the study period, 26 (8.6%) of these were males giving a male: female ratio of 1:10.6 [135]. Similarly, a review of all cases of MBC seen at LAUTECH Teaching Hospital Osogbo, Nigeria between January 2004 and December 2006 indicated that 7 (8.8%) out of 79 cases of breast cancers seen are males. Stage IV disease was most commonly encountered (43.8%) and (68.8%) patients had modified radical mastectomy. Previous report indicates a MBC prevalence of 9% reported from Zaria [137], 8.6% from Jos [135]. Similarly, prevalence of 1.4% was observed in Nnewi and 2.5% in Benin. The prevalence of male breast cancer in Nigeria varies from 1.2% in Enugu [134] to 2.4% in Ibadan, 3.7% in North Eastern Nigeria, 3.7% in Ibadan [138], 8.6% in Jos [135] and 9.0% in Zaria [137]. Incidence rates in Egypt were 12-times that of the United States but the current incidence rate (1.4%) is only slightly higher than the U.S. rate. In a previous report in India, 8 out of 1200 (0.7%) male cancer diagnoses in a pathology review represented breast cancer [139].

Male breast cancer tends to be diagnosed at a more advanced stage. Of the 91 male breast cancer patients diagnosed between 2000 and 2013 and retrospectively identified, 33% presented with stage 1 disease, 39% with stage 2 disease, 22% with stage 3 disease and 4% with metastatic disease. Nigerian male patients with breast cancer like their female counterparts present with advanced disease which is associated with poor outcome of treatment [140]. The prevalence of MBC among Nigerian men who presented with advanced breast cancer to Ahmadu Bello University Hospital in Zaria, Nigeria over the 15-year period 1975–1989 was 9% [137]. In sub-Saharan Africa, patients with MBC present late with advanced disease and associated comorbidity. These patients often seek non-orthodox treatment because of poor

Table 6.1 Prevalence of male breast cancer in different part of Nigeria.

Location	Prevalence (%)	Authors
Ibadan	3.75	Ihekwaba [138]
Zaria	9	Hassan et al. (1995)
North East Nigeria	3.7	Dogo et al. [141]
Jos	8.6	Kidmas et al. [135]
Enugu	1.2	Ezeome et al. [134]
Ibadan	2.4	Ogundiran et al. (2008)

awareness, sociocultural or religious reasons. In addition, whilst surgical therapy is readily available, other resources for breast cancer treatment may be lacking or very limited. These factors may be responsible for the poor treatment outcome among the patients [135] (Table 6.1).

In sub-Saharan Africa, patients with MBC present late with advanced disease and associated comorbidity [136, 138]. Evidence from previous reports indicate that a significant number of MBC cases present in stage III and stage IV. Other studies from Africa reported stage IV disease in 43.8%–67.1% of their patients [136]. These patients often seek non-orthodox treatment because of poor awareness, unaffordability, sociocultural or religious reasons. In addition, surgical therapy is not readily available particularly in rural areas coupled with the fact that other resources for breast cancer treatment may be lacking or very limited. This often results in poor outcome of treatment [137]. In this series, the 5-year survival rate was 50% for stage-II disease and 20.8% for advanced disease. Other studies from Nigeria indicate overall survival ranging from 6 months to 3 years [134, 140]. In the study from LAUTECH 57% of patients died from 1 week to 7 months after diagnosis while an overall 3-year survival of 27.2% was reported from Enugu [134]. The 5-year OS in the patients was 22.8%. Similar poor survival rates were reported from other studies in low-income countries [136]. In high-income countries, the 5-year OS rates for all stages of breast cancer in men range from 36 to 66%, and 10-year survival rates range from 17 to 52% [142, 143].

The rarity of MBC results in paucity of prospective randomized studies validating the efficacy of various treatment strategies for MBC. MBC remains an inadequately characterized disease particularly in developing countries because of lack of specifically designed randomized clinical trials. Current evidence for treatment is derived from female breast cancer and from data derived in the developed world among Caucasians. There is need to generate data from developing countries on MBC by way of RCTs.

References

1. Chalmers TC, Smith H Jr, Blackburn B, Silverman B, Schroeder B, Reitman D, Ambroz A (1981) A method for assessing the quality of a randomized control trial. Control Clin Trials 2(1):31–49
2. Avins AL (1998) Can unequal be more fair? Ethics, subject allocation, and randomized clinical trials. J Med Ethics 24(6):401–408

3. Buyse ME (1989) Analysis of clinical trial outcomes: some comments on subgroup. Analyses 10(4):187S–194S
4. Chan R, Hemeryck L, O'Regan M, Clancy L, Feely J (1995) Oral versus intravenous antibiotics for community acquired lower respiratory tract infection in a general hospital: open, randomized controlled trial. BMJ 310(6991):1360–1362
5. Fukase K, Kato M, Kikuchi S, Inoue K, Uemura N, Okamoto S, Terao S, Amagai K, Hayashi S, Asaka M, Japan Gast Study Group (2008) Effect of eradication of helicobacter pylori on incidence of metachronous gastric carcinoma after endoscopic resection of early gastric cancer: an open-label, randomised controlled trial. Lancet 372(9636):392–397
6. Marson AG, Al-Kharusi AM, Alwaidh M, Appleton R, Baker GA, Chadwick DW et al (2007) The SANAD study of effectiveness of valproate, lamotrigine, or topiramate for generalized and unclassifiable epilepsy: an unblinded randomised controlled trial. Lancet 369(9566):1016–1026
7. Anand S, Ravaillon M (1993) Human development in poor countries: on the XX private incomes and public services. J Econ Perspect 7(1):133–150
8. Bekelman JE, Li Y, Gross CP (2003) Scope and impact of financial conflicts of interest in biomedical research: a systematic review. J Am Med Assoc 289(4):454–465
9. Cremieux P, Ouellette P, Pilon C (1999) Health care spending as determinants of health outcomes. Health Econ 8(7):627–639
10. Ihezue CH, Ugwu BT, Nwana EJ (1994) Breast cancer in highlanders. Nigerian J Surg Sci 4:1–4
11. Gukas ID, Jennings BA, Leinster SJ, Harvey I (2005) A theme issue by, for, and about Africa: collaborative work between Nigeria and UK on breast cancer has been successful. BMJ 331(7519):779
12. Gukas ID, Jennings BA, Mandong BM et al (2005) Clinicopathological features and molecular markers of breast cancer in Jos, Nigeria. West Afr J Med 24:209–213
13. Erhabor O, Adias TC (2011) Challenges of meeting the blood transfusion requirements in sub-Saharan Africa: the need for the development of alternatives to allogenic blood. J Blood Med 2:7–21
14. Akinbami A, Popoola A, Adediran A, Dosunmu A, Oshinaike O, Adebola P, Ajibola S (2013) Full blood count pattern of pre-chemotherapy breast cancer patients in Lagos, Nigeria. Caspian J Intern Med 4(1):574–579
15. Adebamowo CA, Famooto A, Ogundiran TO et al (2008) Immunohistochemical and molecular subtypes of breast cancer in Nigeria. Breast Cancer Res Treat 110:183–188
16. Angell M (1997) The ethics of clinical research in the third world. N Engl J Med 337:847–849
17. Gbolade BA (1997) Exploitative collaborative research must be discouraged. Br Med J 314(7090):1347
18. Levine RJ (1986) Ethics and regulation of clinical research, 2nd edn. Urban & Schwarzenberg, Baltimore
19. Forget P, Vandenhende J, Berliere M, Machiels JP, Nussbaum B, Legrand C, De Kock M (2010) Do intraoperative analgesics influence breast cancer recurrence after mastectomy? A retrospective analysis. Anesth Analg 110:1630–1635
20. Demicheli R, Retsky MW, Hrushesky WJ, Baum M, Gukas ID, Jatoi I (2007) Racial disparities in breast cancer outcome: insights into host-tumor interactions. Cancer 110: 1880–1888
21. Forget P, Machiels JP, Coulie PG, Berliere M, Poncelet AJ, Tombal B, Stainier A, Legrand C, Canon JL, Kremer Y, De Kock M (2013) Neutrophil: lymphocyte ratio and intraoperative use of ketorolac or diclofenac are prognostic factors in different cohorts of patients undergoing breast, lung, and kidney cancer surgery. Ann Surg Oncol 20:S650–S660
22. Ikpatt OF, Ndoma-Egba R (2003) Oestrogen and progesterone receptors in Nigerian breast cancer: relationship to tumour histopathology and survival of patients. Cent Afr J Med 49:122–126
23. Adebamowo CA, Akarolo-Anthony S (2009) Cancer in Africa: opportunities for collaborative research and training. Afr J Med Med Sci 38(2):5–13

24. Anyanwu SN (2000) Breast cancer in eastern Nigeria: a ten-year review. West Afr J Med 19(2):120–125
25. Anyanwu SN (2000) Survival following treatment of primary breast cancer in eastern Nigeria. East Afr Med J 77(10):539–543
26. Dent RTM, Pritchard KI, Hanna WM et al (2007) Triple-negative breast cancer: clinical features and patterns of recurrence. Clin Cancer Res 13:4429–4434
27. Dawood S, Broglio K, Gonzalez-Angulo AM, Kau SW, Islam R, Hortobagyi GN et al (2008) Prognostic value of body mass index in locally advanced breast cancer. Clin Cancer Res 14(6):1718–1725
28. Kroenke CH, Chen WY, Rosner B, Holmes MD (2005) Weight, weight gain, and survival after breast cancer diagnosis. J Clin Oncol 23(7):1370–1378
29. Ewertz M, Jensen MB, Gunnarsdottir KA, Hojris I, Jakobsen EH, Nielsen D et al (2011) Effect of obesity on prognosis after early-stage breast cancer. J Clin Oncol 29(1):25–31
30. Majed B, Moreau T, Senouci K, Salmon RJ, Fourquet A, Asselain B (2008) Is obesity an independent prognosis factor in woman breast cancer? Breast Cancer Res Treat 111(2):329–342
31. Adisa CA, Eleweke N, Alfred AA, Campbell MJ, Sharma R, Nseyo O, Tandon V, Mukhtar R, Greninger A, Risi JD, Esserman LJ (2012) Biology of breast cancer in Nigerian women: a pilot study. Ann Afr Med 11(3):169–175
32. Jemal A, Fedewa SA (2012) Is the prevalence of ER-negative breast cancer in the US higher among Africa-born than US-born black women? Breast Cancer Res Treat 135(3):867–873
33. Huo D, Ikpatt F, Khramtsov A, Dangou JM, Nanda R, Dignam J, Zhang B, Grushko T, Zhang C, Oluwasola O, Malaka D, Malami S, Odetunde A, Adeoye AO, Iyare F, Falusi A, Perou CM, Olopade OI (2009) Population differences in breast cancer: survey in indigenous African women reveals over-representation of triple-negative breast cancer. J Clin Oncol 27(27):4515–4521
34. Agboola AO, Banjo AA, Anunobi CC, Ayoade BA, Deji-Agboola AM, Musa AA, Abdel-Fatah T, Nolan CC, Rakha EA, Ellis IO, Green AR (2014) Molecular profiling of breast cancer in Nigerian women identifies an altered p53 pathway as a major mechanism underlying its poor prognosis compared with British counterpart. Malays J Pathol 36(1):3–17
35. Bowen RL, Duffy SW, Ryan DA et al (2008) Early onset of breast cancer in a group of British black women. Br J Cancer 98:277–281
36. Campone M, Valo I, Jézéquel P, Moreau M, Boissard A, Campion L, Loussouarn D, Verriele V, Coqueret O, Guette C (2015) Prediction of recurrence and survival for triple-negative breast cancer by a protein signature in tissue samples. Mol Cell Proteomics 14(11):2936–2946. doi:10.1074/mcp.M115.048967
37. Allain JP, Anokwa M, Casbard A, Owusu-Ofori S, Dennis-Antwi J (2004) Sociology and behaviour of west African blood donors: the impact of religion on human immunodeficiency virus infection. Vox Sang 87(4):233–240
38. Kasper CK (2002) Conduct of clinical trials in developing countries. Haemophilia 8:166–169
39. Ajekigbe AT (1991) Fear of mastectomy: the most common factor responsible for late presentation of carcinoma of the breast in Nigeria. Clin Oncol 3(2):78–80
40. Gullatte MM, Phillips JM, Gibson LM (2006) Factors associated with delays in screening of self-detected breast changes in African-American women. J Natl Black Nurses Assoc 17(1):45–50
41. Kene TS, Odigie VI, Yusufu LM, Yusuf BO, Shehu SM, Kase JT (2010) Pattern of presentation and survival of breast cancer in a teaching hospital in north western Nigeria. Oman Med J 25(2):104–107
42. Ibrahim NA, Oludara MA (2012) Socio-demographic factors and reasons associated with delay in breast cancer presentation: a study in Nigerian women. Breast 21(3):416–418
43. Gibson LM, Hendricks CS (2006) Integrative review of spirituality in African American breast cancer survivors. ABNF J 17(2):67–72
44. Adisa AO, Gukas ID, Lawal OO, Adesunkanmi AR (2010) Breast cancer in Nigeria: is non-adherence to chemotherapy schedules a major factor in the reported poor treatment outcome? Breast J 16(2):206–207

45. Gullatte MM, Brawley O, Kinney A, Powe B, Mooney K (2010) Religiosity, spirituality, and cancer fatalism beliefs on delay in breast cancer diagnosis in African American women. J Relig Health 49(1):62–72
46. Ali R, Mathew A, Rajan B (2008) Effects of socio-economic and demographic factors in delayed reporting and late-stage presentation among patients with breast cancer in a major cancer hospital in South India. Asian Pac J Cancer Prev 9(4):703–707
47. Ezeome ER (2010) Delays in presentation and treatment of breast cancer in Enugu, Nigeria. Niger J Clin Pract 13(3):311–316
48. Ikpatt OF, Ndoma-Egba R, Collan Y (2002) Influence of age and prognosis of breast cancer in Nigeria. East Afr Med J 79(12):651–657
49. Adebamowo CA (2012) Cancer incidence in Nigeria: a report from population-based cancer registries. Cancer Epidemiol 36(5):e271–e278
50. Abudu EK, Banjo AA, Izegbu MC, Agboola AO, Anunobi CC, Musa OA (2007) Malignant breast lessons at Olabisi Onabanjo university teaching hospital (O.O.U.T.H), Sagamu-a histopathological review. Niger Postgrad Med J 14(1):57–59
51. Ekanem VJ, Aligbe JU (2006) Histopathological types of breast cancer in Nigerian women: a 12-year review (1993–2004). Afr J Reprod Health 10(1):71–75
52. Adewuyi SA, Ajekigbe AT, Campbell OB, Mbibu NH, Oguntayo AO, Kolawole AO et al (2012) Pattern of oncologic emergencies seen in adult cancer patients attending the radiotherapy and oncology Centre, Ahmadu Bello University teaching hospital, Zaria—Nigeria. Niger Postgrad Med J 19(4):208–214
53. Forae G, Nwachokor F, Igbe A (2014) Histopathological profile of breast cancer in an African population. Ann Med Health Sci Res 4(3):369–373
54. Anyanwu SN, Egwuonwu OA, Ihekwoaba EC (2011) Acceptance and adherence to treatment among breast cancer patients in eastern Nigeria. Breast 20(2):S51–S53
55. Adesunkanmi AR, Lawal OO, Adelusola KA, Durosimi MA (2006) The severity, outcome and challenges of breast cancer in Nigeria. Breast 15:399–409
56. Makanjuola SB, Popoola AO, Oludara MA (2014) Radiation therapy: a major factor in the five-year survival analysis of women with breast cancer in Lagos, Nigeria. Radiother Oncol 111(2):321–326
57. Forder PM, Gebski VJ, Keech AC (2005) Allocation concealment and blinding: when ignorance is bliss. Med J Aust 182(2):87–89
58. Lexchin J (2011) Those who have the gold make the evidence: how the pharmaceutical industry biases the outcomes of clinical trials of medications. Sci Eng Ethics 18(2):247–261
59. Lo B, Field MJ (2009) Conflict of interest in medical research, education, and practice. National Academies Press, Washington, DC
60. Jørgensen AW, Hilden J, Gøtzsche PC (2006) Cochrane reviews compared with industry supported meta-analyses and other meta-analyses of the same drugs: systematic review. BMJ 333:782
61. Drazen JM, de Leeuw PW, Laine C, Mulrow C, DeAngelis CD, Frizelle FA et al (2010) Toward more uniform conflict disclosures. JAMA 304:212–213
62. Kjaergard LL, Als-Nielsen B (2002) Association between competing interests and authors' conclusions: epidemiological study of randomised clinical trials published in the BMJ. BMJ 325(7358):249
63. Blumenthal D, Campbell EG, Causino N, Louis KS (1996) Participation of life-science faculty in research relationships with industry. N Engl J Med 335(23):1734–1739
64. Gasparyan AY, Ayvazyan L, Akazhanov NA, Kitas GD (2013) Conflicts of interest in biomedical publications: considerations for authors, peer reviewers, and editors. Croat Med J 54(6):600–608
65. Emanuel EJ, Wendler D, Grady C (2000) What makes clinical research ethical? JAMA 283:2701–2711
66. Glickman SW, McHutchison JG, Peterson ED, Cairns CB, Harrington RA, Califf RM, Schulman KA (2009) Ethical and scientific implications of the globalization of clinical research. N Engl J Med 360:816–823

67. Kelleher F (2004) The pharmaceutical industry's responsibility for protecting human subjects of clinical trials in developing nations. Columbia J Law Soc Probl 38:67–106
68. Arai RJ, Mano MS, De Castro G Jr, Diz Mdel P, Hoff PM (2010) Building research capacity and clinical trials in developing countries. Lancet Oncol 11:712–713
69. Mano MS, Rosa DD, Dal LL (2006) Multinational clinical trials in oncology and post-trial benefits for host countries: where do we stand? Eur J Cancer 42:2675–2677
70. Benatar SR (2000) Avoiding exploitation in clinical research. Camb Q Healthc Ethics 9:562–565
71. Lederer S (1995) Subjected to science: human experimentation in America before the second world war. Johns Hopkins University Press, Baltimore
72. Lilienfeld AM (1982) Ceteris paribus: the evolution of the clinical trial. Bull Hist Med 56:1–18
73. Harris J (1992) Wonder woman and superman: the ethics of human biotechnology. Oxford University Press, Oxford, pp 118–139. Commercial exploitation
74. Emanuel EJ (2000) Protecting communities in biomedical research. Science 289:1142–1144
75. Karim QA, Karim SSA, Coovadia HM, Susser M (1998) Informed consent for HIV testing in a South African hospital: is it truly informed and truly voluntary? Am J Public Health 88:637–640
76. Helsinki Declaration (2012) 1964, as most recently amended at the 59th World Medical Association General Assembly, Seoul, October 2008
77. Forster HP, Emanuel E, Grady C (2001) The 2000 revision of the Declaration of Helsinki: a step forward or more confusion? Lancet 358:1449–1453
78. Ferlay J, Shin HR, Bray F, Forman D, Mathers C, Parkin DM (2010) Estimates of worldwide burden of cancer in 2008: GLOBOCAN 2008. Int J Cancer 127(12):2893–2917
79. Jack RH, Davies EA, Møller H (2009) Breast cancer incidence, stage, treatment and survival in ethnic groups in South East England. Br J Cancer 100:545–550
80. American Cancer Society (2007) Global cancer facts & figures 2007. American Cancer Society, Atlanta
81. Lohr KN, Steinwachs DM (2002) Health services research: an evolving definition of the field. Health Serv Res 37(1):15–17
82. Jack RH, Davies EA, Renshaw C et al (2013) Differences in breast cancer hormone receptor status in ethnic groups: a London population. Eur J Cancer 49:696–702
83. Azubuike S, Okwuokei S (2013) Knowledge, attitudes and practices of women towards breast cancer in Benin City, Nigeria. Ann Med Health Sci Res 3:155–160
84. Harris B, Goudge J, Ataguba JE, McIntyre D, Nxumalo N, Jikwana S, Chersich M (2011) Inequities in access to health care in South Africa. J Public Health Policy 32(1):S102–S123
85. Jones CEL, Maben J, Jack RH et al (2014) A systematic review of barriers to early presentation and diagnosis with breast cancer among black women. BMJ Open 4:e004076
86. Lasserson DS, Chandratheva A, Giles MF et al (2008) Influence of general practice opening hours on delay in seeking medical attention after transient ischaemic attack (TIA) and minor strike: prospective population based study. BMJ 337:a1569
87. Livingston J (2012) Improvising medicine: an African oncology ward in an emerging cancer epidemic. Duke University Press, Durham, pp 1–52
88. Lamyian M, Hydarnia A, Ahmadi F, Faghihzadeh S, Aguilar-Vafaie ME (2007) Barriers to and factors facilitating breast cancer screening among Iranian women: a qualitative study. East Mediterr Health J 13(5):1160–1169
89. Leong SP, Shen ZZ, Liu TJ, Agarwal G, Tajima T, Paik NS, Sandelin K, Derossis A, Cody H, Foulkes WD (2010) Is breast cancer the same disease in Asian and western countries? World J Surg 34(10):2308–2324
90. Wong JC, Fernandes KA, Amin S, Lwin Z, Krzyzanowska MK (2014) Involvement of low- and middle-income countries in randomized controlled trial publications in oncology. Glob Health 10:83
91. Devasenapathy N, Singh K, Prabhakaran D (2009) Conduct of clinical trials in developing countries: a perspective. Curr Opin Cardiol 24(4):295–300

92. Dumville JC, Torgerson DJ, Hewitt CE (2006) Reporting attrition in randomised controlled trials. BMJ 332:969–971
93. Fewtrell MS, Kennedy K, Singhal A, Martin RM, Ness A, Hadders-Algra M, Koletzko B, Lucas A (2008) How much loss to follow-up is acceptable in long-term randomised trials and prospective studies? Arch Dis Child 93:458–461
94. Kristman V, Manno M, Cote P (2004) Loss to follow-up in cohort studies: how much is too much? Eur J Epidemiol 19:751–760
95. Ashery RS, McAuliffe WE (1992) Implementation issues and techniques in randomised controlled trials of outpatient psychosocial treatments for drug abusers. Recruitment of subjects. Am J Drug Alcohol Abuse 18:305–329
96. Hayasaka E (2005) Approaches vary for clinical trials in developing countries. J Natl Cancer Inst Monogr 97(19):1401–1403
97. Lang TA, White NJ, Tran HT, Farrar JJ, Day NP, Fitzpatrick R, Angus BJ, Denis E, Merson L, Cheah PY, Chilengi R, Kimutai R, Marsh K (2010) Clinical research in resource-limited settings: enhancing research capacity and working together to make trials less complicated. PLoS Negl Trop Dis 29(6):e619
98. Greenwood BM, Bhasin A, Bowler CH, Naylor H, Targett GA (2006) Capacity strengthening in malaria research: the gates malaria partnership. Trends Parasitol 22(7):278–284
99. Kilama WL, Chilengi R, Wanga CL (2007) Towards an African-driven malaria vaccine development program: history and activities of the African malaria network trust (AMANET). AmJTrop Med Hyg 77(6):282–288
100. Kitua AY, Corrah T, Herbst K, Nyirenda T, Agwale S, Makanga M, Mgone CS (2009) Strengthening capacity, collaboration and quality of clinical research in Africa: EDCTP networks of excellence. Tanzan J Health Res 11(1):51–54
101. Global Health Clinical Trials. http://ght.globalhealthehub.org/. Accessed 9 June 2011
102. Atela M, Bakibinga P, Ettarh R, Kyobutungi C, Cohn S (2015) Strengthening health system governance using health facility service charters: a mixed methods assessment of community experiences and perceptions in a district in Kenya. BMC Health Serv Res 15:539
103. European Commission, DG Research and Innovation (2012). Responsible research and innovation: Europe's ability to respond to societal challenges. European Union: Publications Office. p 4
104. Bull S, Cheah PY, Denny S, Jao I, Marsh V, Merson L, Shah More N, Nhan le NT, Osrin D, Tangseefa D et al (2015) Best practices for ethical sharing of individual-level health research data from low- and middle-income settings. J Empir Res Hum Res Ethics 10(3):302–313
105. Carr D, Littler K (2015) Sharing research data to improve public health: a funder perspective. J Empir Res Hum Res Ethics 10(3):314–316
106. Jao I, Kombe F, Mwalukore S, Bull S, Parker M, Kamuya D, Molyneux S, Marsh V (2015) Involving research stakeholders in developing policy on sharing public health research data in Kenya: views on fair process for informed consent, access oversight, and community engagement. J Empir Res Hum Res Ethics 10(3):264–277
107. Cohen M (2006) Breast cancer early detection, health beliefs, and cancer worries in randomly selected women with and without a family history of breast cancer. Psychooncology 15(10):873–883
108. Hajian S, Vakilian K, Najabadi KM, Hosseini J, Mirzaei HR (2011) Effects of education based on the health belief model on screening behavior in high risk women for breast cancer, Tehran, Iran. Asian Pac J Cancer Prev 12(1):49–54
109. Bowen DJ, Burke W, Yasui Y, McTiernan A, McLeran D (2002) Effects of risk counselling on interest in breast cancer genetic testing for lower risk women. Genet Med 4(5):359–365
110. Knaul FM, Bhadelia A, Gralow J, Arreola-Ornelas H, Langer A, Frenk J (2012) Meeting the emerging challenge of breast and cervical cancer in low- and middle-income countries. Int J Gynaecol Obstet 119(1):S85–S88
111. Coreil J, Wilke J, Pintado I (2004) Cultural models of illness and recovery in breast cancer support groups. Qual Health Res 14:905–923

112. Hughes C, Fasaye GA, LaSalle VH et al (2003) Sociocultural influences on participation in genetic risk assessment and testing among African American women. Patient Educ Couns 51:107–114
113. Kreuter MW, Haughton LT (2006) Integrating culture into health information for African American women. Am Behav Sci 49:794–811
114. Ashing-Giwa KT, Padilla G, Tejero J et al (2004) Understanding the breast cancer experience of women: a qualitative study of African American, Asian American, Latina and Caucasian cancer survivors. Psychooncology 13:408–428
115. Bowie J, Sydnor KD, Granot M (2003) Spirituality and care of prostate cancer patients: a pilot study. J Natl Med Assoc 95:951–954
116. Krupski TL, Kwan L, Fink A et al (2006) Spirituality influences health related quality of life in men with prostate cancer. Psychooncology 15:121–131
117. Emanuel EJ (2008) Benefits to host countries. In: Emanuel EJ, Grady C, Crouch RA, Lie RK, Miller FG, Wendler D (eds) The Oxford textbook of clinical research ethics. Oxford University Press, New York, pp 719–728
118. Madsen S, Holm S, Riis P (1999) Ethical aspects of clinical trials: the attitudes of the public and out-patients. J Intern Med 245(6):571–579
119. Catania C, De Pas T, Goldhirsch A, Radice D, Adamoli L, Medici M et al (2008) Participation in clinical trials as viewed by the patient: understanding cultural and emotional aspects which influence choice. Oncology 74(3–4):177–187
120. Hussain-Gambles M (2004) South Asian patients' views and experiences of clinical trial participation. Fam Pract 21(6):636–642
121. Loh SY, Lee SY, Quek KF, Murray L (2012) Barriers to participation in a randomized controlled trial of qigong exercises amongst cancer survivors: lessons learnt. Asian Pac J Cancer Prev 13(12):6337–6342
122. Kanavos P (2006) The rising burden of cancer in the developing world. Ann Oncol 17(8):815–823
123. Hanna TP, Kangolle AC (2010) Cancer control in developing countries: using health data and health services research to measure and improve access, quality and efficiency. BMC Int Health Hum Rights 10:24
124. Lu F, Suda KJ, Marks KE (2013) Geographic location of antineoplastic agent clinical trials conducted in developed and developing countries. Int J Clin Pharm 35:87–91
125. Krzyzanowska MK, Kaplan R, Sullivan R (2011) How may clinical research improve healthcare outcomes? Ann Oncol 22(7):vii10–vii15
126. Landis SH, Murray T, Bolden S, Wingo PA (1999) Cancer statistics 1999. CA Cancer J Clin 49:8–31
127. Contractor KB, Kaur K, Rodrigues GS, Kulkarni DM, Singhal H (2008) Male breast cancer: is the scenario changing. World J Surg Oncol 6:58
128. Gradishar W (2000) Male breast cancer. In: Harris J, Lippman M, Morrow M, Osborne C (eds) Diseases of the breast, 2nd edn. Lippincott Williams & Wilkins, Philadelphia, pp 661–667
129. Jepson AS, Fentiman IS (1998) Male breast cancer. Int J Clin Pract 52:571–576
130. Friedman LS, Gayther SA, Kurosaki T et al (1997) Mutation analysis of BRCA1 and BRCA2 in a male breast cancer population. Am J Hum Genet 60:313–319
131. Korde LA, Zujewski JA, Kamin L et al (2010) Multidisciplinary meeting on male breast cancer: summary and research recommendations. J Clin Oncol 28(12):2114–2122
132. Bevier M, Sundquist K, Hemminki K (2012) Risk of breast cancers in families of multiple affected women and men. Breast Cancer Res Treat 132:723–728
133. Atalay MK, Altinok M (2003) Prognostic factors affecting survival in male breast cancer. J Exp Clin Cancer Res 22(1):29–33
134. Ezeome ER, Emegoakor CD, Chianakwana GU, Anyanwu SNC (2010) The pattern of male breast cancer in eastern Nigeria: a 12-year review. Niger Med J 51:26–29
135. Kidmas AT, Ugwu BT, Manasseh AN, Iya D, Opaluwa AS (2005) Male breast malignancy in Jos University teaching hospital. West Afr J Med 24(1):36–40

136. Bhagwandin S (1972) Carcinoma of the male breast in Zambia. East Afr Med J 49:176–199
137. Hassan I, Mabogunje O (1995) Cancer of the male breast in Zaria, Nigeria. East Afr Med J 72(7):457–458
138. Ihekwaba FN (1994) Breast cancer in men in black Africa: a report of 73 cases. J R Coll Surg Edinb 39(6):344–347
139. Kalyani R, Days S, Bindra Singh MS, Kumar H (2010) Cancer profile in Kolar: a ten years' study. Indian J Cancer 47(2):160–165
140. Ihekwaba FN (1993) The management of male breast cancer in Nigerians. Postgrad Med J 69(813):562–565
141. Dogo D, Pindiga PU, Yawe T (2000) Pattern of breast lesions in north eastern Nigeria. Tropical J Med Res 3:14–17
142. Fogh S, Hirsch AE, Langmead JP et al (2011) Use of tamoxifen with postsurgical irradiation may improve survival in estrogen and progesterone receptor-positive male breast cancer. Clin Breast Cancer 11(1):39–45
143. Liukkonen S, Saarto T, Mäenpää H, Sjöström-Mattson J (2010) Male breast cancer: a survey at the Helsinki University Central Hospital during 1981–2006. Acta Oncol 49(3):322–327

Chapter 7
Do Breast Cancer Patients Benefit from Surgery? Hypotheses, Mathematical Models and False Beliefs

Leonid Hanin

Abstract Although much is known about the molecular biology and genomics of breast cancer at the subcellular level, clinical manifestations of the disease and its diagnosis, prognosis and treatment continue to pose major challenges. This chapter is an attempt at critical review and analysis of a few principal hypotheses about the natural history of invasive breast cancer and the effects of surgery. We address a fundamental question regarding the universality of benefits of surgery and whether it should be dropped for some categories of breast cancer patients. We present a mathematical model of metastasis that allows for evaluating the post-surgery dynamics of the metastatic cascade. We show that statistical inference from the results of clinical trials may lead to false knowledge and irreproducible results. Finally, we make a case for identification of the categories of breast cancer patients that could benefit from surgery through a model-based analysis of post-surgery metastatic relapse times. The mathematical model could also serve as an *in silico* surrogate for clinical trials comparing various breast cancer treatments with and without surgery.

Keywords Breast cancer • Front loading principle • Linear progression theory • Mammography • Mathematical modeling • Metastasis • Statistical inference from clinical trials • Surgery

7.1 Linear Progression Theory: The Central Dogma of Oncology

Empirical observations of breast cancer over at least 2000 years have led to a paradigm of its linear progression. It posits that the development of a solid cancer is irreversible and follows its anatomic spread from the primary tumor site to local and

---

L. Hanin (✉)
Department of Mathematics and Statistics, Idaho State University, 921 S. 8th Avenue, Stop 8085, Pocatello, ID 83209-8085, USA
e-mail: hanin@isu.edu

M.W. Retsky, R. Demicheli (eds.), *Perioperative Inflammation as Triggering Origin of Metastasis Development*, DOI 10.1007/978-3-319-57943-6_7

regional lymph nodes and later through metastatic dissemination to distant organs and tissues. Accordingly, treatment of breast cancer since the late nineteenth century was primarily focused on resection of the primary tumor and as many affected lymph nodes and surrounding tissues as possible and practicable. This has led to a sequence of increasingly radical surgeries designed, practiced and advocated by William Halsted and his numerous followers.

The principal challenges to the linear progression theory came from three unrelated sources. The first was extensive clinical and experimental studies by Bernard Fisher and his coworkers in the 1950s–1970s reviewed in [1]. Based on the results of this work, Bernard Fisher hypothesized that in many cases, contrary to the linear progression postulate, breast cancer may become systemic long before primary tumor is detected and spreads to local lymph nodes.

The second challenge originated from the pioneering work of Judah Folkman on tumor angiogenesis that spanned more than three decades 1970s–2008 [2]. It resulted in a discovery that a malignant tumor cannot grow beyond a certain microscopic size of about 1–2 mm unless it induces angiogenesis that enables its further growth [3]. Once the tumor develops a capillary network, it can get additional supply of nutrients, oxygen and growth factors that cannot be delivered by means of diffusion alone. If such an angiogenic switch does not occur, the tumor maintains its size due to a dynamic equilibrium between cell proliferation, apoptosis and quiescence. Judah Folkman's discovery has two profound implications for understanding the natural history of solid cancers and their treatment.

1. It points to the possibility that a primary tumor may start shedding bloodborne metastases before it reaches detectable size. Thus, breast cancer and other malignancies may become systemic well before its primary source is discovered, which provides a biological underpinning to Fisher's hypothesis. The time window for metastasis seeding while the disease is still subclinical can be quite long. For example, assuming that the initial size of a spherical vascular tumor is 1.5 mm, the minimum detectable size is 5 mm and that the tumor grows exponentially with the doubling time of 100 days (a typical value for moderately aggressive primary breast tumors [4]) we find that the time between the start of the tumor's vascular growth and detection is at least 1.4 years.
2. It suggests a mechanism by which small primary tumors and micrometastases may remain dormant [5]. As emphasized in [6], metastatic dormancy is central to explaining various experimental, clinical and epidemiological findings related to breast cancer.

A significant clinical implication of Bernard Fisher's systemic theory of breast cancer is that the extent of surgery would have only minor impact on disease-free and overall survival of patients with invasive breast cancer. To validate this striking hypothesis, Bernard Fisher initiated and directed in 1970s–1990s numerous clinical trials conducted by the Pittsburgh-based National Surgical Adjuvant Breast and Bowel Project (NSABBP). Results of these trials confirmed the tested hypothesis unequivocally [7]. This landmark finding places the long-term outcome of primary breast tumor resection squarely into the hands of the state of metastasis at, or immediately after, surgery. If no metastases are present then most likely the patient will be cured. If, on the other hand, at the time of primary tumor resection solitary metastatic cancer cells or avascular micrometastases are already lodged at secondary sites in the state of dormancy or slow growth, then the patient's survival response to surgery will depend on whether these metastases will ever progress to the stage of vascular, aggressively growing secondary tumors over the patient's lifetime. Finally, if at the time of surgery at least one metastasis has already progressed to vascular stage then the patient will most likely develop metastatic relapse. The Fisher's alternative theory of breast cancer implies that many clinical variables pertaining to the stage of the disease, such as the number of affected lymph nodes, whether resected or not, and the event of primary tumor recurrence, that have long been thought of bearing long-term prognostic significance, are mostly associated with loco-regional short-term treatment outcomes.

The definitive outcomes of NSABBP trials have led to scaling back the extent of surgery for primary breast cancer by limiting it, when appropriate, to lumpectomy augmented with adjuvant or neoadjuvant systemic treatments, mostly chemo-, immuno- and hormonal therapies. In his review paper of 1999 Bernard Fisher prophesied about the future of breast cancer treatment: "... it is likely that surgery for the disease will continue to diminish in importance..." [7].

While the first two challenges to the linear progression theory came from the new insights into the natural history of breast cancer (and other solid cancers) as well as their clinical and epidemiological manifestations, the third one, discussed in the next section, emerged from public health programs aimed at early detection of breast cancer. The linear progression theory was challenged on other fronts as well, see e.g. a seminal early paper [8]. However, due to its simplicity, intuitive appeal and an entrenched network of exponents, it largely remains to this day one of the central dogmas of practical oncology, and so are the therapeutic approaches it informs.

7.2 The Mammography Debacle

The idea of mammographic screening is based on a plausible belief, rooted in the linear progression theory, that early detection and treatment of breast cancer will increase the probability of cure and reduce mortality. The reality of mammographic screening, however, diverged dramatically from these expectations. Numerous large-scale trials conducted in the 1970s–1990s consistently showed little or no benefit of mammography relative to the control (no-mammography) group. Moreover, analysis of the results of these trials revealed the "mammography paradox" whereby early detection of breast cancer may actually *increase* mortality for certain groups of women. As one striking example, a thorough meta-analysis of seven large randomized mammography trials found that women aged 40–49 years at study entry had higher cumulative mortality than in the control group for 10 years of follow-up in a row [9].

The stark departure of the observed effects of mammography from theoretical predictions presented an imminent threat to pro-mammography professional and advocacy groups and their vested interests. Their fierce resistance has led to almost three decades of "mammography wars" described in detail in [10] (for a particularly vivid report from the "battlefield," see [11]). While the "war" was still raging, mass mammography has continued unabated causing a major public health disaster. Due to massive overdiagnosis hundreds of thousands women received unnecessary, disfiguring and debilitating treatments [12]. Recall that overdiagnosis in this context means discovery of a breast lesion that (1) may disappear on its own; (2) is benign; (3) is malignant but indolent or non-invasive; or (4) is invasive but growing and disseminating so slowly that it would never surface during the patient's lifetime. As a result, the highly vaunted and expensive mass screening program is being gradually reduced and refocused on a relatively small fraction of women who may actually stand to benefit from it, most notably those with family history of breast cancer or carrying specific mutations in BRCA1 and BRCA2 genes.

7.3 The Front Loading Principle

Taken collectively, the ideas of early cancer detection and early aggressive treatment of primary tumor and metastases constitute a paradigm that can be called the *Front Loading Principle*. It insists on discovering cancer as soon as possible and hitting it as hard and early as possible. The principle seems self-evident, for it has ostensibly the greatest chance of preventing the cancer's further proliferation and spread over any alternative strategy. It is worth noting that in the setting of fractionated cancer radiotherapy, the Front Loading Principle can be rigorously proved under very general assumptions [13–15]. In cases where considerations of radiation-induced normal tissue toxicity can be reduced to imposing certain fixed upper limits on the total dose and dose per fraction, it implies optimality of the uniform fractionation schedules [15].

The Front Loading Principle dominates the thinking of oncologists and cancer patients alike. What is seldom realized is that this principle is deeply rooted in the linear progression paradigm. Therefore, every challenge to the latter is likely to casts a doubt on the Front Loading Principle as well.

Is the Front Loading Principle actually true in the case of breast cancer? To answer this question, we will have to analyze its hidden foundations. In doing so we will follow Henri Poincaré, a genius French mathematician, theoretical physicist and philosopher of the nineteenth and early twentieth century, who was the first to keenly understand the fundamental importance of hypotheses and assumptions for the validity of scientific research [16]. Apparently his ideas appeared so much ahead of their time that even more than a century later they have not been fully recognized and taken to heart by the scientific community.

What are the hypotheses underlying the Front Loading Principle as applied to breast cancer detection and treatment? Its validity rests on several implicit assumptions: (1) early breast cancer does not regress spontaneously; (2) primary breast tumor and/or its metastases will manifest clinically during a patient's lifetime; (3) biopsy at an early stage of breast cancer can yield a reliable diagnosis; (4) breast cancer does not metastasize before primary tumor detection; and (5) existing breast cancer treatments do not exacerbate the disease. It has been known long ago that, as general statements, all these assumptions are false.

First, although spontaneous regression of cancer is hard to observe systematically, such clinical cases have been reported and brought into the medical mainstream as early as in the 1960s [17, 18]. Indirect estimates of the rate of early breast cancer regression based on epidemiological models put it as high as 22% [19]. Thus, in certain cases early breast cancer may be reversible, and so are some other types of cancer as well [20]. This constitutes one source of overdiagnosis and overtreatment of breast cancer brought about by mammography. Sporadic cancer regression is enabled by the regulatory role of tumor microenvironment that modulates tumor evolution. A large body of experimental evidence reviewed and analyzed in [21–23] suggests that normal microenvironment can inhibit cancer progression and even reprogram cells with malignant phenotype back into normal cells.

Second, the above-discussed Folkman's theory suggests that the primary and secondary tumors may remain indefinitely in a dormant or indolent subclinical state. That this possibility is very real in the case of breast cancer was confirmed in an autopsy study [24] that discovered breast tumors in 25.3% of women who died from various causes unrelated to breast cancer. This is more than twice the lifetime probability to be diagnosed with breast cancer in the general American female population.

Third, by its sampling nature, needle biopsy is unreliable; moreover, as every pathologist knows, distinguishing between various benign lesions, breast carcinoma *in situ*, and invasive breast cancer as well as scoring the histological grade in the early stages of the disease may prove difficult, which may lead to false positive and false negative diagnoses that contribute to overdiagnosis and increased mortality, respectively. Most importantly, no methods are currently available to reliably tell an aggressive, life-threatening early stage breast cancer from the one that can be safely ignored.

Fourth, as was discussed above, the work of Bernard Fisher and his colleagues has proven beyond reasonable doubt that in a large fraction of patients with invasive breast cancer by the time primary breast tumor becomes clinically detectable it has already metastasized. Mathematical modeling based on the analysis of site-specific volumes of metastases in real patients points to the same conclusion [25, 26].

For women who fall into the "Fisher effect" category, mammography has no impact, except for unnecessary exposure to carcinogenic radiation. Thus, for many patients with invasive breast cancer, who were initially supposed to benefit from mammography the most, detection of their disease comes way too late.

Finally, in the next section we will briefly discuss the evidence and putative mechanisms by which resection of the primary tumor may exacerbate the disease. This phenomenon is of paramount importance, and it furnishes a compelling explanation of the mammography paradox.

Were the above hidden assumptions underlying mammography screening carefully formulated and closely scrutinized, the disastrous rush to total mammographic screening would have been stemmed and research focused instead on the search for those categories of women for whom the benefits of mammography outweigh the risks.

7.4 The Independence Principle: Yet Another Dogma of Oncology

The *Independence Principle* states that different primary and secondary tumors evolve independently. It is a curious historical fact that, although the validity of this postulate was questioned more than a century ago, it still remains a cornerstone of mainstream clinical oncology.

Investigation of the interactions between various tumors started in the beginning of the twentieth century with a pioneering work of Paul Ehrlich published in 1906 [27] (see also a 1907 paper [28]). The main conclusion of these and subsequent experimental studies was that large tumors suppress the growth of smaller ones. See a comprehensive review [29]. Not surprisingly, then, resection of a large primary tumor could lead to accelerated growth of metastases. This phenomenon was observed in numerous animal experiments and reported in many published clinical case studies, see comprehensive reviews [30, 31]. Many details about the patterns of metastasis dynamics following surgery have recently emerged. In particular, it was shown that accelerated growth of liver metastases after resection of human colorectal carcinoma is mostly due to decreased apoptosis rather than increased proliferation [32] (interestingly, the same is true for accelerated tumor repopulation following radiation [33]). Another recent work [34] found that variation of the number and sizes of metastases at the time of relapse can serve as a quantitative measure of the effects of primary breast tumor excision on metastasis. Finally, an experimental angiogenesis biomarker study [35] showed that breast tumor excision leads to a transient spike in angiogenic activity. In summary, a vast body of experimental, clinical and epidemiological evidence amassed over the last century has proven that surgical resection of the primary tumor may trigger escape from metastatic dormancy, promote angiogenesis and boost the growth of vascular secondary tumors.

Several non-mutually exclusive mechanisms explaining these effects of surgery on metastasis have been proposed:

1. According to Richmond Prehn [36] each tumor produces both growth and angiogenesis factors as well as inhibitors of these processes. These factors and their inhibitors have different biochemical properties: while the former are easily degradable and spread mostly locally by diffusion the latter are more stable and when shed into the blood stream may reach distant sites and suppress metastatic progression. When primary tumor is excised, supply of the inhibitors is abrogated. This causes vascularization of metastases and boosts their growth.
2. Resection of the primary tumor (and any other surgery for that matter [37]) initiates local and systemic production of growth and angiogenesis factors required for effective wound healing. As they are captured by dormant or slowly growing metastases, angiogenesis and growth processes are accelerated.
3. The idea that cancer is associated with inflammation was advanced by Rudolf Virchow in 1863 and is supported by numerous clinical and experimental studies. As one example, tumors are routinely found to be infiltrated by various cells of the immune system including T-lymphocytes, macrophages, natural killer cells and neutrophils [38]. A related hypothesis is that surgery-induced systemic inflammation fuels metastasis. One of many ways in which this may occur is due to the increase in blood vessel permeability caused by inflammation, which facilitates both intravasation of cancer cells shed off the primary tumor and extravasation of circulating tumor cells. A dramatic, if only indirect, evidence of a strong metastasis-promoting effect of surgery-related inflammation was recently found by a group of Belgian anesthesiologists who discovered that the use of ketorolac, a non-steroidal anti-inflammatory analgesic, during surgery for primary breast cancer led to a fivefold drop in the number of short-term (i.e. within the first 5 years post-surgery) relapses, as compared to analgesics without anti-inflammatory activity [39]. The explanation of this finding, the promise it holds for the improvement of breast cancer therapy and a proposal for a randomized phase III clinical trial were explicated in [40–43].

7.5 Do Breast Cancer Patients Benefit from Surgery?

The principal cause of mortality from breast cancer is distant metastases that typically spread to bone, brain, liver and lungs. If such metastases are clinically manifest at presentation then resection of primary tumor is rarely performed unless primary tumor poses live-threatening risks unrelated to metastasis. Otherwise the main reason for surgery is to prevent metastasis. Given that metastatic disease in subclinical form may already be present and that surgery may exacerbate the course of the disease, a fundamental question arises: *Will resection of the primary tumor benefit a particular breast cancer patient?*

The benefits of any treatment can only be assessed against the background of survival of untreated patients who receive palliative care alone. Such a benchmark was established in a remarkable study [44]. It analyzed a group of 250 untreated breast cancer patients who were observed for the entire duration of their residual lifespan since admission to the Middlesex Hospital in England between 1805 and 1933. Ninety-five percent of these patients succumbed with distant metastases and/or extensive local breast cancer; the rest died as a result of intercurrent disease. The mean survival since onset of symptoms was 3 years. The fractions of surviving patients at 5, 10 and 15 years were 18%, 3.6% and 0.8%, respectively. The longest survival was 18 years and 3 months. In 86 cases seen between 1902 and 1933 post-mortem examination was performed. It revealed that histological grade was highly correlated with survival. Specifically, the average survival since onset of symptoms for patients with grades I, II and III was 47, 39 and 22 months, respectively.

Thus, the decision on resecting a primary breast tumor at a given time depends critically on the answers to following three questions:

(A) Are there subclinical metastases lodged at various secondary sites?
(B) What would be the effects of surgery on metastatic progression?
(C) How likely is it that surgery itself will produce metastases?

A traditional way to conduct a comparative study of survival effects of surgery for primary breast cancer is to run a randomized clinical trial where standard treatments involving surgery would be compared with the same treatments without the surgery. However, implementation of this approach faces two major difficulties: (1) The no-surgery option may be viewed as "unethical" making approval of the trial problematic; and (2) Because breast cancer is notorious for late recurrences appearing as late as 20–25 [45, 46] or even 40 years [47] post-treatment, obtaining conclusive results would necessitate a very long trial time. Additionally, and perhaps much more importantly, we show in the next section that statistical inference from any clinical trial may produce misleading results. Thus, although clinical trials may be used for empirical comparisons between various treatments, inference on unobservable biomedical processes based on the results of clinical trials should be discouraged.

7.6 Statistical Inference from Clinical Trials: A Source of False Knowledge and Irreproducible Results?

Theoretical statistics, like all mathematical sciences, is based on theorems that consist of assumptions and conclusions. The validity of the arguments by which the conclusions are derived from the assumptions is there for anyone to verify. In applied statistics, statistical methods and tests resulting from these theorems are used to draw inferences about natural processes based on empirical data. But are the assumptions behind the methods and tests valid?

The most fundamental assumption that underlies virtually every application of statistics in natural sciences and medicine is that a set of observations, say $x_1, x_2, \ldots, x_n$, is a random sample from a certain probability distribution. Informally, this means that the observed values result from independent replications of the same random experiment, just like a sequence of "heads" and "tails" results from flips of a coin or numbers 1–6 result from rolls of a die. Critically, the assumptions that these random variables are stochastically independent and identically distributed (the *iid property*) cannot be verified empirically, for each of these random variables is represented by a *single* value. Thus, in all applications the most basic assumption that underlies statistical inference from data is necessarily and invariably taken on faith.

The question as to whether a given data set can be viewed as a random sample can be quite subtle. For example, suppose $x_1, x_2, \ldots, x_n$ are the volumes of metastases measured at a given time t in a particular secondary site (such as lungs, bones, liver, etc.) through analysis of CT and PET images taken for an individual patient. Among a large number of metastases shed off the primary tumor, these n metastases survived, reached their target site and after some dormancy period started to grow, induced angiogenesis and by time t reached a detectable size. The rate of metastasis shedding off the primary tumor depends on its volume and is therefore a function of time. Because the detected metastases were almost surely shed by the primary tumor at different times, the rates of metastasis shedding at those times were also different. Thus, the volumes of the detected metastases cannot be thought of as resulting from replication of the same random experiment, and so $x_1, x_2, \ldots, x_n$ cannot be viewed as a random sample from a probability distribution! It is interesting to note, however, that in one important particular case, namely when metastasis shedding is governed by a Poisson process with arbitrary time-dependent rate, the lack of the iid property can be mitigated. Specifically, in this case the set of ordered volumes of detected metastases is equidistributed, conditional on their number, with the set of order statistics of a random sample from a certain probability distribution that can be computed in closed form [48–50]. An important practical implication is that various unobservable quantities descriptive of metastatic cancer progression in an individual patient can be estimated from the observed volumes of metastases through the use of symmetric (i.e. permutation-invariant) statistics, e.g. by using the method of maximum likelihood [25, 26]. We emphasize that such inference is enabled by the above "quasi-iid" property resulting from (1) the assumed Poisson nature of the process of metastasis shedding and (2) conditioning on the random number, n, of detectable metastases at time t.

To see how justified is the reliance on the iid property in clinical trials, consider a hypothetical randomized controlled clinical trial comparing survival or disease-free survival of stage I–III breast cancer patients under traditional treatment involving surgery and a certain combination of cytotoxic chemotherapy, adjuvant radiation and hormonal therapy on the one hand and the same treatment without the surgery on the other hand. Because the most significant factors that largely determine survival outcomes (specifically, the state of metastasis at the beginning of treatment, intrinsic aggressiveness of the disease and the strength of the patient's immune system and other natural defenses against cancer) are either unobservable or hard to formalize and quantify, the patients' survival in the trial should be related to surrogate explanatory variables, some of which may be unobservable or only partially observable. They include (1) patient's susceptibility to developing metastasis; (2) age at presentation; (3) stage of the disease at the beginning of treatment; (4) extent of nodal involvement; (5) menopausal status at study entry; (6) histological grade of the disease; (7) estrogen and progesterone receptor status; (8) presence of specific mutations in BRCA1 or BRCA2 genes; (9) family history of breast cancer; (10) individual history of other malignancies; (11) death of causes other than breast cancer over the observation period; and (12) censoring.

Even this rough and incomplete set of clinical variables creates a large number of categories of women whose survival and disease-free survival responses in the experimental and control groups could be potentially very different. Note that randomization won't eliminate such heterogeneity; it will only reduce the difference in the extent of the heterogeneity between the experimental and control groups. The inter-subject heterogeneity is quite typical of clinical trials (as opposed to biological experiments with tightly controlled inter-subject variation) and has profound implications for the validity of statistical inference from their results. First, the distributions of individual survival response variables for subjects in both groups cannot be even approximately viewed as identical. Second, regardless of the sample size, each group will contain many categories with known or unknown numbers of subjects. Moreover, both the number of such categories in each group and the numbers of their representatives are dependent random variables with unknown distributions. Therefore, the most basic assumptions underlying any kind of statistical analysis are not met.

Thus, even for large-scale randomized controlled clinical trials commonly viewed as the gold standard of biomedical research, the "heterogeneity curse" makes statistical inference a dubious proposition and will quite likely lead to false knowledge generation. Furthermore, variation in the number of categories and the number of subjects representing each category between different trials would make their results potentially irreproducible.

There is one case, however, where the heterogeneity problem is non-existent, namely when a sample consists of just one subject. A great advantage of individual case studies is that learning everything that is there to know is quite feasible and that inference from this knowledge is not confounded by inter-subject variation. If one believes that biomedical processes are governed by natural laws and have causes, mechanisms and effects, then studying a single subject thoroughly should be very informative. Doing so for many individual patients will eventually reveal all the important characteristics of the disease and effects of various interventions. This is the way medicine gained enormous empirical knowledge over many centuries, and there is no reason to believe that this same approach won't work well in the future.

7.7 A Mathematical Model of Post-surgery Metastatic Progression

The three questions (A–C) about the state of metastasis at surgery and the effects of surgery on subsequent metastatic progression that we posed in Section 5 deal with unobservable events that are separated from observable clinical outcomes by months, years or even decades. That is why the only way to answer these questions is through mathematical modeling. Described below is a very general mathematical model of post-surgery evolution of metastases that is rooted in the biology of metastasis but avoids a detailed mechanistic description that would make the model mathematically intractable and its numerous parameters inestimable. We assume that at the time of surgery distant metastases, if present, are in a subclinical state. For more details about the model, see [51].

Parameters of the model described below can be estimated from a data base of breast cancer patients that contains information on the time of post-surgery metastatic relapse which may include censoring. Additionally, the data base should preferably contain information on the patient-specific mechanism of metastatic relapse. In fact, for some patients, relapse may occur spontaneously as a result of surfacing of clinical symptoms while for other patients, metastatic relapse may be detected in the course of pre-scheduled medical exams for which dates should be available. These two mechanisms imply different size thresholds for metastasis detection and thus affect the time between surgery and metastatic relapse. Ideally, for the purpose of efficient parameter estimation, a subset of patients to be analyzed should be as homogeneous as possible with respect to the clinical variables described in Section 6 and to the treatment they received post-surgery; however, it should still contain sufficiently many subjects.

The main focus of the model is on describing evolution of metastasis. The latter is a complex and highly selective multi-stage process. These stages include: (a) separation of a cancer cell from the primary tumor; (b) migration to a blood vessel; (c) intravasation; (d) free circulation; (e) adhesion to a blood vessel wall and extravasation; (f) invading a secondary site; (g) dormancy or slow avascular growth at the site in question; (h) induction of angiogenesis and vascularization; and finally (i) aggressive growth leading to a clinically detectable secondary tumor. This metastatic cascade is quite inefficient in that only a tiny fraction of cancer cells shed off the primary tumor give rise to viable clinically significant metastatic lesions.

To model post-surgery evolution of metastases mathematically, we aggregate the above stages of the metastatic cascade into the following three successive states of metastases:

1. solitary cancer cells that were shed into the bloodstream during surgery or were already present at the time of surgery as either circulating tumor cells or quiescent cancer cells lodged at various secondary sites;
2. avascular dormant or slowly growing micrometastases;

3. vascularizing or vascular metastases that had started their aggressive growth prior to surgery but are still subclinical at the time of surgery.

A similar classification of metastatic states was considered in [6].

The unobservable snapshot of the metastatic cascade immediately after surgery serves as the initial state of the post-surgery evolution of metastases while metastatic relapse represents its observable endpoint. In what follows we assume that metastatic relapse is due to metastases that were present at, or formed as a result of, surgery only. In particular, the effects of secondary metastasis (that is, "metastasis of metastasis") and of metastases originating from the recurring primary tumor, in case such a recurrence happens, are presumed negligible.

7.7.1 The Model

Our model deals with *viable* metastases, i.e. those metastases that are bound to develop into detectable secondary tumors. The time, counted from surgery, when a viable metastasis reaches the size that potentially makes it clinically detectable will be called *progression time*. The observed time of metastatic relapse, then, is the smallest among progression times of viable metastases present immediately after surgery.

It is assumed that viable metastases in a given patient evolve independently of each other and that the variation of the number, N_k, of viable metastases in state k at surgery within the population of interest follows a Poisson distribution with expected value λ_k, $k = 1, 2, 3$. Additionally, random variables N_k, $k = 1, 2, 3$, are thought of as stochastically independent. Therefore, the total number of viable metastases at surgery has Poisson distribution with the expected value $\lambda_1 + \lambda_2 + \lambda_3$. Denote by T_k the duration of state k, with the understanding that state 3 is terminated when metastasis becomes clinically detectable. We assume that sojourn times T_k, $k = 1, 2, 3$, are stochastically independent and absolutely continuous, and denote by g_k, $k = 1, 2, 3$, the respective probability density functions (pdf's).

Let U be the progression time of a viable metastasis. If such metastasis was in state 3 at surgery then $U = T_3$ and hence the pdf of random variable U is $f_3 := g_3$. If the state of a viable metastasis at surgery was 2 then $U = T_2 + T_3$ and therefore pdf of U is the convolution of pdf's g_2 and g_3 which we denote f_2:

$$f_2(t) = \int_0^t g_2(u)g_3(t-u)du$$

Finally, if a viable metastasis was in state 1 at surgery then $U = T_1 + T_2 + T_3$ so that pdf, f_1, of random variable U is the convolution of pdf's g_1, g_2 and g_3. Denote by F_i the cumulative distribution function (cdf) corresponding to the pdf f_i, and let $\bar{F}_i = 1 - F_i$ be the corresponding survival function, $i = 1, 2, 3$.

The observed time, T, from surgery to metastatic relapse is the minimum of the progression times over all viable metastases present at surgery (if a patient was metastasis-free at surgery then we set $T = \infty$). It follows from our assumptions that for any $t > 0$

$$\Pr(T > t | N_1 = n_1, N_2 = n_2, N_3 = n_3) = \overline{F}_1^{n_1}(t)\overline{F}_2^{n_2}(t)\overline{F}_3^{n_3}(t)$$

Then for the survival function, $\overline{G}(t) = \Pr(T > t)$, of random variable T we have

$$\begin{aligned}\overline{G}(t) &= \sum_{n_1=0}^{\infty}\sum_{n_2=0}^{\infty}\sum_{n_3=0}^{\infty} e^{-(\lambda_1+\lambda_2+\lambda_3)} \frac{\lambda_1^{n_1}}{n_1!}\frac{\lambda_2^{n_2}}{n_2!}\frac{\lambda_3^{n_3}}{n_3!}\overline{F}_1^{n_1}(t)\overline{F}_2^{n_2}(t)\overline{F}_3^{n_3}(t) \\ &= \exp\{-[\lambda_1 F_1(t) + \lambda_2 F_2(t) + \lambda_3 F_3(t)]\}\end{aligned} \tag{7.1}$$

Note that

$$\overline{G}(\infty) = \exp\{-(\lambda_1 + \lambda_2 + \lambda_3)\}$$

represents the probability that a patient is metastasis-free at surgery.

Finally, we denote by 1-p the probability that a patient is insusceptible to developing clinically detectable metastatic relapse and set for such patients $T = \infty$. Therefore, the overall survival function for the time to relapse is represented as a mixture model

$$S(t) = 1 - p + p\overline{G}(t) \tag{7.2}$$

Observe that the time of metastatic relapse for a given patient may be missing in the database due to the following non-mutually exclusive reasons: (1) the patient is insusceptible to metastatic relapse due to her genetic make-up, strength of the immune system, high levels of circulating growth and angiogenesis inhibitors or other intrinsic reasons; (2) no viable metastases were present immediately after surgery; (3) the patient was lost to follow-up during the observation period (censoring); (4) the time span over which the data was collected was insufficient for clinical manifestation of metastatic relapse; and (5) the patient died from a cause other than metastatic breast cancer before the end of the observation period.

The model depends on parameters p, λ_1, λ_2, λ_3 as well as parameters built into the distributions of the sojourn time in states 1, 2 and 3. The most natural way to estimate all these parameters is to use the method of maximum likelihood. If metastatic relapse in a patient was spontaneous and occurred at time t post-surgery then the contribution of such patient to the model-based log-likelihood function is

$$L = \log p - \lambda_1 F_1(t) - \lambda_2 F_2(t) - \lambda_3 F_3(t) + \log[\lambda_1 f_1(t) + \lambda_2 f_2(t) + \lambda_3 f_3(t)]$$

If metastatic relapse in a patient was detected through a pre-scheduled medical exam at time t then

$$L = \log p + \log H(t)$$

where $H(t) = G(t) - G(t - \tau)$ if the previous exam given to the patient at time τ was negative and $H(t) = G(t)$ if metastatic relapse was detected by the first exam; here G(t) is the cdf corresponding to the survival function (7.1). Finally, if a patient was censored at time C then

$$L = \log\{1 - p + p\exp\{-[\lambda_1 F_1(C) + \lambda_2 F_2(C) + \lambda_3 F_3(C)]\}\}$$

Based on the model, one can compute the probability, P_k, that the observed metastatic relapse originated from a metastasis in state k at surgery, k = 1, 2, 3, given that the patient was not metastasis-free at surgery. We will call these important quantities *attribution probabilities*. As shown in [51],

$$P_k = \frac{\lambda_k \int_0^\infty \exp\{-[\lambda_1 F_1(t) + \lambda_2 F_2(t) + \lambda_3 F_3(t)]\} f_k(t)dt}{1 - \exp\{-(\lambda_1 + \lambda_2 + \lambda_3)\}}, \quad k = 1,2,3 \tag{7.3}$$

Clearly, $P_1 + P_2 + P_3 = 1$.

7.7.2 An Example

The simplest hypothesis about transition rates from metastatic states 1, 2, 3 is that these rates are constant in time. This leads to the exponential distribution of sojourn times in states 1, 2, 3 considered in [51]. Specifically, we assumed that the distribution of sojourn time T_k is exponential $Exp(\beta_k)$ with the expected value β_k^{-1}, k = 1, 2, 3. Parameters β_1 and β_2 represent post-surgery rates of transition from state 1 to state 2 and from state 2 to state 3, respectively, while parameter β_3 can be interpreted as the rate at which metastases in state 3 reach detectable size. Then for the pdf, f_k, of the progression time of a viable metastasis that was in state k at surgery we have [51]:

$$f_3(t) = \beta_3 e^{-\beta_3 t}, \quad f_2(t) = \frac{\beta_2\beta_3}{\beta_2 - \beta_3}(e^{-\beta_3 t} - e^{-\beta_2 t})$$

and

$$f_1(t) = \frac{\beta_2\beta_3}{(\beta_1-\beta_2)(\beta_1-\beta_3)}\beta_1 e^{-\beta_1 t} + \frac{\beta_1\beta_3}{(\beta_2-\beta_1)(\beta_2-\beta_3)}\beta_2 e^{-3_2 t}$$
$$+\frac{\beta_1\beta_2}{(\beta_3-\beta_1)(\beta_3-\beta_2)}\beta_3 e^{-\beta_3 t}$$

The corresponding survival functions are

$$\overline{F}_3(t) = e^{-\beta_3 t}, \quad \overline{F}_2(t) = \frac{\beta_2 e^{-\beta_3 t} - \beta_3 e^{-\beta_2 t}}{\beta_2 - \beta_3}$$

and

$$\overline{F}_1(t) = \frac{\beta_2\beta_3}{(\beta_1-\beta_2)(\beta_1-\beta_3)} e^{-\beta_1 t} + \frac{\beta_1\beta_3}{(\beta_2-\beta_1)(\beta_2-\beta_3)} e^{-\beta_2 t} + \frac{\beta_1\beta_2}{(\beta_3-\beta_1)(\beta_3-\beta_2)} e^{-\beta_3 t}$$

In the case of exponentially distributed sojourn times model (7.1), (7.2) depends on seven parameters: λ_1, λ_2, λ_3, β_1, β_2, β_3, p. Note that if some of the rates β_1, β_2, β_3 are equal then the above formulas have to be replaced with the corresponding limiting expressions.

Pdf of the exponential distribution is a decreasing function, which means that larger sojourn times occur with smaller probabilities. To explore more flexible patterns while keeping the model as parsimonious as possible, it was assumed in [51] that metastasis sojourn time in state k = 1, 2, 3 follows an Erlang distribution $E(n_k, \beta)$, where n_k is a natural number and $\beta > 0$ is assumed the same for all three states. Recall that Erlang distribution $E(n, \beta)$ with the pdf

$$f(x) = \frac{\beta^n}{(n-1)!} x^{n-1} e^{-\beta x}, \quad x \geq 0$$

is a gamma distribution with integer shape parameter n and scale parameter β. In the case n = 1 Erlang distribution reduces to the exponential distribution $Exp(\beta)$, while for n > 1 its pdf is unimodal and asymmetrically bell-shaped with the mode $(n - 1)/\beta$ and mean n/β. Thus, progression time distributions for metastases in states 1, 2, 3 at surgery are $E(n_1 + n_2 + n_3, \beta)$, $E(n_2 + n_3, \beta)$ and $E(n_3, \beta)$, respectively. A distinct advantage of the Erlang distribution $E(n, \beta)$ over the more general gamma distribution is that its cdf can be computed in closed form:

$$F(x) = 1 - e^{-\beta x} \sum_{k=0}^{n-1} \frac{(\beta x)^k}{k!}, \quad x \geq 0$$

For Erlang distributed sojourn times, the resulting model depends on eight parameters: λ_1, λ_2, λ_3, n_1, n_2, n_3, β, p.

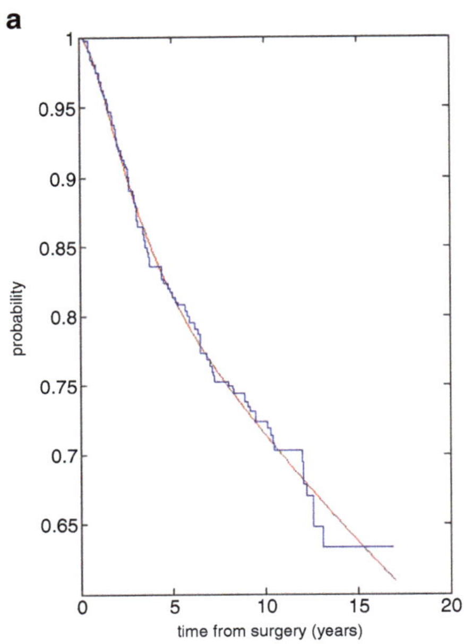

Fig. 7.1 (**a**, **b**) Fit between the empirical (step-wise curve) and theoretical (continuous curve) survival functions for all 673 patients under scenario 1 for the exponential model (panel **a**) and Erlang model (panel **b**). Theoretical survival function is given by formulas (7.1), (7.2) while empirical survival function is the Kaplan-Meier estimator. Optimal values of model parameters are given in Tables 1 and 2 of [51]. Reproduced from [51] with permission from Elsevier

The above-described model with exponential or Erlang sojourn times was applied to a database of 673 breast cancer patients treated with surgery [51]. Briefly, the mean age at surgery was 59.6 years (range 32–88 years). The event of metastatic relapse was recorded in 164 patients (24.6%) while for all other 509 patients, metastasis-free survival time, i.e. the time of the last observation, was reported. The mean recorded time to metastatic relapse counted from surgery was 49 months (range: 3 months–13 years) while the largest metastasis-free survival time (i.e. the length of the observation period) was 16.85 years. Finally, 62.5% of the patients were given adjuvant Tamoxifen while all other patients received surgery alone.

The data base in question did not contain information on the metastasis detection mechanism. To overcome this difficulty, two extreme scenarios were assumed in [51]: (1) metastasis surfaced spontaneously in all patients who experienced metastatic relapse; and (2) detection of metastatic relapse in all patients was due to periodic medical exams given every 3 or 6 months. Accordingly, reported below are conclusions that were common to both extreme scenarios and both exam periodicities under scenario 2. This makes it plausible that the same conclusions would hold for the unknown actual (and most likely patient-specific) detection mechanism. Also, we report only those results that are common for both exponential and Erlang sojourn time distributions. In both cases the model with likelihood-maximizing parameters, that were computed without any supervision or calibration, produced an amazingly good fit to the data under scenario 1 (see Fig. 7.1), which testifies to model adequacy. Given that the exponential model had triple degeneration ($\lambda_3 = 0$, $\beta_2 = \beta_3$, $p = 1$), this seems especially remarkable. Note that under scenario 2 the relapse times are not well-defined, and so is the fit to data.

1. *Early metastatic dissemination.* According to the model, among the 673 breast cancer patients analyzed, many already had either avascular dormant micrometastases or growing vascular secondary tumors at the time of surgery. This means that in many patients the onset of metastasis had occurred before their primary tumor became clinically detectable. This finding supports Bernard Fisher's theory of early metastatic dissemination of invasive breast cancer.
2. *Metastatic dormancy.* At the time of surgery, a significant fraction of patients had dormant single cell metastases or dormant avascular micrometastases. Furthermore, the majority of solitary cancer cells remained dormant after the surgery. These results support the notion of metastatic dormancy [5, 46, 52–55] and confirm clinical significance of the dormancy-based paradigm of breast cancer proposed in [6]. Because of the short half-life of circulating cancer cells, in a few days after surgery their surviving fraction will reach the target secondary sites. Thus, the population of dormant state 1 metastases lodged at various secondary sites forms a pool that fuels the metastatic pipeline.
3. *Metastatic stages at surgery and their durations.* In the above model, metastases were classified into three categories: state 1 (solitary cancer cells), state 2 (avascular micrometastases) and state 3 (vascular secondary tumors). It was found that both the abundance of viable metastases in various states at surgery and the duration of those states decrease with the state number. In particular, it was estimated in [51] that, while viable metastases may reside in state 1 for decades post-surgery, their vascularization and growth until detection take just a few months or years.
4. *State attribution of metastatic relapse.* Although metastases in earlier states were found to be more numerous than in later states, they are father away in time from the end of metastatic pipeline. The outcome of this competition depends on the assumed sojourn time distributions for the three metastatic states, see Eq. (7.3). In particular, it was found in [51] that under the Erlang model all three states are likely to contribute significantly to the observed metastatic relapse while in the case of exponential model this is true for states 1 and 2 only.
5. *Does surgery lead to dissemination of metastases?* While not excluding this possibility, the analysis in [51] suggested that formation and dissemination of new metastases during surgery is unlikely to be the principal cause of metastatic relapse of breast cancer.
6. *Surgery-induced acceleration of metastasis.* If surgery were neutral with regard to metastatic dormancy, then metastases that were dormant at surgery would most likely remain dormant thereafter. This would suggest that the contribution of metastases in state 1 and 2 at surgery to the observed metastatic relapse is minor accounting only for their spontaneous transition to the next state; in other

words, the relapse would mostly be due to the growth of state 3 metastases. However, this was found not to be the case [51]. In fact, under the model with exponentially distributed sojourn times virtually all metastatic relapses were attributed to state 1 or 2 metastases while under the Erlang model 36–46% of relapses were estimated to result from state 1 or 2 metastases. A natural explanation of this finding is that surgery itself triggers processes that cause metastases to escape from dormancy and propels them through the metastatic pipeline thus enlarging the pool of actively growing vascular secondary lesions. In summary, the results of model-based data analysis support the well-documented notion that surgery has threefold effect on metastasis:

(a) it promotes intra- and extravasation of solitary cancer cells thus facilitating their entrance into and progression through state 1;
(b) it stimulates growth of metastases enabling their transition from state 1 into state 2, propelling them through state 2 and accelerating their growth in state 3; and
(c) it triggers production of angiogenesis factors while at the same time reducing concentration of angiogenesis inhibitors, which turns on angiogenesis and thus promotes transition from state 2 into state 3.

7.7.3 Model Extension

The above model developed in [51] can be extended in several directions. First, the model may accommodate a more detailed classification of the states of the metastatic cascade that will provide more information about the kinetics of metastasis pipeline and the effects of surgery. Second, it may explore more complex and flexible sojourn time distributions than those belonging to the exponential and Erlang families. Third, it may account for arbitrary patient-specific schedules of post-surgery follow-up exams if these data are available. Fourth, the model may be applied to cohorts of patients with a specific site of metastatic relapse. Finally, the model may incorporate the effects of primary tumor recurrence on the dynamics of metastasis.

7.8 Breast Cancer, Its Diagnosis and Treatment: The Mystery Remains

Breast cancer has baffled medical doctors and scientists for at least 2000 years. The advent of molecular biology and genomics has furthered our understanding of the biological nature and subtypes of the disease (in particular, through discovery of the role of estrogen and progesterone receptors, mutations in BRCA1 and BRCA2 genes, and especially through detection and characterization of breast cancer stem cells [56–58]). However, there remains an enormous gap between what we know about breast cancer at the molecular, genetic and subcellular levels and how the disease manifests in a given patient clinically at the systemic level.

Two aspects of the natural history of breast cancer have been established with great certainty through extensive experimental, clinical and epidemiological work: (1) heterogeneity of the disease and (2) the fundamental role of dormancy in the dynamics of primary and secondary tumors. It was found that breast cancer encompasses a great spectrum of conditions ranging from non-invasive indolent and even spontaneously regressing forms to invasive but slowly progressing types to aggressively growing and fast metastasizing variants of the disease. It is generally recognized that invasive breast cancer is incurable by contemporary therapeutic means and may remain subclinical for many years or even decades before and after treatment [4]. Most unfortunately for the patients, no early detection protocols that could accurately position a given case within this spectrum of disease gravity have been developed so far. One of the reasons is that the lion's share of effort and funding in breast cancer research (and oncology in general) went into molecular biological and genomic studies rendering many traditional approaches (including cytological, histological and biochemical) unattractive and underfunded. This is especially bewildering given that the reductionist approach centered on a single cancer cell, its genome and sub-cellular processes is well-known to have inherent diagnostic and prognostic limitations. As a result, diagnostic potential of several other avenues of research has not been fully investigated. One of them is the study of the tumor microenvironment that wields the power of exacerbating the disease, maintaining its dormancy or even reversing it. Another one is analyzing in depth the markers of tumor-immune system interaction. An additional early diagnostic tool for the estrogen and progesterone receptor positive types of the disease consists of monitoring the endocrine system and accounting for patients' reproductive history that is known to be an important modifier of the risks of breast cancer. Finally, there is little doubt that intrinsic differences between breast cancer cells may also manifest in their different geometric shapes and physical properties including membrane elasticity and adhesion forces. However, their diagnostic value has not been adequately explored.

Another fundamental problem in diagnosing breast cancer is the absence of assays for detection of occult metastases at various secondary sites. Together with assays for circulating tumor cells, this would put staging of the disease on a solid empirical foundation. By contrast, the conventional breast cancer staging system registers an apparent rather than actual state of the disease, which may lead to an overly optimistic assessment of the extent of cancer spread in a subset of cancer patients and mislead their doctors regarding the required treatment and prognosis. In its present form, the breast cancer staging system has more to do with the sensitivity of various tests and imaging technologies as well as chance factors associated with biopsy than with unobservable yet clinically and prognostically critical characteristics of metastasis.

The uncertainty in diagnosis translates into low efficacy of treatment. For stage I-III breast cancer patients, the first line of treatment is typically surgery followed by a combination of adjuvant radio-, chemo- or hormonal therapies. In the case of non-invasive or invasive indolent disease, resection of the primary is in most cases unnecessary and may even accelerate the disease by producing a transient spike in growth, angiogenesis and pro-inflammation factors combined with partial abrogation of growth and angiogenesis inhibitors. But in the case of more aggressive invasive breast cancer surgery is given too late and may pose even a greater risk of exacerbating the course of the disease. Thus, the "window of opportunity" for surgery may in reality be fairly narrow mostly consisting of those cases where the benefits of local and systemic relief as well as prevention of further dissemination outweigh the risks of aggravating the course of the already systemic but not yet clinically manifest disease.

How to identify those categories of patients who stand to benefit from surgery? One way to determine them is to apply the above-described mathematical model to various virtual cohorts of patients defined by certain combinations of clinical variables described in Section 6 and similar treatment protocols based on the existing databases with known metastatic relapse or post-surgery censoring times. This would allow one to estimate model parameters and uncover the distributional characteristics of the state of metastatic cascade at surgery or any time thereafter and assess the effects of surgery on metastasis. This would also enable computing the expected metastasis-free survival time for any new group of patients with the same clinical variables and treatment plans. Implementing this strategy relies on the size and quality of databases, a point eloquently made in [59]. In particular, such data bases should ideally contain information on metastasis detection mechanism for each individual patient and relapse site. A similar analysis can be also performed for similar no-surgery cohorts for which metastatic relapse time data is available, thus allowing for *in silico* clinical trials requiring no waiting time and approval.

Surgery for primary breast cancer remains the last unchallenged redoubt of the Halstedian linear progression theory. Its continued presence within the landscape of breast cancer oncology should be predicated on credible proof of specific benefits rather than historical tradition alone.

References

1. Fisher B (1980) Laboratory and clinical research in breast cancer: a personal adventure. The David A. Karnofsky memorial lecture. Cancer Res 40:3863–3874
2. Cooke R (2001) Dr. Folkman's war: angiogenesis and the struggle to defeat cancer. Random House, New York
3. Folkman J (1974) Tumor angiogenesis factor. Cancer Res 34:2109–2113
4. Moiseenko VM (2002) "Natural history" of breast cancer growth. Pract Oncol 3(1):6–14 (in Russian)
5. Holmgren K, O'Reilly MS, Folkman J (1995) Dormancy of micrometastases: balanced proliferation and apoptosis in the presence of angiogenesis suppression. Nat Med 1:149–153
6. Demicheli R, Retsky MW, Swartzendruber DE, Bonadonna G (1997) Proposal for a new model of breast cancer metastatic development. Ann Oncol 8:1075–1080
7. Fisher B (1999) From Halsted to prevention and beyond: advances in the management of breast cancer during the twentieth century. Eur J Cancer 35:1963–1973
8. Douglas JRS (1971) Significance of the size distribution of bloodborne metastases. Cancer 27:379–390

9. Cox B (1997) Variation in the effectiveness of breast screening by year of follow-up. JNCI Monographs 22:69–72
10. Gøetsche P (2012) Mammography screening: truth, lies and controversy. Radcliffe Publishing, London
11. Baines CJ (2011) Rational and irrational issues in breast cancer screening. Cancers 3:252–266
12. Welch HG, Black WC (2010) Overdiagnosis in cancer. JNCI 102(9):605–613
13. Sachs RK, Heidenreich WF, Brenner DJ (1996) Dose timing in tumor radiotherapy: considerations of cell number stochasticity. Math Biosci 138:131–146
14. Fakir H, Hlatky L, Li H, Sachs R (2013) Repopulation of interacting tumor cells during fractionated radiotherapy: stochastic modeling of the tumor control probability. Med Phys 40(12):121716
15. Hanin L, Zaider M (2014) Optimal schedules of fractionated radiation therapy by way of the *greedy* principle: biologically-based adaptive boosting. Phys Med Biol 59:4085–4098
16. Poincaré H (1952) Science and hypothesis. Dover Publications, New York
17. Boyd W (1966) The spontaneous regression of cancer. Thomas, Springfield, IL
18. Everson TC, Cole WH (1966) Spontaneous regression of cancer. Saunders, Philadelphia, PA
19. Zahl P-H, Mæhlen J, Welch HG (2008) The natural history of invasive breast cancer detected by screening mammography. Arch Intern Med 168:2311–2316
20. Smithers DW (1967) Spontaneous regression of cancer. Ann R Coll Surg Engl 41(Suppl):160–162
21. Sonnenschein C, Soto AM (2000) Somatic mutation theory of carcinogenesis: why it should be dropped and replaced. Mol Carcinog 29:205–211
22. Soto AM, Sonnenschein C (2004) The somatic mutation theory of cancer: growing problems with the paradigm? BioEssays 26:1097–1107
23. Sonnenschein C, Soto AM (2008) Theories of carcinogenesis: an emerging perspective. Semin Cancer Biol 18:372–377
24. Andersen J, Nielsen M, Jensen J (1985) Essential histological findings in the female breast at autopsy. In: Zander J, Baltzer J (eds) Early breast cancer. Berlin, Springer, pp 52–63
25. Hanin L, Rose J (2016) Uncovering the natural history of cancer from post mortem cross-sectional diameters of hepatic metastases. Math Med Biol 33(4):397–416
26. Hanin L, Seidel K, Stoevesandt D (2016) A "universal" model of metastatic cancer, its parametric forms and their identification: what can be learned from site-specific volumes of metastases. J Math Biol 72(6):1633–1662
27. Ehrlich P (1906) Experimentelle Karzinomstudien an Mäusen. Arch Koiglichen Inst Exp Ther Frankfurt am Main 1:65–103
28. Bashford E, Murray J, Cramer W (1907) The natural and induced resistance of mice to the growth of cancer. Proc R Soc Lond 79:164–187
29. Gorelik E (1983) Concomitant tumor immunity and resistance to a second tumor challenge. Adv Cancer Res 39:71–120
30. Demicheli R, Retsky M, Hrushesky WJ, Baum M, Gukas ID (2008) The effects of surgery on tumor growth: a century of investigations. Ann Oncol 19:1821–1828
31. Retsky M, Demicheli R, Hrushesky W, Baum M, Gukas I (2010) Surgery triggers outgrowth of latent distant disease in breast cancer: an inconvenient truth? Cancers 2:305–337
32. Peeters CFJM, de Waal RMW, Wobbes T, Westphal JR, Ruers TJM (2006) Outgrowth of human liver metastases after resection of the primary colorectal tumor: a shift in the balance between apoptosis and proliferation. Int J Cancer 119:1249–1253
33. Ang KK, Thames HD, Jones SD, Jiang G-L, Milas L, Peters LJ (1988) Proliferation kinetics of a murine fibrosarcoma during fractionated irradiation. Radiat Res 116:327–336
34. Dillekås H, Transeth M, Pilskog M, Assmus J, Straume O (2014) Differences in metastatic patterns in relation to time between primary surgery and first relapse from breast cancer suggests synchronized growth of dormant micrometastases. Breast Cancer Res Treat 146:627–636
35. Georgiu GK, Igglezou M, Sainis I, Vareli K, Batsis H, Briasoulis E, Fatouros M (2013) Impact of breast cancer surgery on angiogenesis circulating biomarkers: a prospective longitudinal study. World J Surg Oncol 11:213

36. Prehn RT (1993) Two competing influences that may explain concomitant tumor resistance. Cancer Res 53:3266–3269
37. Maida V, Ennis M, Kuziemsky C, Corban J (2009) Wounds and survival in cancer patients. Eur J Cancer 45:3237–3244
38. Lanca T, Silva-Santos B (2012) The split nature of tumor-infiltrating leukocytes. Implications for cancer surveillance and immunotherapy. Oncoimmunology 1(5):717–725
39. Forget P, Vandenhende J, Berliere M, Machiels JP, Nussbaum B, Legrand C, DeKock M (2010) Do intraoperative analgesics influence breast cancer recurrence after mastectomy? A retrospective analysis. Anesth Analg 110(6):1630–1635
40. Retsky M, Rogers R, Demicheli R, Hrushesky WJ, Gukas I, Vaidya JS, Baum M, Forget P, DeKock M, Pachmann K (2012) NSAID analgesic ketorolac used perioperatively may suppress early breast cancer relapse: particular relevance to triple negative subgroup. Breast Cancer Res Treat 134(2):881–888
41. Retsky M, Demicheli R, Hrushesky WJM, Forget P, DeKock M, Gukas I, Rogers R, Baum M, Pachmann K, Vaidya JS (2012) Promising development from translational or perhaps anti-translational research in breast cancer. Clin Transl Med 1:17
42. Retsky M, Demicheli R, Hrushesky WJM, Forget P, DeKock M, Gukas I, Rogers RA, Baum M, Sukhatme V, Vaidya JS (2013) Reduction of breast cancer relapses with perioperative non-steroidal anti-inflammatory drugs: new findings and a review. Curr Med Chem 20(33):4163–4176
43. Demicheli R, Osaro E, Retsky M, Forget P, Vaidya JS, Bello SO (2016) Protocol for a randomised, multicentre, double blinded phase III study of perioperative ketorolac in women of African descent with operable breast cancer. Jacobs J Intern Medicine 2(1):017
44. Bloom H, Richardson W, Harries E (1962) Natural history of untreated breast cancer (1805–1933). British Med J 2:213–221
45. Brinkley D, Haybittle J (1975) The curability of breast cancer. Lancet 2(7925):95–97
46. Karrison TG, Ferguson DJ, Meier P (1999) Dormancy of mammary carcinoma after mastectomy. J Natl Cancer Inst 91:80–85
47. Rutqvist L, Wallgren A (1985) Longterm survival of 458 young breast cancer patients. Cancer 55:658–665
48. Hanin LG, Rose J, Zaider M (2006) A stochastic model for the sizes of detectable metastases. J Theor Biol 243:407–417
49. Hanin LG (2008) Distribution of the sizes of metastases: mathematical and biomedical considerations. In: Tan WY, Hanin LG (eds) Handbook of cancer models with applications. World Scientific, Singapore, pp 141–169
50. Hanin L, Zaider M (2011) Effects of surgery and chemotherapy on metastatic progression of prostate cancer: evidence from the natural history of the disease reconstructed through mathematical modeling. Cancers 3:3632–3660
51. Hanin L, Pavlova L (2016) A quantitative insight into metastatic relapse of breast cancer. J Theor Biol 394:172–181
52. Hadfield G (1954) The dormant cancer cell. Br Med J 2:607–610
53. Sugarbaker EV, Ketcham AS, Cohen AM (1971) Studies of dormant tumor cells. Cancer 28:545–552
54. Meltzer A (1990) Dormancy and breast cancer. J Surg Oncol 43:181–188
55. Demicheli R (2001) Tumour dormancy: findings and hypotheses from clinical research on breast cancer. Semin Cancer Biol 11:297–306
56. Dick JE (2003) Breast cancer stem cells revealed. PNAS 100(7):3547–3549
57. Al-Hajj M, Wicha MS, Benito-Hernandez A, Morrison SJ, Clarke MF (2003) Prospective identification of tumorigenic breast cancer cells. PNAS 100(7):3983–3988
58. Kai K, Arima Y, Kamiya T, Saya H (2010) Breast cancer stem cells. Breast Cancer 17:80–85
59. Retsky M, Demicheli R (2014) Multimodal hazard rate for relapse in breast cancer: quality of data and calibration of computer simulation. Cancers 6:2343–2355

Chapter 8
The Impact of Wound Inflammation on Cancer Progression: Studies in Fish and Patients

Marie Louise Bønnelykke-Behrndtz, Henrik Schmidt, Yi Feng, and Paul Martin

Abstract There is a long history of literature suggesting parallels between wound healing and cancer growth, and similarly, much anecdotal evidence that tissue damage may impact on the growth and progression of cancers. In our recent studies we have investigated the association between wound-induced inflammation, as might be triggered post biopsy or surgery, and the subsequent proliferation and migratory tumour cell characteristics in zebrafish and human ulcerated melanoma. The translucent zebrafish allowed us to live visualise the behaviour of inflammatory cells around a wound, which we made in the vicinity of clones of early pre-neoplastic cells. These studies showed that neutrophils and macrophages are sequentially recruited to sites of tissue wounding, and subsequently distracted from the wound by competing attractants from the nearby pre-neoplastic cells. The interaction

M.L. Bønnelykke-Behrndtz, M.D., Ph.D. (✉)
Department of Plastic and Breast Surgery, Aarhus University Hospital,
Nørrebrogade 44, 8000 Aarhus, Denmark
e-mail: mariboen@rm.dk

H. Schmidt, M.D., Dr.Med.
Department of Oncology, Aarhus University Hospital, Aarhus, Denmark

Department of Clinical Medicine, Aarhus University, Aarhus, Denmark
e-mail: henrschm@rm.dk

Y. Feng
MRC Centre for Inflammation Research, University of Edinburgh, Edinburgh, UK
e-mail: yi.feng@ed.ac.uk

P. Martin
School of Biochemistry, University of Bristol, Bristol, UK

School of Physiology and Pharmacology, University of Bristol, Bristol, UK

School of Medicine, University of Cardiff, Cardiff, UK
e-mail: paul.martin@bristol.ac.uk

M.W. Retsky, R. Demicheli (eds.), *Perioperative Inflammation as Triggering Origin of Metastasis Development*, DOI 10.1007/978-3-319-57943-6_8

between inflammatory cells, largely neutrophils, and pre-neoplastic cells directly led to increased proliferation of the pre-neoplastic cells, through release of trophic/growth factors including prostaglandin (PGE2). Complementary clinical data showed that the density of infiltrating neutrophils correlates with increasing size of wound, in this instance extent of ulceration, and with tumour-cell proliferation in human melanoma, whilst there was no correlation between infiltrating macrophages and proliferation or prognosis. In addition to the demonstrated inflammation induced tumour-cell proliferation we showed an independent prognostic link between neutrophil influx and melanoma specific survival, supporting the hypothesis that wound-induced inflammation may be detrimental to patient survival. Reactivation of developmental and migratory cell behaviours of melanocytes may be an essential link between inflammation and tumour progression, equivalent to what is conventionally described as epithelial to mesenchymal transition (EMT) in epithelial-derived tumours. In what has been found from zebrafish studies, both melanoblasts and mature melanocytes migrate towards sites of tissue wounding, under the influence of innate immune cells. In ulcerated melanomas, the infiltration of neutrophils in ulcerated areas is associated with migratory tumour cell characteristics such as spindle shaped morphology and loss of e-cadherin expression and extravascular migratory metastasis (angiotropism), linking inflammation to a pro-migratory microenvironment.

Keywords Melanoma • Zebrafish • Neutrophils • Proliferation • Migration

8.1 Inflammatory Cells Are Attracted to the Site of Tissue Injury but Rapidly Drawn Out from the Wound by Competing Signals from Nearby Pre-neoplastic Cells

Damage to tissue initiates a cascade of events that under normal circumstances leads to tissue repair and scarring. These events are influenced by a plethora of chemokines, cytokines and growth factors, produced by resident- and recruited cells, leading to a robust inflammatory response [1]. Under normal acute inflammatory situations the inflammatory response is self-limiting and immune cells resolve by apoptosis or return to the circulation [1]. However, in some cases, inflammation does not resolve and may become chronic and maintained for a prolonged time [2]. In 1863 Rudolph Virchow described the presence in tumour tissues of a leukocyte infiltrate and suggested that infiltration of inflammatory cells reflected the origin of cancer at sites of chronic inflammation. He concluded that a functional connection ought to exist between inflammation and cancer. Cancers consequently have been referred to as ‘wounds that do not heal’ [3].

To further our understanding of the behavior of innate immune cells around pre-neoplastic cells in the vicinity of a wound, we turned to a model of cancer in the zebrafish which has several advantages over other models including its genetic tractability and its translucency which allows imaging of inflammatory cells as they interact with cancer cells [4–6]. Different de novo cancers can be modeled in zebrafish by driving expression of human mutant oncogenes under particular tissue specific promoters; in this instance we used zebrafish, expressing oncogenic $HRas^{G12V}$-eGFP (RASV12 here after) under the kita promoter which expresses in the notochord and melanoblast and goblet cell lineages to model melanoma ($RASV12^{+}$ in melanocytes) and carcinoid tumours ($RASV12^{+}$ in mucus secreting cells) in the skin. These transgenes were co-expressed with fluorescent marker genes (GFP or RFP) in zebrafish lines that were also expressing complementary fluors in either neutrophils or macrophages. This made it possible to observe how the two innate immune cell lineages interacted with the pre-neoplastic cells from the "birth" of the cancer clones. We observed that neutrophils were generally recruited toward pre-neoplastic cells, from when they are a single cell or just a doublet, and certainly well before these cells divide to form larger clones [7].

Standardly, when wild type zebrafish larval skin is wounded, innate immune cells are rapidly recruited to the wound and retained within the wound for 6 h or so before they resolve. However, if the same wound is made to a $RASV12^{+}$ fish, then the innate immune cells first drawn to the wound as part of an acute inflammatory wound response are rapidly distracted away from the wound by competing signals from the near-by pre-neoplastic cells (Fig. 8.1A–D); this migration on towards pre-neoplastic cells begins as soon as 1 h post wounding. This was most clearly visualised by the "footprints" of neutrophils in the time period 1–3 h post-wounding which extended well beyond the wound site in fish carrying a pre-neoplastic cell burden (Fig. 8.1C″, D″). Because wounding draws more neutrophils to the flank of the fish than would otherwise normally be present (Fig. 8.1E), $RASV12^{+}$ cells received significantly more contact with innate immune cells when in close proximity to a wound compared to non-wounded $RASV12^{+}$ fish (64% versus 26%, 2 h post-wounding) (Fig. 8.1F). When neutrophil- and macrophage recruitment were followed for up to 5 days post-wounding (Fig. 8.1G–O) the number of neutrophils recruited to pre-neoplastic cells in wounded RasV12+ larvae was significantly higher ($p = 0.007$) than in unwounded RasV12+ larvae (Fig. 8.1P), while there was trend but no significant difference in macrophage recruitment over the total time course ($p = 0.10$) (Fig. 8.1Q). Overall, we observed a significant increase in the number of pre-neoplastic cells receiving contact from immune cells, a contact that was maintained for at least 3 days after wounding (Fig. 8.1R).

8.2 The Interaction Between Inflammatory Cells and Pre-neoplastic Cells Led to Increased Proliferation of the Pre-neoplastic Cells

To determine the possible effect of the increased inflammation due to wounding on pre-neoplastic cell proliferation, we counted the number of pre-neoplastic cells 3 days post wounding. A significant local increase in pre-neoplastic cell number was

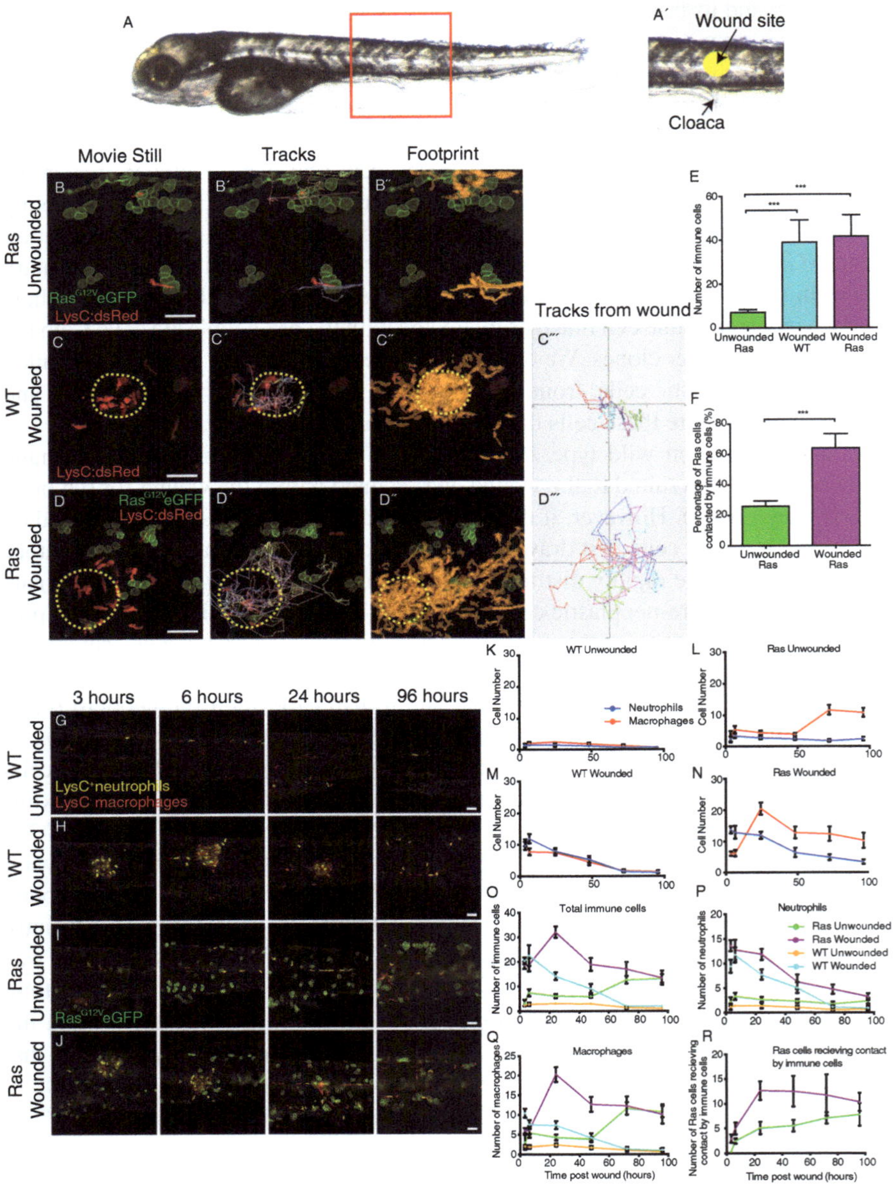

Fig. 8.1 Live imaging reveals neutrophils distracted away from wounds due to competing signals from adjacent pre-neoplastic cells. (**A**, **A′**) Five-days post-fertilisation larva illustrating the region of flank where we image and wound (**A**). Wounds (*yellow circle*) are made in the centre of the flank just above the cloaca (*arrow*) in all larval experiments (**A′**). (**B**–**B″**) Stills from a time-lapse movie of a larva with RasG12VeGFP pre-neoplastic cell clones but no wound. (**C**–**C‴**) Equivalent time-lapse stills of a control, laser-wounded larva with no pre-neoplastic cell clones at 90 min post-wounding (wound indicated with *yellow dotted line*). (**D**–**D‴**) Stills from a time-lapse movie of a larva with RasG12VeGFP pre-neoplastic cell clones (*green*), again wounded. (**E**) Graph comparing

demonstrated in comparison to equivalent flank regions of unwounded larvae (Fig. 8.2A–E). This suggests that wound-associated inflammation triggers proliferation of pre-neoplastic cells. To further test the role of macrophages and neutrophils, normal development of the two cell lineages was transiently delayed by injection of morpholinos (PU.1 and GCSFR) at the 1-cell embryo stage (Fig. 8.2F–K). This led to an almost complete depletion of neutrophils and macrophages for up to 4 days, and an almost complete reduction in wound associated pre-neoplastic proliferation (Fig. 8.2L). It is also possible to manipulate neutrophil and macrophage numbers individually and if we delay the development of neutrophils significantly then we see considerably depleted pre-neoplastic cell numbers, with no observed increase in pre-neoplastic cell number after wounding (Fig. 8.2N). However, when macrophages were depleted, there was only a partial reduction in the number of pre-neoplastic cells (Fig. 8.2O) and an increase was observed after wounding; there is, unfortunately an unavoidable complication with regard to the latter experiment because the method we use to reduce macrophages leads to a partial compensatory increase in neutrophil numbers.

These zebrafish experiments show that the acute inflammatory response triggered by wounding results in a pool of cells from which some are recruited by competing signals from any nearby pre-neoplastic cells. The exposure to innate immune cells that is amplified is associated with increased proliferation of pre-neoplastic cells, which appears largely dependent upon innate immune cells, and it seems as if the major player may be the neutrophil.

Fig. 8.1 (continued) the number of LysC:dsRed+ neutrophils recruited over a 2-h period to the equivalent flank region of unwounded RasG12VeGFP larvae (n = 11), versus wounded WT larvae (n = 3), wounded RasG12VeGFP larvae (n = 5) and wounded RasG12VeGFP larvae treated with DPI inhibitor (n = 7). ***P ≤ 0.001. (**F**) Graph comparing the percentage of Ras+ pre-neoplastic cells that receive contacts with neutrophils during the 2-h period of the movie in unwounded (n = 11) versus wounded (n = 5) larvae. ***P ≤ 0.001. (**G–J**) Unwounded WT sibling; LysC:dsRed+ larva (n = 10 per time point) for comparison of clone growth with (**H**) laser wounded WT sibling: LysC:dsRed+ larva (n = 15 per time point), (**I**) unwounded Ras+; LysC:dsRed+ larvae (n = 15 per time point) and (**J**) laser-wounded Ras+; LysC:dsRed+ (n = 20 per time point). Larvae were harvested and fixed between 3 dpf and 7 dpf (i.e. between 3 and 96 h post-wounding), and stained with anti-L-plastin and anti-RFP antibodies to distinguish neutrophils (*yellow*) and macrophages (*red*). (**K–N**) Graphs showing the numbers of neutrophils and macrophages in the flanks of unwounded WT siblings (**K**), unwounded Ras+ larvae (**L**), wounded WT siblings (**M**) and wounded Ras+ larvae (**N**). (**O–Q**) Graphs indicating the total number of innate immune cells (**O**), macrophages (**P**) and neutrophils (**Q**) recruited over time in wounded and unwounded WT and unwounded and wounded Ras+ larvae. (**R**) Graph showing the number of pre-neoplastic cells receiving contact by immune cells in unwounded/wounded larvae over time (P = 0.0052 for 5 days post-wound). Data information: In (**K–R**) x-axes denote time post-wound (h). All scale bars represent 50 lm. (**B, C** and **D**) Show stills of the time-lapse movie; (**C′** and **D′**) show tracks of five immune cells as they migrate after entering the wound; (**B″**, **C″** and **D″**) show the footprints of all LysC:dsRed immune cells throughout the movie. (**C‴** and **D‴**) Illustrate the migration of neutrophils from when they enter the centre of the wound. All graphs display mean SEM

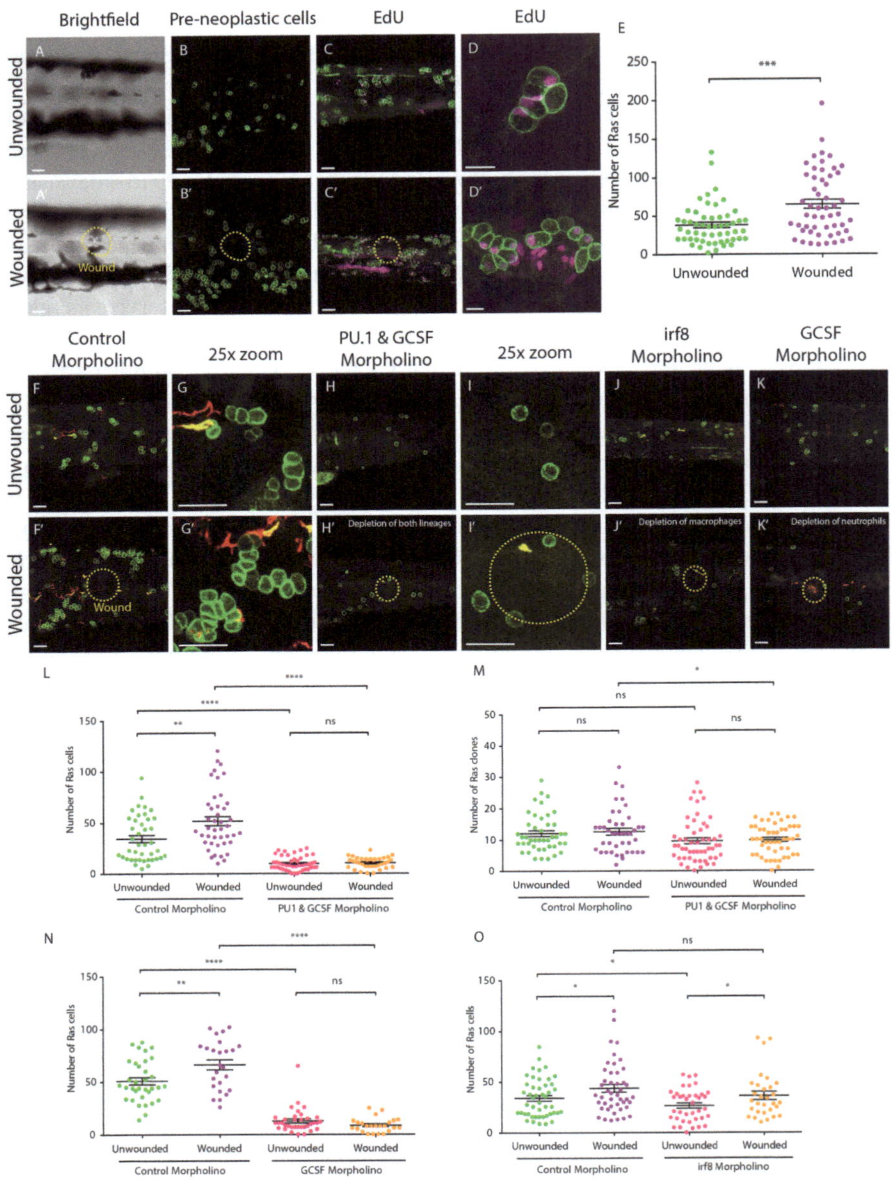

Fig. 8.2 Wounding leads to increased proliferation of pre-neoplastic cells. (**A–D′**) RasG12VeGFP larvae were left unwounded (**A–D**) or laser-wounded (yellow dotted line) at 2 dpf just dorsal to the cloaca (**A′–D′**). Larvae were left to grow for 3 days before being fixed and analysed for pre-neoplastic cell number (n = 30 larvae in each group). EdU accumulation (*purple*) is shown at low magnification (**C** and **C′**) and a representative pre-neoplastic cell clone is shown (**D** and **D′**). (**E**) Graph illustrating pre-neoplastic cell numbers in unwounded versus wounded larvae (n = 27 of each group). Data from three independent experiments showed the same level of significance. $^{***}P \leq 0.001$.

From additional zebrafish studies, prostaglandin (PGE2) has been shown to be released by both neutrophils and macrophages and function as one—presumably of several—trophic signals that are beneficial for pre-neoplastic cell growth [8].

To test the impact of prostaglandins in wound-induced tumour cell proliferation, larvae were immersed in Cox-2 inhibitor, which blocks prostaglandin synthesis, and compared with control untreated larvae. The number of pre-neoplastic cells analysed 2 days post laser wounding indicates that Cox-2 inhibitors significantly reduce pre-neoplastic cell number post wounding, although our data make it clear that prostaglandins are not the only source of growth signals.

8.3 In Ulcerated Melanoma There Is a Correlation Between Infiltration of Neutrophils and Tumour-Cell Proliferation

To investigate whether our observations in zebrafish might extend into patients, and if innate immune cells are associated with tumour cell proliferation in humans, we turned to ulcerated melanoma, which is a subgroup of melanoma with a superimposed chronic wound. Our cohort included 385 patients with cutaneous melanoma, in which all tumours were sectioned and stained with immunohistochemistry and antibodies detecting neutrophils (cd66b), macrophages (cd163) and proliferating melanoma cells (MelanA/Ki67) (Figs. 8.3A–C and 8.4A–F). From these complementary clinical data we saw a strong correlation between tumour-cell proliferation and infiltration of neutrophils ($p = 0.0002$) (Fig. 8.3D). Although infiltration of neutrophils was correlated with tumour-cell proliferation in ulcerated melanoma, statistical analysis showed that the association between neutrophils and tumour cell proliferation appeared strongest up to minimal/moderate ulceration, and plateaued out for larger ulcers. This could reflect the pathogenesis of melanoma, which seems to reach a proliferative plateau when first ulcerated; indeed, an excessive and necrotic melanoma is a rare event and even thin melanomas can harbor the ability to metastasize.

While we observed a significant correlation between tumour-cell proliferation and infiltration of neutrophils, we could not demonstrate a correlation between

Fig. 8.2 (continued) (**F–G′**) Images of larvae injected with control morpholino at the one-cell stage, and either left unwounded (**F**, high magnification: **G**) or laser-wounded at 3 dpf (**F′**, high magnification: **G′**) and fixed at 5 dpf. (**H–J′**) Larvae injected with a combination of PU-1 and GCSF morpholinos at the one-cell stage, left unwounded (**H**, high magnification: **I**) or laser-wounded at 3 dpf (**H′**, high magnification: **I′**) and fixed at 5 dpf. Images of larvae injected with irf8 morpholino, and either unwounded (**J**) or laser-wounded at 3 dpf (**J′**) before subsequent fixation at 5 dpf. (**K, K′**) Larvae injected with GCSF morpholino, and either left unwounded (**K**) or laser-wounded at 3 dpf (**K′**) and fixed at 5 dpf. (**L, M**) Graphs to show the total number of Ras+ cells and clones (respectively) at 5 dpf after PU-1 and GCSF morpholinos. (**N, O**) Graphs showing the number of Ras+ cells at 5 dpf after irf8 morpholino (**N**) or after GCSF morpholino injection (**O**). Data information: All scale bars represent 50 lm except (**D**) and (**D′**) which represent 15 lm. n = 15–20 larvae in each group (**L–O**). All graphs display mean SEM

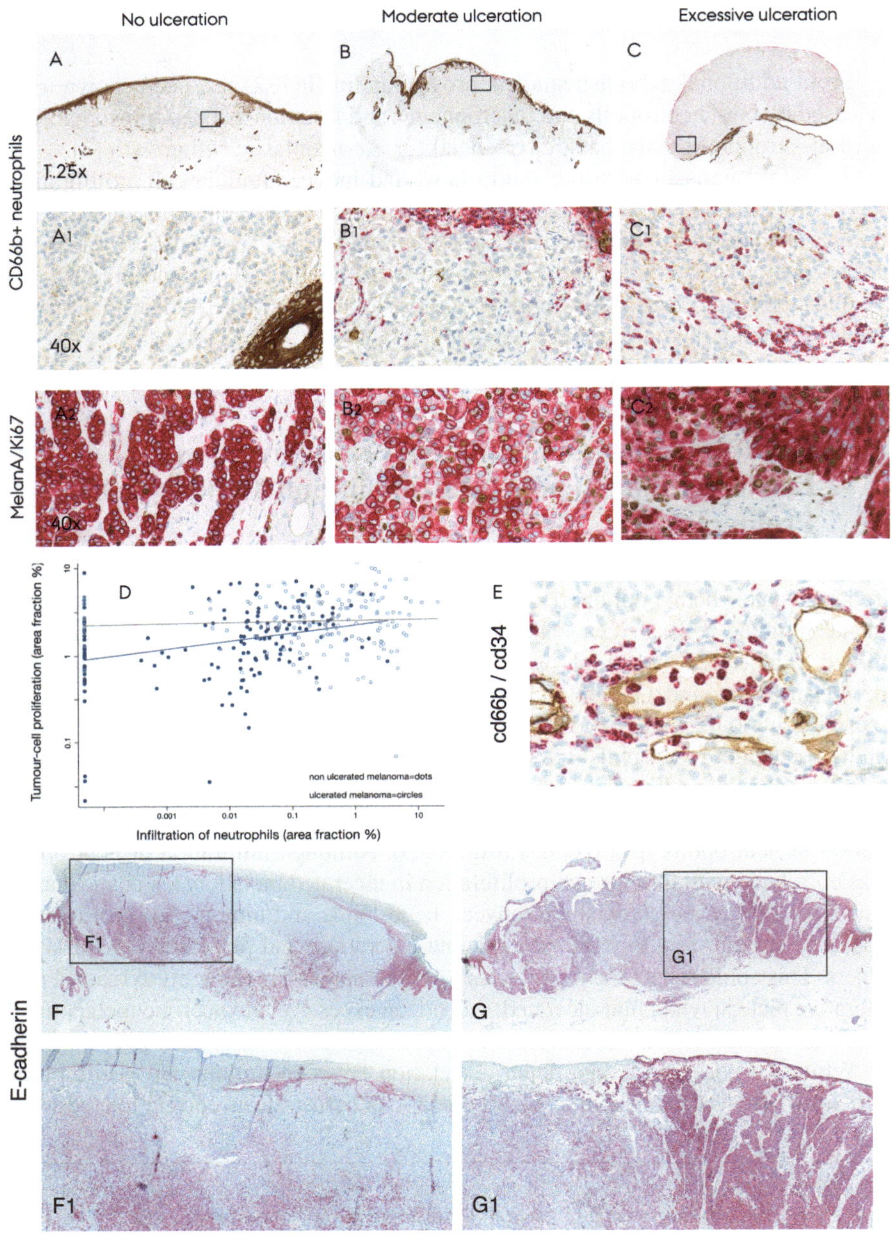

Fig. 8.3 Ulcerated human melanomas show a correlation between level of neutrophil influx, tumour cell proliferation and migratory tumour cell characteristics (**A**–**C**″). Typical non-ulcerated, moderate and excessively ulcerated melanomas, respectively, all immunostained for pancytokeratin to illustrate epidermal wound margins (**A**′, **B**′ and **C**′). High magnification details from (**A**, **B** and **C**) costained for CD66b to illustrate neutrophil accumulation. (**A**″, **B**″ and **C**″). Parallel sections from the same patient blocks, but stained for MelanA and Ki67 to determine proliferating melanoma cells. (**D**) Graph illustrating the extent of correlation between neutrophil influx and tumour cell proliferation (P = 0.002; R2 = 0.17). *Solid dots* are from non-ulcerated lesions and show a good correlation, whereas *circles* represent ulcerated melanomas. (**E**) Image stained with cd34+ (endothelial marker) and cd66b+ (neutrophil marker) illustrating neutrophil-associated

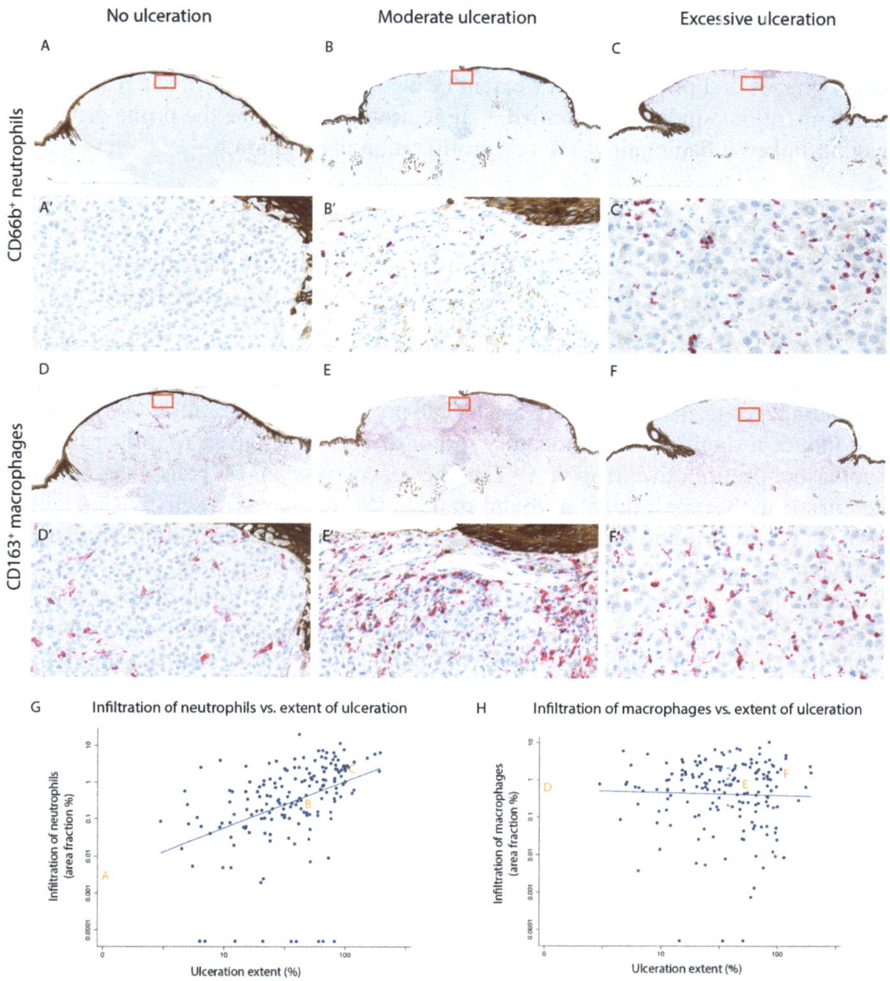

Fig. 8.4 Neutrophil, but not macrophage, recruitment is correlated to the presence and to the extent of ulceration in human melanoma. (**A**–**C′**) Typical non-ulcerated, moderate and excessively ulcerated melanomas, respectively, all immunostained for pancytokeratin (*brown*) to illustrate epidermal wound margins. (**A′**, **B′** and **C′**). High magnification details from (**A**, **B** and **C**) (highlighted by *red boxes*) co-stained for CD66b to illustrate neutrophil accumulation. (**D**–**F′**) Parallel sections from the same patient blocks as in (**A**–**C′**), but stained for CD163 and pan-cytokeratin to illustrate macrophage influx. (**G**) Graph showing the correlation between extent of ulceration and extent of neutrophil influx ($P < 0.0001$; $R2 = 0.19$). **A**, **B** and **C** indicate the patient points from whom corresponding neutrophil immunostaining data are shown. (**H**) In contrast to (**G**), no correlation between extent of ulceration and extent of macrophage influx was observed ($P = 0.9$; $R2 = 0.0004$). **D**, **E** and **F** indicate the patient points from whom corresponding macrophage immunostaining data are shown. Data information: Scale bars represent 3 mm (**A** and **D**), 6 mm (**B**, **C**, **E** and **F**) and 200 lm (**A′**, **B′**, **C′**, **D′**, **E′** and **F′**)

Fig. 8.3 (continued) angiotropism (extravascular migratory metastasis) in an ulcerated melanoma. The presence of angiotropism, defined as clustering of tumor cells (*blue*) around the external vessel walls (*brown*), which is clearly associated with neutrophils (*red*) (magn. ×40). (**F**–**G**) Ulcerated melanoma demonstrating loss of E-cadherin (magn. ×1.25); in the superficial part of the lesion (**F**) and ulcerated part of the lesion (**G**). High magnification details from (**F1** and **G1**) (magn. ×5)

macrophages and proliferation or extent of ulceration (Fig. 8.4H), suggesting that, much as for our studies in zebrafish, that neutrophils might be the prime drivers of wound-linked inflammation-induced proliferation in melanoma.

8.4 Only Larger Wounds Trigger a Significant Inflammatory Response, Which Drives Tumour-Cell Clones Rather Than Initiating New Clones

Wounding, per se, does not lead to cancer cell progression in zebrafish. Only wounds that induce a significant inflammatory response over 48 h appear to trigger the pre-neoplastic proliferative response. The increased number of cells that are pre-neoplastic in the proximity of a wound could be due to increased cell division within clones or increased initiation of new clones, or contributions from both of these. It is clear however that the numbers of clones counted at the 2 day point after wounding are generally unaltered by comparison to unwounded fish; rather, the increase in pre-neoplastic cell number is almost entirely due to increase in the size of individual clones (Fig. 8.2M). Depleting innate immune cells leads to similar numbers of clones—usually around ten clones within the region of the wound however a number of these remain as single cells even after wounding. Rather than delivering factors that initiate new clones, this suggests strongly that indeed innate immune cells, drawn from the wound deliver trophic signals to clones of pre-neoplastic cells thus encouraging proliferation.

Moreover, the effect of the wound-induced proliferation is local, rather than systemic, because no increase in numbers of $HRasV12^{+}$ cells was seen in the epithelium overlying the yolk or in the head.

The importance of a threshold size of wound and the extent of the inflammatory response was also demonstrated in our clinical data, as the density of infiltrating neutrophils increases 15 times ($p < 0.0001$) from non-ulcerated to minimal ulcerated lesions and 100 times ($p < 0.0001$) from non-ulcerated to excessive ulcerated lesions (Fig. 8.4G). In addition, tumour-cell proliferation rates were 1.7 times higher ($p = 0.0004$) for melanomas with minimal ulcerations, and two times higher ($p = 0.0001$) for melanomas with excessive ulceration, by comparison to melanomas with no ulceration as reference.

8.5 The Density of Tumour Infiltrating Neutrophils Is Correlated with Poor Melanoma Specific Survival in Human Melanoma

Tumour associated macrophages and neutrophils can constitute a large proportion of the tumour mass and has been associated with poor prognosis in early-stage human melanomas [9, 10]. To date, macrophages have generally been considered the lead players, at least of the innate immune cells of the cancer microenvironment, and have been extensively linked with a proliferative and invasive microenvironment [11]. However, our data suggests a key role for neutrophils in damaged tissue associated with a tumour, as the only cell to be significantly associated with proliferation of tumour cells. Additionally, regarding the suggested inflammation-induced tumour-cell proliferation, we also found an independent prognostic link between neutrophil influx and melanoma specific survival ($p < 0.0001$), while we saw no correlation between macrophage infiltration and survival. Our data show that the extent of ulceration is a stronger prognostic marker than the mere presence versus absence of ulceration [12], which we hypothesize, might be, in part, due to a strong correlation between increasing extent of ulceration and increasing neutrophil density (Fig. 8.4G). These results support the hypothesis that inflammation may be detrimental to patient survival, with neutrophils as the suggested prime driver in ulcerated lesions.

It has been suggested that some of the embryonic properties of migratory cells might be reactivated during wound healing and metastasis in adults [13]. This reactivation might explain the association between wound-induced inflammation and the observed poor survival in patients with ulcerated melanoma. Epithelial to mesenchymal transition (EMT) is an important developmental process whereby epithelial cells that normally possess strong cell-to-cell adhesion with their neighbours and interaction with the basement membrane, lose their polarization and gain invasive properties. EMT is associated with increased production of matrix degradative factors (NE and MMP9), spindle-shaped morphology and loss of cell-to-cell, largely adherens (e-cadherin-based) adhesions [14].

8.6 Mature Melanocytes Migrate Towards Tissue Wounding, Indicating That Innate Immune Cells Have an Essential Role in Melanocyte Migration

Transition towards a migratory phenotype is reflected in the normal repair process and re-epithelialisation, as keratinocytes migrate towards each other to close up a wound. In unwounded skin, keratinocytes adhere closely to each other and to the basement membrane in the epidermis. However, during wound re-epithelialisation the advancing keratinocytes lose their adherens junctions but not desmosomal junctions and this "loosening" or partial EMT allows them to migrate [1, 15]. These processes are under the influence of the Eph family of tyrosine kinase receptors, as well as pro-inflammatory cytokines, inflammation-linked transcription factors and proteases [16]. However, not only do keratinocytes respond to inflammatory signals; inflammation also causes migration of melanocytes, as demonstrated from earlier zebra fish experiments [17]. In this study Levesque et al. observed that hyperpigmentation of wounds which is often seen in clinical patients could be modelled in zebrafish and was a consequence of melanocytes migrating to site of tissue wounding [17]. With transient knockdown of innate immune cells, melanoblast and melanocyte migration towards wounds was halted, suggesting that innate immune cells play an essential role in melanocyte migration.

8.7 Ulcerated Melanoma Is Associated with Loss of e-Cadherin and Gain of Spindle Shaped Morphology, Tumour Cell Characteristics Indicating a Migratory Potential

In human melanoma, neutrophils are largely located within the superficial and ulcerated part of the tumour, while tumour-associated macrophages infiltrate the tumour stroma throughout the tumour section and show no significant pattern linked with the region of ulcerated lesion [18]. While the literature provides ample evidence for a role of macrophages as inducers of EMT [19], little is known about a role for neutrophils in this regard. Interestingly, a few in vitro studies have shown that neutrophils can degrade cadherin-based adhesions via elastase in both pancreatic and liver cell lines [20, 21]. In a zebrafish model where skin cells are transformed by HRASV12, neutrophils have been shown to induce EMT through triggering MMP9 and snail expression in HRASV12+ cells [22]. MMP9 has been found to be an important factor for degradation of extracellular matrix and basement membrane, but is naturally and usually rapidly degraded and regulated by the linked tissue inhibitor of metalloproteinase-1 (TIMP-1) in the cancer microenvironment [23, 24]. Importantly, inflammation-recruited and activated neutrophils possess a TIMP-1-free, MMP9 that is rapidly activated and unable to be inhibited by TIMP-1. This TIMP-1-free MMP9 is regarded as a potent source of MMP9 in the cancer microenvironment [25]. From serial sections and co-staining with immunohistochemistry, we observed that cd66b+ granulocytes expressed both MMP9 and neutrophil elastase (NE), which suggests that these tumour-associated innate immune cells are activated neutrophils.

MMP9 and NE have also been demonstrated to cleave the e-cadherin based junctions [21], that not only provide epidermal stability but also anchor melanocytes and melanoma cells to one another and to the nearby keratinocytes [26]. As a result of inflammation and up-regulation of MMP9 and NE, tumour cells that lose their E-cadherin become more responsive to EMT induction by various growth factors, and inflammation sustains this positive feedback loop [13]. Degradation of extracellular matrix and loss of cell-to-cell adhesion are crucial events, which enhance cell migration.

In our study cohort, E-cadherin immunostaining showed considerable intratumoural heterogeneity with loss of expression typically associated with the ulcerated areas (Fig. 8.3F, G). We estimated the weakest stained tumour area (1 × 1 mm), and referred to it as weak-spot score. A low weak-spot score correlated with the presence of ulceration ($p = 0.0004$) and the extent of ulceration ($p = 0.0013$). We observed 28% of the non-ulcerated, 42% of the minimal/moderately ulcerated- and 53% of the excessively ulcerated tumours to have low e-cadherin scores. In addition, we calculated the presence of spindle cell morphology and found it associated with ulcerated areas and lesions ($p = 0.021$). Spindle cell morphology may therefore be an important histopathological marker of inflammation-induced EMT.

8.8 Extravascular Migratory Metastasis Associates with Ulcerated Human Melanoma and Infiltrating Neutrophils

"Extravascular migratory metastasis" or EVMM as it has been termed was recently described as an additional potential mechanism by which melanoma might spread. This mechanism involves tumour cells travelling along the external surfaces of vessels rather than within the lumen, as has been demonstrated in animal models [27, 28]. Histopathologically, this concept is referred to as angiotropism [29]. Angiotropism has been defined as accumulation of tumour cells around the external surface of vessels and it is presumed that this marks a site of EVMM. This phenomenon is observed after ultraviolet-radiation-induced inflammation of melanomas in mice and in ulcerated human melanomas stained with H&E and cd31 for vessel location [30]. In our study we verify that angiotropism is associated with ulcerated lesions and is often located at the ulcerated and superficial areas of the tumour. In addition to the clustering of tumour cells, we observed large numbers of neutrophils associated with these extravascular melanoma cells (Fig. 8.3E). This is evidenced by double stains of cd34+ vessels and cd66+ neutrophils (Fig. 8.3E). This suggests that neutrophils may play an important role in extravascular migratory metastasis.

8.9 Implications of These Studies for Clinical Management of Melanoma and Other Cancers, Particularly with Respect to Biopsy and Cancer Surgery

Since cancer surgery clearly necessitates making a wound in the vicinity of a growing cancer we wondered how a single wound might impact these cancer cells. The acute wound inflammatory response is clearly triggered at any site of tissue injury. We decided to investigate how this might attract immune cells to the location of the cancer cells and to determine what the result might be.

Our earlier studies had been on larval zebrafish and small clones of pre-neoplastic cells, but what about fish that are adult? Then a small percentage of these clones develop into invasive melanomas. By surgically removing a segment of melanoma from the tail fin of adult zebrafish, and subsequently examining an in situ remaining portion of the tumour 3 days later, we observed increased numbers of both neutrophils and macrophages in the wound area. The increase in neutrophil numbers in the wounded cancer tissue spatially correlates with increased phospho-H3 immunostaining suggesting that local tissue proliferation might be triggered at the site of surgery because of the associated inflammatory cell influx.

In the local cancer microenvironment, the inflammatory response may be modulated in a more chronic and pro-tumoural direction, as Rudolph Virchow first described in the late 1800s [31]. In contrast there is considerable anecdotal evidence that an inflammatory response can be instrumental in killing cancer cells. More recently there are reports suggesting neutrophils can also eliminate hypoxic tumour cells [32, 33]. William Coley reported spontaneous tumour regression after a post-operative infection, and subsequently treated some of his inoperable sarcoma patients with a bacterial toxin taking advantage of an acute fever response [34]. Taking a lead from Coley and his toxins, one potential therapeutic approach might be to take advantage of an enhanced recruitment of inflammatory cells and modulate these cells to kill rather than nurture the cancer cells. This may be part of the explanation as to why patients with ulcerated melanoma tend to show improved survival when treated with interferon-α, provided that an inflammatory phenotype follows on to the corresponding metastasis or that inflammatory signals are the prominent drivers of these disseminated cell clones. Studies have demonstrated that macrophages can be switched from expressing markers of a pro-tumoural to an anti-tumoural phenotype depending on the microenvironment [35]. In addition, MMP9 expression can be reversed and e-cadherin expression restored after treatment with interferon-α in bladder cancer cell lines and murine models, restoring the MMP9/e--cadherin balance [36]. It is not yet clear whether neutrophil phenotypes in the cancer microenvironment can be altered or whether patients with ulcerated melanoma show increased therapy benefit from other immunotherapies, due to an active inflammatory microenvironment, but this is currently being investigated.

Surgery has long been accepted as the most effective means to treat human solid cancers if they have not yet metastasized [37]. However, tissue damage is implicated as a possible trigger in the development of various cancers [38–40], and a niche that is favourable for reoccurrence may be inadvertently provided [41], as well as facilitating the growth of pre-existing micro-metastases [42], suggesting that surgery may have clinical consequences beyond simply removing the primary cancer [43].

Surgery is naturally linked with an acute inflammatory response. Since the acute wound inflammatory response is transient, and rapidly can be reversed in a tumour supportive way, another approach would be to block the delivery of trophic signals to cancer cells from the inflammatory cells at the time of surgery, particularly if there might be remnant tumour cells in the sentinel node basin or at the site of the primary surgery. Zebrafish experiments show that blocking PGE2, one of the likely trophic signals encouraging growth of these pre-neoplastic cells, at the time of wounding can partially dampen the inflammation-dependent proliferative effect [44]. In the clinic, just as long term, low dose intake of prostaglandin inhibitors, have proven to be good preventatives of several cancers [45], they may also serve as potential preventatives for remnant cells during melanoma surgeries.

Growth factors, among them PDGF and EGF, are clearly also associated with inflammation and have been generally accepted as drivers of both proliferation and invasion. However, Muinonen-Martin et al. have recently challenged this dogma [46]. Their work suggests that growth factors play only a negligible chemotactic role; rather, they potentiate the lipid lysophoshatic acid (LPA), which is demonstrated as a remarkably strong attractant. It is suggested that melanoma cells rapidly break down LPA and create their own LPA gradient in the local microenvironment.

Since melanoma cells are attracted by LPA, this gradient serves as a self-generated migratory signal that allows melanocytes to travel for significant distances. Importantly, inflammatory cells are a principle source of LPA, and so this may be another way in which ulceration-induced inflammation and possibly surgery might function as initiators of melanoma dispersal.

Our recent studies in zebrafish and humans have linked wound-induced inflammation, in particular neutrophils, with tumour cell proliferation and migratory tumour cell characteristics in melanoma. Our work contributes to the understanding of ulcerated melanoma, but more importantly highlights the importance of determining key trophic and chemotactic signals and migratory drivers originating from wounds and wound recruited immune cells, before considering how to modulate these behaviours in ways that may benefit cancer patients, particularly those undergoing biopsy or surgery procedures.

References

1. Martin P, Leibovich SJ (2005) Inflammatory cells during wound repair: the good, the bad and the ugly. Trends Cell Biol 15(11):599–607
2. Wilgus TA, Roy S, McDaniel JC (2013) Neutrophils and wound repair: positive actions and negative reactions. Adv Wound Care (New Rochelle) 2(7):379–388
3. Dvorak HF (1986) Tumors: wounds that do not heal. Similarities between tumor stroma generation and wound healing. N Engl J Med 315(26):1650–1659
4. Ceol CJ, Houvras Y, White RM, Zon LI (2008) Melanoma biology and the promise of zebrafish. Zebrafish 5(4):247–255
5. Martin P, Feng Y (2009) Inflammation: wound healing in zebrafish. Nature 459(7249):921–923
6. White R, Rose K, Zon L (2013) Zebrafish cancer: the state of the art and the path forward. Nat Rev Cancer 13(9):624–636
7. Feng Y, Santoriello C, Mione M, Hurlstone A, Martin P (2010) Live imaging of innate immune cell sensing of transformed cells in zebrafish larvae: parallels between tumor initiation and wound inflammation. PLoS Biol 8(12):e1000562
8. Feng Y, Renshaw S, Martin P (2012) Live imaging of tumor initiation in zebrafish larvae reveals a trophic role for leukocyte-derived PGE(2). Curr Biol 22(13):1253–1259
9. Jensen TO, Schmidt H, Moller HJ, Hoyer M, Maniecki MB, Sjoegren P et al (2009) Macrophage markers in serum and tumor have prognostic impact in American Joint Committee on Cancer stage I/II melanoma. J Clin Oncol 27(20):3330–3337
10. Jensen TO, Schmidt H, Moller HJ, Donskov F, Hoyer M, Sjoegren P et al (2012) Intratumoral neutrophils and plasmacytoid dendritic cells indicate poor prognosis and are associated with pSTAT3 expression in AJCC stage I/II melanoma. Cancer 118(9):2476–2485
11. Lewis CE, Pollard JW (2006) Distinct role of macrophages in different tumor microenvironments. Cancer Res 66(2):605–612
12. Bonnelykke-Behrndtz ML, Schmidt H, Christensen IJ, Damsgaard TE, Moller HJ, Bastholt L et al (2014) Prognostic stratification of ulcerated melanoma: not only the extent matters. Am J Clin Pathol 142(6):845–856
13. Kalluri R, Weinberg RA (2009) The basics of epithelial-mesenchymal transition. J Clin Invest 119(6):1420–1428
14. Kalluri R (2009) EMT: when epithelial cells decide to become mesenchymal-like cells. J Clin Invest 119(6):1417–1419

15. Nunan R, Campbell J, Mori R, Pitulescu ME, Jiang WG, Harding KG et al (2015) Ephrin-Bs Drive Junctional Downregulation and actin stress fiber disassembly to enable wound re-epithelialization. Cell Rep 13(7):1380–1395
16. Lopez-Novoa JM, Nieto MA (2009) Inflammation and EMT: an alliance towards organ fibrosis and cancer progression. EMBO Mol Med 1(6–7):303–314
17. Levesque M, Feng Y, Jones RA, Martin P (2013) Inflammation drives wound hyperpigmentation in zebrafish by recruiting pigment cells to sites of tissue damage. Dis Model Mech 6(2):508–515
18. Bønnelykke-Behrndtz ML et al (2017) Loss of E-cadherin as part of a migratory phenotype in melanoma is associated with ulceration. Am J Dermatopathol. doi:10.1097/DAD.0000000000000750
19. Bonde AK, Tischler V, Kumar S, Soltermann A, Schwendener RA (2012) Intratumoral macrophages contribute to epithelial-mesenchymal transition in solid tumors. BMC Cancer 12:35, 2407-12-35
20. Grosse-Steffen T, Giese T, Giese N, Longerich T, Schirmacher P, Hansch GM et al (2012) Epithelial-to-mesenchymal transition in pancreatic ductal adenocarcinoma and pancreatic tumor cell lines: the role of neutrophils and neutrophil-derived elastase. Clin Dev Immunol 2012:720768
21. Gaida MM, Steffen TG, Gunther F, Tschaharganeh DF, Felix K, Bergmann F et al (2012) Polymorphonuclear neutrophils promote dyshesion of tumor cells and elastase-mediated degradation of E-cadherin in pancreatic tumors. Eur J Immunol 42(12):3369–3380
22. Freisinger CM, Huttenlocher A (2014) Live imaging and gene expression analysis in zebrafish identifies a link between neutrophils and epithelial to mesenchymal transition. PLoS One 9(11):e112183
23. Ardi VC, Van den Steen PE, Opdenakker G, Schweighofer B, Deryugina EI, Quigley JP (2009) Neutrophil MMP-9 proenzyme, unencumbered by TIMP-1, undergoes efficient activation in vivo and catalytically induces angiogenesis via a basic fibroblast growth factor (FGF-2)/FGFR-2 pathway. J Biol Chem 284(38):25854–25866
24. Bekes EM, Schweighofer B, Kupriyanova TA, Zajac E, Ardi VC, Quigley JP et al (2011) Tumor-recruited neutrophils and neutrophil TIMP-free MMP-9 regulate coordinately the levels of tumor angiogenesis and efficiency of malignant cell intravasation. Am J Pathol 179(3):1455–1470
25. Ardi VC, Kupriyanova TA, Deryugina EI, Quigley JP (2007) Human neutrophils uniquely release TIMP-free MMP-9 to provide a potent catalytic stimulator of angiogenesis. Proc Natl Acad Sci U S A 104(51):20262–20267
26. Pla P, Moore R, Morali OG, Grille S, Martinozzi S, Delmas V et al (2001) Cadherins in neural crest cell development and transformation. J Cell Physiol 189(2):121–132
27. Lugassy C, Wadehra M, Li X, Corselli M, Akhavan D, Binder SW et al (2013) Pilot study on "pericytic mimicry" and potential embryonic/stem cell properties of angiotropic melanoma cells interacting with the abluminal vascular surface. Cancer Microenviron 6(1):19–29
28. Lugassy C, Vernon SE, Busam K, Engbring JA, Welch DR, Poulos EG et al (2006) Angiotropism of human melanoma: studies involving in transit and other cutaneous metastases and the chicken chorioallantoic membrane: implications for extravascular melanoma invasion and metastasis. Am J Dermatopathol 28(3):187–193
29. Barnhill R, Dy K, Lugassy C (2002) Angiotropism in cutaneous melanoma: a prognostic factor strongly predicting risk for metastasis. J Invest Dermatol 119(3):705–706
30. Bald T, Quast T, Landsberg J, Rogava M, Glodde N, Lopez-Ramos D et al (2014) Ultraviolet-radiation-induced inflammation promotes angiotropism and metastasis in melanoma. Nature 507(7490):109–113
31. Balkwill F, Mantovani A (2001) Inflammation and cancer: back to Virchow? Lancet 357(9255):539–545
32. Blaisdell A, Crequer A, Columbus D, Daikoku T, Mittal K, Dey SK et al (2015) Neutrophils oppose uterine epithelial carcinogenesis via debridement of hypoxic tumor cells. Cancer Cell 28(6):785–799

33. Granot Z, Henke E, Comen EA, King TA, Norton L, Benezra R (2011) Tumor entrained neutrophils inhibit seeding in the premetastatic lung. Cancer Cell 20(3):300–314
34. Hoption Cann SA, van Netten JP, van Netten C, Glover DW (2002) Spontaneous regression: a hidden treasure buried in time. Med Hypotheses 58(2):115–119
35. Porcheray F, Viaud S, Rimaniol AC, Leone C, Samah B, Dereuddre-Bosquet N et al (2005) Macrophage activation switching: an asset for the resolution of inflammation. Clin Exp Immunol 142(3):481–489
36. Slaton JW, Karashima T, Perrotte P, Inoue K, Kim SJ, Izawa J et al (2001) Treatment with low-dose interferon-alpha restores the balance between matrix metalloproteinase-9 and E-cadherin expression in human transitional cell carcinoma of the bladder. Clin Cancer Res 7(9):2840–2853
37. Ceelen W, Pattyn P, Mareel M (2014) Surgery, wound healing, and metastasis: recent insights and clinical implications. Crit Rev Oncol Hematol 89(1):16–26
38. Lee JW, Shahzad MM, Lin YG, Armaiz-Pena G, Mangala LS, Han HD et al (2009) Surgical stress promotes tumor growth in ovarian carcinoma. Clin Cancer Res 15(8):2695–2702
39. Kasper M, Jaks V, Are A, Bergstrom A, Schwager A, Svard J et al (2011) Wounding enhances epidermal tumorigenesis by recruiting hair follicle keratinocytes. Proc Natl Acad Sci U S A 108(10):4099–4104
40. Senet P, Combemale P, Debure C, Baudot N, Machet L, Aout M et al (2012) Malignancy and chronic leg ulcers: the value of systematic wound biopsies: a prospective, multicenter, cross-sectional study. Arch Dermatol 148(6):704–708
41. Hofer SO, Shrayer D, Reichner JS, Hoekstra HJ, Wanebo HJ (1998) Wound-induced tumor progression: a probable role in recurrence after tumor resection. Arch Surg 133(4):383–389
42. Bogden AE, Moreau JP, Eden PA (1997) Proliferative response of human and animal tumours to surgical wounding of normal tissues: onset, duration and inhibition. Br J Cancer 75(7):1021–1027
43. Kuraishy A, Karin M, Grivennikov SI (2011) Tumor promotion via injury- and death-induced inflammation. Immunity 35(4):467–477
44. Neil JR, Johnson KM, Nemenoff RA, Schiemann WP (2008) Cox-2 inactivates Smad signaling and enhances EMT stimulated by TGF-beta through a PGE2-dependent mechanisms. Carcinogenesis 29(11):2227–2235
45. Rothwell PM, Fowkes FG, Belch JF, Ogawa H, Warlow CP, Meade TW (2011) Effect of daily aspirin on long-term risk of death due to cancer: analysis of individual patient data from randomised trials. Lancet 377(9759):31–41
46. Muinonen-Martin AJ, Susanto O, Zhang Q, Smethurst E, Faller WJ, Veltman DM et al (2014) Melanoma cells break down LPA to establish local gradients that drive chemotactic dispersal. PLoS Biol 12(10):e1001966

Chapter 9
Long Term Consequences of Acute Inflammation in Cancer Surgery

Patrice Forget and Marc De Kock

Abstract Perioperative inflammation assessment can be used to screen and stratify the perioperative status of the cancer patient. Biomarkers such as the neutrophil-to-lymphocyte ratio help clinicians and researchers develop and apply new screening and monitoring strategies. To control the perioperative inflammatory reaction, and to promote early resolution, pharmacological interventions such as NSAIDs are proposed as promising. One of their applications is the prevention of the early peak of recurrence, seen in the first few years after surgery. Additionally, to progress toward the development of new options a combined role of database analyses and incorporation of biomarkers is proposed.

Keywords Inflammation • Surgery • Cancer • Neutrophil-to-lymphocyte ratio • Non-steroidal anti-inflammatory drugs • Perioperative

9.1 Introduction

Perioperative inflammation has become considered not only as a therapeutic target but also included in new screening strategies, patient stratification, and preoperative optimization, especially for the surgical cancer patient. The goal of this chapter is to propose a specifically perioperative vision of the inflammatory response to surgery in the cancer patient. Some perspectives to adopt adequate strategies are discussed.

P. Forget, M.D., Ph.D. (✉)
Anesthesiology and Perioperative Medicine, Vrije Universiteit Brussel (VUB), Universitair Ziekenhuis Brussel (UZ Brussel), Laarbeeklaan 101, 1090 Brussels, Belgium
e-mail: forgetpatrice@yahoo.fr

M. De Kock, M.D., Ph.D.
Anesthesiology, Centre Hospitalier de Wallonie Picarde (CHWAPI), Tournai, Belgium

M.W. Retsky, R. Demicheli (eds.), *Perioperative Inflammation as Triggering Origin of Metastasis Development*, DOI 10.1007/978-3-319-57943-6_9

9.2 Acute Inflammation in Cancer Surgery

Acute inflammation is clearly associated with cancer's natural history [1]. At least for solid tumors, surgery can cure some of these patients. Unfortunately, rapid recurrences can occur after surgery sometimes with evidence of accelerated growth of metastases, probably linked to an acute perioperative inflammatory reaction [2]. More than 10 years ago, a bimodal frequency of postoperative cancer relapse has been observed. This was shown in breast cancer patients treated only by mastectomy by different teams [3]. Analysis of these databases showed an early peak of relapses during the first 3 years. Most of the relapses (50–80%) occurred during this early peak. The time of occurrence of early relapses seemed chronologically correlated to surgery. Is it surprising? Probably not so much if we remember that surgery induces some pro-inflammatory pathways that are not only associated with the essential mechanisms of wound healing but are also typically described as part of the cancer pathophysiology [4] (Fig. 9.1).

9.3 The Vision

9.3.1 The Neutrophil-to-Lymphocyte Ratio as a Screening and a Stratification Tool

Various inflammatory markers are proposed for use in both cancer and non-cancer patients such as white blood cell count (WBC), C-Reactive Protein (CRP) level, neutrophil-to-lymphocyte ratio (NLR), platelets-to lymphocyte ratio (PLR), the modified Glasgow prognostic score (mGPS), Prognostic Index (PI), and Prognostic Nutritional Index (PNI) [5].

In perioperative settings, NLR has been shown to be interesting in breast, lung, and kidney cancer surgery. However a dysregulation of the inflammatory response is probably not specific to cancer patients. Indeed, in non-cancer patients, similar observations exist in elderly patients after hip fracture. The main causes of death at 3 months after hip fracture are cardiovascular complication and chest infection [6]. Indeed, many recent studies suggest NLR as a "new cardiovascular risk factor" that might improve patient screening. A recent observational study including diabetic patients with a follow-up of 4 years, showed NLR as an independent predictor of major cardiac events [7]. In this cohort, patients with NLR > 2.4 had significantly worse survival (21.4 *vs* 5.3%). This promising role of high NLR to predict cardiovascular outcome as early postoperative mortality has been confirmed by others [8–12].

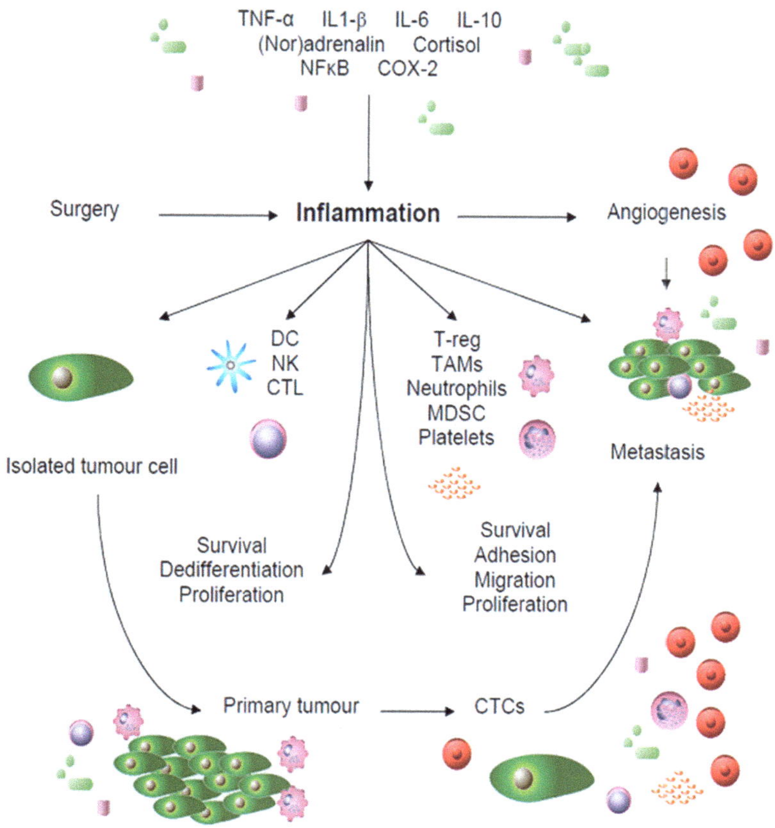

Fig. 9.1 Surgery and inflammation are closely associated, and linked to mechanisms that promote tumor growth. At the time of the extirpation of the tumor, the incidence of circulating tumor cells (CTCs) depends on several mechanisms including the inflammatory environment around the tumor itself. Inflammation promotes escape into the bloodstream and also growth of metastases. By adhesion mechanisms and/or by the synthesis of mediators, platelets can be involved in this dissemination process. Immune cells could both participate in the elimination of cancer cells (*CTL* cytotoxic T lymphocytes, *NK* Natural Killer cells, *DC* dendritic cells) or to the suppression of the immune response (T regulator lymphocytes, T reg, *MDSC* myeloid-derived suppressor cells, tumor-associated macrophages and neutrophils). COX-2 is over-expressed in tumor cells and in immune suppressor cells such as macrophages. PGE2 could directly and indirectly promote tumor growth through suppression of cell-mediated immunity. The cytokines IL1-beta, TNF-alpha and IL-6 can also directly suppress the activity of immune cells and increase the number and activation of suppressor cells. Other factors, increased by surgery, accentuate this phenomenon, including (nor) adrenalin and cortisol levels. Anesthesia *per se,* or through its impact against the surgery-induced inflammatory process, is able to interfere with many of these mechanisms. Non-steroidal anti-inflammatory drugs have an effect on all steps of this cascade, resulting in their potential anticancer effects. With permission, adapted from [7].

9.3.2 Inflammatory Scores Are Useful for Secondary Stratification, but Are Not Interchangeable

The interest of these scores is increasing before and after surgery. For example, as NLR is proposed as an objective risk factor (of mortality, cardiovascular morbidity and infections in the early and late postoperative days), we can postulate that the inflammatory scores could help stratify the patients. Nevertheless, if inflammatory biomarkers and scores, like CRP, WBCs, NLR, and PNI are modified after surgery, the absence of concordance among the inflammatory scores shows that these are not interchangeable during the perioperative period and should not be interpreted as such. For example, performance of NLR and CRP seem to differ following different kinetics after surgery.

To select the best score to be used during the perioperative period, the time course description of their evolution is an important step. Inflammatory biomarkers and scores are differently modified after surgery. Changes appear not to be parallel, and concordance analyses show clear discordance between the inflammatory scores. Interchangeability hypotheses can therefore reasonably be rejected.

9.3.3 The Interest of the NLR

What is the reason to propose the use of NLR in addition to the more canonical CRP? Before surgery, we already know that those parameters do not necessarily reflect the same phenomenon, since these depend at least in part on different mechanisms. After surgery, these differences are evident, as evolution of NLR and CRP are not parallel. An analysis of a cohort of patients undergoing major abdominal surgery showed correlation between CRP and NLR was moderate before surgery and at postoperative day + 7 ($R^2 = 0.40$ and 0.38, $P < 0.05$). In contrast, even if statistically significant, correlation was poor at day + 1 and +2 ($R^2 = 0.06$ and 0.10, $P < 0.05$) [9]. Interestingly, at day + 7, an increased NLR was the only independent parameter associated with more complications ($P < 0.001$). In other words, complications are associated with a greater inflammatory response to abdominal surgery and this is better reflected by a significantly higher NLR, 7 days after the surgery, than by the CRP level. It is noted that NLR remains elevated in patients developing complications post-operatively compared with non-complicated outcome patients. In a multivariate analysis, the NLR value at D + 7 was the only factor associated with postoperative complications.

CRP levels have delayed kinetics compared to NLR, increasing at D + 2 and not normalizing at D + 7 whether there are complications or not. This confirms previous observation of Vaugan-Shaw et al. and Cook et al. [10, 11]. The importance of a persisting high NLR value after 1 week has been associated not only with short term morbidity (septic and cardiovascular) but also with higher long term mortality after lung cancer surgery and orthopaedic surgery for hip fracture.

9.3.4 There Is Still a Need for Further Inflammatory Biomarkers

As inflammation is a complex and ubiquitous phenomenon, efficient parameters are important in many situations, and not only as screening and stratification tools. Two examples exist, successful or not, and are interesting to discuss, even if not directly linked to cancer outcome. Postoperative neuropathy pathophysiology has been at least partially elucidated, by studies focusing on inflammatory processes. A second example is the lack until now of effective immune monitoring in immunonutrition programs.

In postoperative neuropathy, a significant study from Mayo Clinic in 2010 showed how inflammation plays an important role [12]. For many years postsurgical neuropathies were attributed to mechanical factors (compression, stretch, contusion or section). In 33 patients, the Mayo authors investigated and characterized neuropathies diagnosed in the first 30 postoperative days. They found that, even if focal and multifocal neuropathies often mimicked mechanical aetiologies, histopathological investigations showed in nearly all cases an inflammatory infiltrate confirmed by magnetic resonance imaging (MRI) findings (abnormally increased T2 nerve signal). This remarkable documentation, including biomarker analyses, permitted clear illustration that not all postsurgical neuropathies are mechanical and that inflammatory mechanisms may be associated and potentially causative in many cases, especially in multifocal neuropathies.

In immunonutrition programs, the problem is different. Pre-existing malnutrition is one of the most important factors affecting postsurgical complications especially in cancer patients. Consequentially, an immune function as an outcome could be reversed by immunonutrition. To help the clinician as the researcher, a routinely available biomarker (derived from clinical or biological data) should be of great importance. Unfortunately, serum markers, such as albumin, transthyretin, white blood cells counts and C-reactive protein are not specific. Composite scores, including the Prognostic Inflammatory and Nutritional Index (PINI), the Nutritional Risk Index (NRI), the modified Glasgow Prognostic Score (mGPS), the neutrophil-to-lymphocyte ratio, CD4 and CD8 lymphocyte counts, the platelet-to-lymphocyte ratio (PLR), the Prognostic Index (PI) and the Prognostic Nutritional Index (PNI) are prognostic factors of outcome, but studies have shown an inability to correlate these to an immunonutrition effect [13]. This shows that there remains a need for an effective and widely available immunonutritional monitoring marker.

In brief, inflammatory biomarkers are not interchangeable and sometimes insufficient in some situations (notably immunonutrition programs), despite a high need to elucidate some perioperative processes such as postoperative neuropathy.

9.4 The Options?

9.4.1 To Control the Inflammatory Reaction

As explained above, there is a strong rationale to test some interventions in the perioperative period that could be associated with an optimal control of the inflammatory reaction to prevent a perioperative disequilibrium in cancer patients leading to postoperative accelerated tumor growth and early relapse [14]. And even if persistence of an inflammatory process is a consequence rather than a cause, investigation of this phenomenon may be interesting as a potential target. In other words, are there pathophysiological mechanisms linking a persisting high NLR value with an outcome that is worse? Could we propose an early therapeutic intervention to improve outcome?

9.4.2 Non-steroidal Anti-inflammatory Drugs in Cancer

Amongst the possible interventions, at least in cancer, one of these, non-steroidal anti-inflammatory drugs (NSAIDs) have been proposed. NSAIDs have been shown to impair the growth of tumors at all the steps described above. In addition to the opiate-sparing effect, NSAIDs present a promising anticancer profile with respect to the pathophysiological steps of tumor proliferation and dissemination [15]. These therapeutic effects of chronic NSAIDs in cancer have been described for various carcinomas, with a great concordance between studies. While the role of NSAIDS in cancer prevention remains somewhat unclear, this is not related to a lack of data on their anticancer effect but, rather, to side effects associated with chronic administration [16, 17]. In surgical animal models, concordant data have been published suggesting a direct specific effect of NSAIDs on perioperative protumoral events, leading circulating tumors cells and/or micrometastasis to survive and proliferate [18, 19]. Unfortunately, in human studies focusing on perioperative interventions to influence postoperative cancer outcome, methodological pitfalls including various endpoints selection and most often unreported NSAIDs use precludes any definitive conclusion [20]. Consequently, additional studies have been conducted, using existing prospective patients listing and high quality databases, in breast, prostate, lung and kidney cancer surgery, and support a possible place for NSAIDs in this field [21].

9.4.3 Time for a Paradigm Shift

Subgroups identification can be important to understand the effects of our interventions. As explained above, it helped us in the comprehension of the effect of NSAIDs in breast cancer patients. Due to the high incidence of early relapse observed after breast cancer surgery especially in triple-negative histological type patients, a selection of patients based on this prognostic biomarker to test the anticancer effect of ketorolac has been proposed. This approach could reduce the high attrition rate and minimise futile exposure of patients to ineffective investigational therapies. Other examples exist where development of drug candidates was stopped whereas it might have been successful. A successful test can focus on patients most likely to benefit from the drug. The incorporation of biomarkers is, at least partially, a response to identify these patients. In our work, incorporation of NLR led to improved understanding and documentation of the relevant biology. It could prevent failure of clinical trials testing drug candidates. In the same direction, we can also propose to use the data of large available series, e.g., the PeriOperative Ischemic Evaluation-2 Trial (POISE-2). This is an example of a large database (10,000 patients) that should be used to monitor the effect on cancer recurrence of aspirin, even if not designed for this goal.

Additionally, and as detailed above, an attractive role of high NLR to identify high-risk patients has been proposed in cancer and in non-cancer settings. It could be assessed in the preoperative period and followed after surgery. We propose that the NLR would be used to screen patients and to monitor their response to cancer and to surgery. This monitoring could be used in clinical practice from diagnosis to the end of postoperative recovery. This could also be used as an inclusion criterion in clinical trials [22].

9.5 Conclusion

Inflammation is a major prognostic factor after cancer surgery as previously shown in nonsurgical settings. Biomarkers like NLR can reflect this process and can now be used in clinical practice and integrated in clinical research. Biomarkers are now proposed in cancer surgery to identify high risk subgroups. Pharmacological interventions such as NSAIDs are proposed in the perioperative period. This illustrates the combined role that database analyses and incorporation of biomarkers can play in clinical research.

References

1. Forget P, De Kock M (2014) Perspectives in anaesthesia for cancer surgery. J Cancer Res Clin Oncol 140(3):353–359
2. Demicheli R, Retsky MW, Hrushesky WJM, Baum M (2007) Tumor dormancy and surgery-driven dormancy interruption in breast cancer: learning from failures. Nat Clin Pract Oncol 4:699–710
3. Retsky MW, Demicheli R, Hrushesky WJ, Baum M, Gukas ID (2008) Dormancy and surgery-driven escape from dormancy help explain some clinical features of breast cancer. APMIS 116(7–8):730–741

4. Forget P, Coulie PG, Retsky M, Demicheli R, Machiels JP, De Kock M (2013) Is there a rationale for an anesthesiologist's role against cancer recurrence? Acta Anaesthesiol Belg 64:15–24
5. Forget P, Rengger N, Berliere M, De Kock M (2014) Inflammatory scores are not interchangeable during the perioperative period of breast cancer surgery. Int J Surg 12(12):1360–1362
6. Roche JJ, Wenn RT, Sahota O, Moran CG (2005) Effect of comorbidities and postoperative complications on mortality after hip fracture in elderly people: prospective observational cohort study. BMJ 331(7529):1374
7. Azab B, Chainani V, Shah N, McGinn JT (2013) Neutrophil-lymphocyte ratio as a predictor of major adverse cardiac events among diabetic population: a 4-year follow-up study. Angiology 64(6):456–465. doi:10.1177/0003319712455216. PubMed PMID: 22904109
8. Forget P, Moreau N, Engel H et al (2015) The neutrophil-to-lymphocyte ratio (NLR) after surgery for hip fracture (HF). Arch Gerontol Geriatr 60(2):366–371
9. Forget P, Dinant V, De Kock M (2015) Is the neutrophil-to-lymphocyte ratio more correlated than C-reactive protein with postoperative complications after major abdominal surgery? PeerJ 3:e713
10. Vaughan-Shaw PG, Rees JR, King AT (2012) Neutrophil lymphocyte ratio in outcome prediction after emergency abdominal surgery in the elderly. Int J Surg 10(3):157–162
11. Cook EJ, Walsh SR, Faroog N, Alberts JC, Justin TA, Keeling NJ (2007) Post-operative neutrophil-lymphocyte ratio predicts complications following colorectal surgery. Int J Surg 5(1):27–30
12. Staff NP, Engelstad J, Klein CJ, Amrami KK, Spinner RJ, Dyck PJ, Warner MA, Warner ME, Dyck PJ (2010) Post-surgical inflammatory neuropathy. Brain 133(10):2866–2880
13. Forget P, Echeverria G, Giglioli S et al (2015) Biomarkers in immunonutrition programme, is there still a need for new ones? A brief review. Ecancermedicalscience 9:546
14. Forget P, Simonet O, De Kock M (2013) Cancer surgery induces inflammation, immunosuppression and neo-angiogenesis, but is it influenced by analgesics? F1000Res 2:102
15. Forget P (2014) A single dose of ketorolac during surgery may suppress cancer relapse: something for nothing? Proc Belg Royal Acad Med 3:53–60
16. Holmes MD, Chen WY, Li L, Hertzmark E, Spiegelman D, Hankinson SE (2010) Aspirin intake and survival after breast cancer. J Clin Oncol 28(9):1467–1472
17. Burn J, Gerdes AM, Macrae F et al (2012) Long-term effect of aspirin on cancer risk in carriers of hereditary colorectal cancer: an analysis from the CAPP2 randomised controlled trial. Lancet 378(9809):2081–2087
18. Forget P, Collet V, Lavand'homme P, De Kock M (2010) Does analgesia and condition influence immunity after surgery? Effects of fentanyl, ketamine and clonidine on natural killer activity at different ages. Eur J Anaesthesiol 27(3):233–240
19. Forget P, De Kock M (2009) Could anaesthesia, analgesia and sympathetic modulation affect neoplasic recurrence after surgery? A systematic review centered over the modulation of natural killer cells activity. Ann Fr Anesth Reanim 28(9):751–768
20. Forget P, Leonard D, Kartheuser A, De Kock M (2011) Choice of endpoint and not reporting all the analgesics used may render inconclusive studies on oncological outcome. Anesthesiology 114(3):717
21. Forget P, Machiels JP, Coulie PG, Berliere M, Poncelet AJ, Tombal B, Stainier A, Legrand C, Canon JL, Kremer Y, De Kock M (2013) Neutrophil:lymphocyte ratio and intraoperative use of ketorolac or diclofenac are prognostic factors in different cohorts of patients undergoing breast, lung, and kidney cancer surgery. Ann Surg Oncol 20(Suppl 3):S650–S660. doi:10.1245/s10434-013-3136-x. PubMed PMID:23884751
22. Forget P, Berlière M, van Maanen A, Duhoux FP, Machiels JP, Coulie PG, Bouche G, De Kock M, Ketorolac in Breast Cancer trial (KBCtrial) group (2013) Perioperative ketorolac in high risk breast cancer patients. Rationale, feasibility and methodology of a prospective randomized placebo-controlled trial. Med Hypotheses 81(4):707–712. doi:10.1016/j.mehy.2013.07.033. PubMed PMID: 23937996

Chapter 10
Cancer: Nurture and Nature

Romano Demicheli

Abstract The currently prevalent somatic mutation theory of carcinogenesis and metastases explicitly assumes that cancer is a cellular disease, i.e. a disease of the control of cell proliferation and/or cell differentiation. Accordingly, explanations should always be sought for at a gene and/or gene product level, regardless of the level of organization at which the phenomenon is observed. Such a reductionist approach characterized the century-old effort to find cancer cell singularities, absent in normal cells, without apparent success, however. More recently alternative views have been put forward, assuming that cancer is a tissue based disease involving disturbed interactions within the tissue architecture.

In this review, selected reports on normal tissue homeostasis and bone marrow contribution to both tumour cells and tumour stroma are reviewed. Regarding normal tissues, the existence of a complex homeostatic system actually involving the whole organism emerges. Regarding tumours, remarkable similarities with normal tissue activities are apparent, providing some evidence that tumours share many biological features and processes with normal tissues. The review supports the concept that cancer is a tissue based disease and that its pathological nature may result from unbalanced/untimely activation of otherwise normal physiological processes.

Keywords Tumour homeostasis • Tumour stroma and cells • Bone marrow • Pre-metastatic niche • Wound healing • Similarities between tumour and normal tissue

---

The text of this chapter is basically extracted from a paper published in Targeted Oncology in 2013: *Demicheli R: Tumours and tissues: similar homeostatic systems? Target Oncol. 2013 Jun;8(2):97–105. doi:10.1007/s11523-013-0277-6.*

R. Demicheli (✉)
Istituto Nazionale Tumori di Milano, Fondazione IRCCS, Milan 20133, Italy
e-mail: romano.demicheli@istitutotumori.mi.it

M.W. Retsky, R. Demicheli (eds.), *Perioperative Inflammation as Triggering Origin of Metastasis Development*, DOI 10.1007/978-3-319-57943-6_10

10.1 Introduction: Homeostasis Traits from Tissue Damage Repair

The early perception of cancer was substantially borrowed from the paradigms of bacterial infections [1–2]. Indeed, cancer was regarded as pathologic phenomenon occurring at cellular level, a genome-driven disease, where the accumulation of a sufficient number of alterations in key genes results in "cell transformation". Transformed cells were viewed as *aliens* intruding a vulnerable idle microenvironment. Cell transformation was believed to be an irreversible process: "Once a cancer cell, always a cancer cell".

Yet, this paradigm was progressively challenged by a number of experimental and clinical findings, highlighting the crucial role of tumour stroma in carcinogenesis, tumour development and clinical behaviour and providing evidence that normal cells may display cancer-like behaviour while, conversely, cancer cells may regain normal cell traits [3–8]. The novel cancer image, where tumours look like pseudo-organ structures more than invading hordes, supported reasonable explanations for clinical findings and suggested new concepts such as tumour dormancy and accelerated metastasis growth due to primary tumour removal [9–10]. It also advocated the occurrence of some kind of homeostatic effect of primary tumour upon distant metastases, apparently mimicking the organ homeostasis that succeeds the growth process. In this review, similarities between normal tissue and tumour behaviours will be examined by a parallel scrutiny of normal homeostatic mechanisms and tumour relationships with the host organism. This survey further supports the concept that tumours share many biological processes with normal tissues, although these "normal" processes are often de-contextualized and result in pathological outcome.

Seminal knowledge on tissue homeostasis emerged from investigations on damage repair, where dramatic reawakening of the tissue building machinery is required. Both parallel processes between wound healing and morphogenesis [11] and the role of growth factors and cytokines [12] have been recognized, as well as the role of bone marrow (BM), which provides inflammatory mature cells to injured tissues. Furthermore, a number of recent reports, in both animals and humans, indicate that bone marrow also supplies cells capable of producing non-hematopoietic tissue. Since the nature of such cells as well as their denomination remain debated, they will be henceforth referred to as bone marrow-derived cells (BMDCs).

10.1.1 Animals

In animals, the contribution of BMDCs to epithelial and stromal cells at steady state conditions is detectable in several organs (skin, lung, liver, gastrointestinal trait), although at different frequencies, with maximum levels into the skin [13–15]. Accordingly, a few cells within the BM, a rare population that can be estimated to represent about 0.001–0.01% of the BM nucleated cells [16], can originate in vivo non-hematopoietic tissue, a phenomenon that is enhanced in tissue damage repair.

Skin wound healing has been extensively investigated [14, 15, 17–21]. Locally, BMDCs increase early, peak after a week and then decrease to a stable level estimated to be 10–20% [15]. Most of them are spindle-shaped dermal fibroblast-like cells [15, 17, 19, 21] that produce type III collagen, not synthesized by skin-resident dermal fibroblasts [15]. A lower fraction originates epithelial cells [13, 14, 18–20], which are detectable in epidermis, hair follicles, and sebaceous glands. Skin damage activates the release of chemokines from the injured site, which interact with BMDC receptors (e.g. CCL21/CCR7) and induce mobilization and local recruitment [17, 20, 22]. A study focused on the role of BMDCs in the local angiogenesis process concluded that they play a major role by paracrine mechanisms without endothelial differentiation [22].

A positive correlation between tissue damage and BMDC homing with contribution to stromal and epithelial cells was ascertained in other organs, including lung and salivary glands [23–26].

10.1.2 Humans

In humans, the conversion of BMDCs into epithelial cells was observed in patients receiving BM or other organ transplantations from gender discordant donors.

In archival specimens, hepatocytes and cholangiocytes from BMDCs ranged from 4 to 43% [27], suggesting that hepatocytes and cholangiocytes derived from circulating BMDCs, which were able to replenish large numbers of hepatic parenchymal cells. In lung transplantations, recipient-derived epithelial cells were detected in bronchial epithelium of the transplanted organ [28]. A markedly higher degree of chimerism was observed in epithelial structures displaying signs of chronic injury, such as squamous metaplasia (24% *versus* 9.5%). Another report [29] confirmed chimerism in up to 6.6% of epithelial cells in bronchial and alveolar tissue, providing evidence that extrapulmonary precursor cells, putatively BMDCs [30], are able to contribute to pulmonary regeneration.

After BM transplantation, BMDCs were identified as differentiated cells in each of the parenchymal components of salivary glands: acini, ducts and stroma (0.65–1.44%) [31]. Higher frequency of microchimerism (~10%) was found in the buccal mucosa of a few patients, suggesting higher BMDC contribution for tissues with higher turnover. A positive association between the proliferative activity and the BMDC epithelial commitment was observed in colonic mucosa as well [32], where BMD epithelial cells frequency was significantly higher in samples indicating non-specific colitis.

A remarkable investigation on the effect of skin injury as inducer of cell mobilization from other body compartments in 44 patients with total body surface burn area of 30–60% and, for comparison, in 23 healthy subjects has been recently published [33]. Cells expressing stem cell-associated markers, such as CD133,

CD34, and CXCR4 as well as small cells expressing profile markers of pluripotent cells (Oct-4$^+$ Nanog$^+$ SSEA-4$^+$ CXCR4$^+$ lin$^-$ CD45$^-$) were detected. Changing serum concentrations of Stroma Derived Factor 1 (SDF-1), Hepatocyte Growth Factor (HGF) and Vascular Endothelial Growth Factor (VEGF) were measured. The mobilization of putative stem cells increased significantly 5 days after skin injury, which may reflect the serum dynamics of chemoactive factors and the time needed to the cell pool amplification.

In conclusion, wound healing, far from being a local process, is basically a systemic process involving complex homeostatic mechanisms that only recently are beginning to be understood.

10.2 Tumours: Wounds That Do Not Heal

10.2.1 Tumour Cells from Bone Marrow

It is well known that a few tumours have haematological origin (e.g. leukaemia). Yet, even non-haematological tumour cells may derive from BM cells. For instance, in recipients of sex mismatched BM, peripheral blood stem cell or organ transplantation, developing a successive solid cancer, BMDCs were found to contribute to tumour cells. In particular, in a few patients with oral squamous cell carcinoma, most, if not all, tumour cells were donor-derived [34–36], indicating that tumours were apparently generated by the transplanted BM cells. The contribution of BM to tumour cells was also detected, although less extensively (1–5%), in other tumours (lung adenocarcinoma, larynx squamous cell carcinoma, glioblastoma, Kaposi sarcoma, mucoepidermoid carcinoma of the parotid gland, breast cancer, papillary thyroid carcinoma and Barrett's adenocarcinoma) [37–40].

A seminal investigation on the possible contribution of BMDCs to tumour cells was performed in murine gastric cancer development from *Helicobacter* infection [41]. After infection, rapid increase of inflammatory BMDCs within gastric tissue was observed, but there was no early engraftment and differentiation as epithelial cells. Engraftment was first seen later and, in chronically infected mice, a large population of BMDCs within the gastric mucosa expressed intestinal-type mucins and displayed phenotype of the metaplastic lineage. Epithelial dysplasia increased in severity over time and eventually resulted in carcinoma. All of the intraepithelial neoplasia cells arose from BM cells.

Somewhat different behaviour was observed for intestinal adenomas in female mice. BM derived columnar-like epithelial cells were detected in the adenomas of all small bowel and colon specimens at a rate of 0.02%. When animals were injected with murine lung cancer the contribution of BMDCs to lung tumours was nearly 1%. In a parallel analysis of human histological specimens of colonic adenoma, skin cancer and squamous cell carcinoma of the lung, none of the skin cancer cells showed BMDC origin, 1–4% of the adenoma epithelial cells and 20% of the lung cancer cells were from BMDCs. Authors propose that BM participates to neoplasia at the level of *developmental mimicry*, whereby BMDCs are called into a neoplastic environment where they respond to developmental cues and adopt phenotypes similar to the surrounding neoplastic epithelial cells [42].

In summary, BMDCs may develop as a constituent of tumour cell populations, generating, in some cases, the entire tumour mass, the same as they may accomplish in wound healing.

10.2.2 Tumour Stroma from Bone Marrow

Inflammatory cells infiltrating tumour bulk, once assumed to act to attenuate tumour development, were successively found to play roles in promoting progression of many types of cancer [43].

A number of reports evaluated the dynamics of BMDC homing and differentiation in tumour stroma. In a human pancreatic cancer cell line transplanted in mice [44], BMDCs appeared early as inflammatory cells accounting for 13% of myofibroblasts and 25% of endothelial cells at 2 weeks. Later, percentages evolved to 40% and 26% respectively, suggesting that BMDCs contribution dynamics is different for endothelial cells and myofibroblasts. Differently, BMDC contribution to tumour endothelial cells appeared substantially lower (about 0.4% or less) in another study on spontaneous adenocarcinoma of the mouse prostate [45]. Detailed analysis of cell position revealed that while BMDCs were discernible in perivascular position in both primary tumour and lung metastases none were at the luminal surface. BM was suggested to be a reservoir for cells that increase tumour angiogenesis via endocrine/paracrine mechanisms, while the tumour endothelium would be derived primarily from the local environment. BMDC contribution to angiogenesis was also comparatively analysed in ischemic retinas, Lewis lung carcinoma (LLC) and B16 melanoma [46]. The spectrum of BM involvement was dependent on model system with SDF-1α as a key permissive trigger. In ischemic retinas, BMDCs provided long-term neovascularization and BMDCs expressing CXCR4 and CD133 participated directly in blood vessel formation. In tumours, LLC had BM-derived neo-vessels (17%) and exhibited both increased SDF-1α serum levels and site-specific expression; whereas B16 melanoma did not show either site-specific SDF-1α expression or BM derived neo-vessels. B16 melanomas still contained little to no BM contribution when growing in an environment of elevated serum SDF-1α level, whereas blood vessels had a density similar to that of LLC tumours, suggesting that tumour neovascularization occurs through redundant mechanisms, possibly tumour type related.

BMDCs contribute considerably to carcinoma-associated fibroblasts (CAFs), which express α-smooth muscle actin (myofibroblasts). In mouse models of inflammation-induced gastric cancer, at least 20% of CAFs originated from BM and their recruitment was blocked by CXCR4 inhibition, while myofibroblasts expansion was reduced by TGF-β inhibition [47]. CAFs are likely to be a special phenotype that BMDCs adopt after recruitment in neoplasias. Indeed, in chronic pancreatitis by caerulein and in carcinogenesis by DMBA [48], cancer-associated, but not pancreatitis-associated BMD stellate cells expressed the cancer related specific marker CELSR3, suggesting that BMDCs can adopt different phenotypes, conceivably responding to the different environmental signals.

Integrin α4β1 promoting the homing of BMDCs to neo-vasculature, tumour derived transforming growth factor β1 (TGF-β1) attracting BMSCs, and BMSC derived IL-17B attracting tumour cells, were suggested as mediators of tumour-stroma interactions [49, 50]. In another remarkable investigation, a human breast cancer cell line yielding vigorously growing tumour xenografts (labelled as "instigator") was implanted in one flank of nude mice, while another indolent cell line (labelled as "responder") was implanted into the contralateral flank [51]. Instigating tumours, even when small (0.08% of total body mass), facilitated the outgrowth of already-established, otherwise-indolent tumour cells located contralaterally. Release of soluble factors (e.g. osteopontin) enabled instigating tumours to communicate and perturb BM, the functional activation of which conveyed activated BMDCs to the stroma of responding tumours, fostering growth. This effect involved also micrometastases and, interestingly, a xenografted human tumour surgical specimen from colon cancer.

The notion that operative injury may worsen the prognosis of cancer patients was supported by a study on the effect of surgery (gastrotomy) on the course of LLC in mice [52]. Twelve days after operation, the tumour volume almost doubled in mice after gastrotomy with significant increase of BMDCs, microvessel density and proliferating cells, while the number of apoptotic cells was significantly reduced in comparison with controls. Interfering with the SDF-1/CXCR4 signalling pathway inhibited the recruitment of BMDCs and negated completely the acceleration in tumour growth after operation. The mobilization of BMDCs, however, could be different after different operative injuries, as this phenomenon was undetectable after hepatectomy.

In summary, BMDCs may play in tumours and in wound healing similar supportive roles in the form of stroma cells that regulate the local "parenchymal" cell population by reacting to microenvironmental signals.

10.2.3 The Pre-metastatic Niche

More recently it was discovered that, before the arrival of tumour cells, adjustments occur in metastatic sites that make them conducive for successive metastasis development. This process results in a metastatic niche providing support to metastasis-initiating cells, by analogy with the physiological niches that support stem cells in healthy tissues. The local tissue tuning before tumour cell arrival has been labelled *pre-metastatic niche* and this cellular 'bookmarking' was first reported for lung metastases from LLC and B16 melanoma in mice [53]. Before tumour implantation, minimal BMDCs were observable in the lungs. By day 14 after tumour implantation, but before the arrival of tumour cells, a remarkable cluster formation of BMDCs was detectable near terminal bronchioles and distal alveoli. On day 16, established BMDC clusters dictated the contours of future metastatic lesions. Individual tumour cells, associated with pre-existing BMDC clusters, were visible by day 18 and progressed to micrometastases by day 23. Intradermal injection of LLC cells resulted in BMDC cluster formation limited to the lung and liver with no clusters in other organs. In contrast, B16 melanoma tumour cells induced the formation of BMDC clusters in multiple tissues such as lung, liver, testis, spleen and kidney. Remarkably, pre-treatment with melanoma derived conditioned medium resulted in redirection of LLC metastasis to sites frequently observed in B16-melanoma. Implanted LLC tumour cells were associated with increased fibronectin expression at the lung pre-metastatic niche, compared with the baseline level. The fully formed pre-metastatic niche ($VEGFR1^+$ BMDCs, fibroblasts and fibronectin) highly expressed SDF-1, creating a chemokine gradient attracting tumour cells that thereby developed a complete metastatic lesion.

Pre-metastatic changes preceding tumour seeding were observed in a mouse model of spontaneous lymph node metastasis, where sentinel lymph nodes were significantly enlarged before detectable metastasis, and were enriched in functional blood vessels, an effect absent in the next lymph nodal station, implying a selective mechanism [54]. Contrasting with cancerous related lymphadenopathy, the morphology of vessels in endotoxin induced lymphadenopathy was unchanged, suggesting nodal reaction by different modalities. In humans, the process of vascularisation in the metastatic versus non-metastatic versus non-cancerous inflamed axillary lymph nodes was consistent with findings in the animal model [54]. Of note, in patients with prostatic cancer, HSCs and cancer cells occupy just the same endosteal niche and compete with each other for niche occupancy on the osteoblast [55].

Factors involved in the pre-metastatic niche development and in the following cancer cell homing and survival include hypoxia-inducible factor-1 [56] and coagulation, which is required for the recruitment to distant sites of monocytes/macrophages [57]. Focal vascular hyper-permeability involvement, with endothelial cell-focal adhesion kinase activity facilitating cancer cell homing to lungs, has been also observed [58]. A few reports point out the prominence of extracellular matrix components, such as tenascin [59] and periostin [60]. In particular, the role of periostin emerges from an elegant and detailed investigation on a mouse breast cancer model with spontaneous lung metastases [60]. Authors provide evidence that (i) the metastatic process is sustained by a subpopulation of tumour initiating cells (TICs), accounting for 3% of all tumour cells in both primary tumour and lung metastases, which are the only cancer cells able to benefit from periostin; (ii) the metastasis efficiency is determined by the stromal periostin production that is upregulated in response to the TGF-β released from cancer cells; (iii) periostin, in a feed-back interaction with Wnt ligands of TICs, boosts Wnt signalling activity that promote cell survival and metastatic colonization. VCAM-1 expression in breast cancer cells was also reported to provide survival advantage to cancer cells [61]. Taken together, these reports indicate that interactions of cancer cells with extracellular matrix components of the metastatic niche, activating pro-survival tumour cell processes, like Wnt, Notch and PI3K pathways, are necessary in order to support the metastatic phase.

10.3 Components of the Homeostatic Process

BM is a source of cells directly supporting the homeostasis of tissues (in steady state conditions and after lesions) and able to originate cells from the three distinct germ-cell layers (ectoderm, mesoderm, and endoderm). Moreover they play a key role in tumour development. Trans-differentiation, cell fusion processes and non-hematopoietic primitive stem cells (SCs) in BM were hypothesized to explain such phenomena. Trans-differentiation and fusion have been questioned as main processes [62, 63], while several populations of non-hematopoietic SCs potentially able to differentiate into given cells in tissues have been described in the BM. In particular, a population of very small embryonic-like stem cells (VSELs) was identified, which are apparently a good candidate for a leading role in tissue homeostasis. VSELs have been firstly purified from murine BM and from several other adult murine organs (e.g., brain, liver, skeletal muscles, heart, and kidney) [64]. A corresponding population of small (4–7 μm) $CD133^{+}$ Lin^{-} $CD45^{-}$ cells that display embryonic-like morphology have been identified in human umbilical cord blood, in mobilized peripheral blood and in adult BM [65]. Human VSELs expressed Oct4 and Nanog in their nuclei and displayed the SSEA-4 antigen. The number of circulating VSELs increased during tissue or organ injuries (e.g., heart infarct, stroke, or acute colitis), as well as after administration of certain drugs mobilizing HSCs into peripheral blood (e.g., G-CSF) [66]. BM-derived VSELs displayed the ability to differentiate in vivo into multiple mesenchymal lineages and generate osseous tissues. When injected into the hearts of mice that had undergone ischemia/reperfusion injury, VSELs induced improved global and regional left ventricular systolic function and attenuated myocyte hypertrophy in surviving tissue [67].

Whatsoever such cellular performers may be, it is crucial to understand how they participate to the collective action by communicating with other participants in this process. Usually it was believed that soluble factors such as cytokines, chemokines, growth factors and bioactive lipids released from a given cell type and circulating through the whole organism are able to induce responses by other cells endowed with specific receptors. Recent research, however, is elucidating a much more complex and efficient communication system, the core of which is a busy trafficking of microvesicles.

Microvesicles (MVs), frequently observed by electron microscopy in the interstitial space of tissues and for long time considered cellular debris, have been recently recognized as functionally relevant [68]. MVs are spherical membrane fragments containing a cargo of cytosol including a distinct and definite combination of lipids, proteins and nucleic acids (mRNA, miRNA and DNA), i.e. a non-random sample of the molecular repertoire of the originating cell [69]. MV surfaces express the adhesion molecules of the cell of origin, allowing specific capture by target cells that recognize them, which may be modified by surface interaction [70]. Most important, MVs may induce epigenetic changes in target cells by transferring selected arrays of mRNA and miRNA associated with ribonucleoproteins. Transferred mRNA can be translated after entering the target cells [69]. For example, human endothelial progenitor cell-derived MVs may activate an angiogenic program in recipient quiescent endothelial cells [71]. MVs not only mediate tissue-specific changes in mRNA by direct delivery of mRNA but also by induction of mRNA from the target cell [72]. Remarkably, some miRNAs are selectively accumulated within MVs released by adult human mesenchymal SCs and absent in the cells after MV release, whereas others are retained within the cells and not secreted in MVs [73]. This suggests a regulated process of miRNA compartmentalization and secretion by MVs.

MVs may have a functional role for tumours. Exposing normal recipient cells to bioactive MVs constitutively shed by certain human cancer cells caused the recipient cells to acquire a transformed phenotype [74]. At pre-metastatic niche level, melanoma-released MVs induced expression of a network of interconnected extracellular matrix factors responsible for tumour cell recruitment, trapping and growth [75]. Tumour-initiating cells from a human renal cell carcinoma released MVs shuttling specific mRNAs and miRNAs that triggered angiogenesis and promoted the formation of a pre-metastatic niche in the lung [76]. Human lung cancer cells changed the genetic phenotype of human BM cells by inducing lung-specific mRNA by exposure to pelleted microvesicles [77]. Of interest, BM cells co-cultured with lung melanoma and sarcoma, expressed lung-specific genes, raising interesting possibilities of bidirectional cross talk between cancers and the normal host tissue. These findings once again suggest that cell structures are less stable than previously considered and that cell phenotype, including cancer phenotype, might be exportable.

10.4 Concluding Remarks

The above reported findings indicate that BM routinely provides a contribution of specific parenchymal cells to various tissues especially after tissue damage. Remarkably, the homing of BMDCs into the damaged tissue is associated, to some extent, with the emergence of gene expression patterns corresponding to phenotypes of stroma and parenchymal cells of the "invaded" tissue (e.g. myofibroblasts and keratinocytes in the skin) (Fig. 10.1). This phenotypic change apparently relies on dominant effects of the tissue microenvironment upon imported cells. This concept is strongly supported by a few focused investigations [78, 79].

Tissue homeostasis in a given organ is apparently a complex and very integrated system actually involving the whole organism. Indeed, progenitor cells with different commitment (e.g., HSCs, MSCs and ESCs) in addition to pluripotent cells (e.g., VSELS) may reside in virtually all organs, among which BM is a main reservoir. When homeostasis alterations occur, signalling pathways (e.g. SDF-1/CXCR4) may

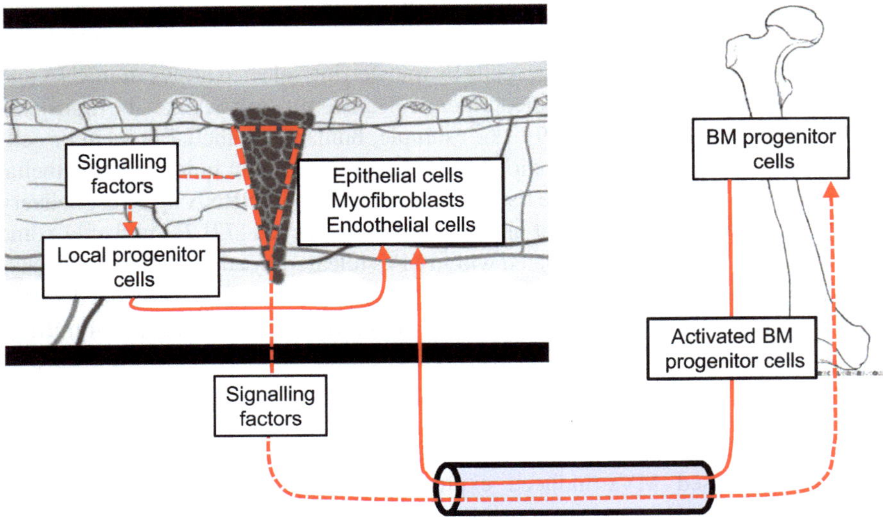

Fig. 10.1 Outline of tissue damage repair. Tissue lesion induces release of signaling factors locally activating progenitor cells and, via blood circulation, reaching bone marrow where they activate and mobilize further progenitor cells quickly homing in the damaged area. Activated progenitor cells originate repair stroma cells (myofibroblasts and endothelial cells) and also epithelial cells, although at different percentages. Bone marrow derived inflammatory cells are also recruited in the wound (not reported in the schematic figure). The coordinated interaction of all cells results in the progressive tissue repair and the following long lasting tissue remodeling

activate and, if needed, mobilize them. Activated SCs secrete a variety of growth factors, cytokines, chemokines and bioactive lipids that regulate their biology and orchestrate interactions with the surrounding microenvironment. In addition to soluble factors, activated SCs also secrete MVs, conveying packaged signalling factors, including genetic information, which may change the phenotype of the target cells, locally or at distance. Thus, one can conceive that, while cellular populations may be relatively stable, transcriptional regulation, a key determinant of the phenotype of a particular cell, may shift between different cell types [80]. What remains stable and, if damaged, induces cellular conversions to re-achieve the original condition is apparently the whole tissue architecture.

In this "normal" landscape, some "hallmarks of cancer" actually appear as familiar traits of normal cell populations. Angiogenesis is a current feature in tissues during physiological conditions and damage repair. The process we label as invasion is usually adopted by non-neoplastic cells that, mobilized from distant organs, enter target tissues. Tumour cell activities, underlying the metastatic process, basically appear as expression of the current cell trafficking network, with which they share molecular mechanisms (e.g. the SDF-1/CXCR4 axis). The tumour ability of creating the "tumour microenvironment" (Fig. 10.2) apparently parallels the ability of tissues of maintaining the "normal microenvironment" or creating the "repair microenvironment" (Fig. 10.1). Moreover, the metastatic development does not

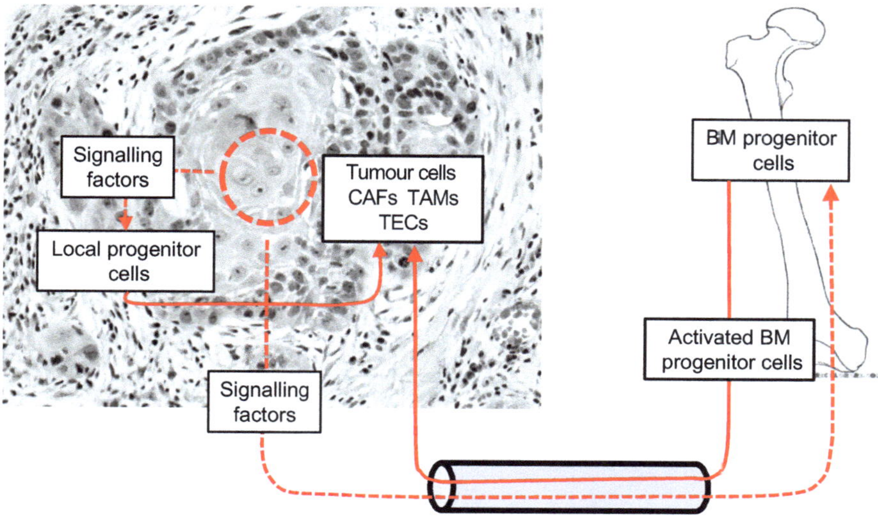

Fig. 10.2 Outline of tumour actions underlying growth. Tumour presence induces release of signalling factors that activate local progenitor cells and, via blood circulation, reach bone marrow where they mobilize and activate further progenitor cells quickly homing in the tumour area. Activated progenitor cells originate tumour stroma cells (CAFs and endothelial cells) and also tumour cells, although at different percentages, while this ability is still undecided for local progenitor cells. Bone marrow derived inflammatory cells are also recruited in the wound (not reported in the schematic figure). The coordinated interaction of all cells results in the tumour further growth

apparently diverge from such a general processing structure and is probably firmly related to inter-tissue connections (Fig. 10.3).

The recently proposed tumour hierarchical structure, including tumour stem/progenitor cells and differential metastatic capacity, further supports the parallelism between tumour and tissue structures, including the presence of stem/progenitor cells at local level and the ability of recruiting stem/progenitor cells from other sites. Furthermore, tumour cell niches are comparable to normal cell niches and are sometimes identical to them, so that both tumour and normal stem cells compete for the same site. Local conducive changes allow for recruitment and homing of stem/progenitor cells in both cases. Tumours, therefore, appear well integrated in the complex physiologic homeostatic network and it is difficult to refute the notion that tumours, far from being harsh invaders hijacking "normal" performances, share most traits with normal cells, although the normal (or normal-like) processes they use are often de-contextualized and result in pathological processes.

Most important, the central tumour hallmark, the *genome instability,* implies a paradigm of normality where lineage pathways are unidirectional and narrowly restricted, because of irreversible inactivation of genes that are required for alternate pathway selection. We are now discovering that not only normal cells could, at certain conditions, jump between lineages, but there are also specific ways to

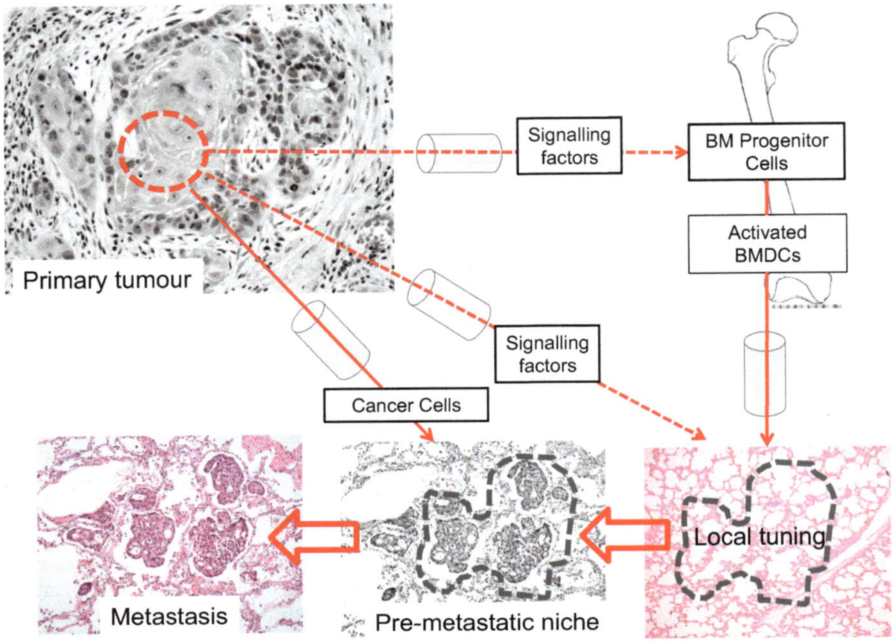

Fig. 10.3 Outline of the metastasis development via the pre-metastatic niche. Primary tumour signals (soluble factors, MVs) act in a manner that before the arrival of tumour cells, adjustments occur in metastatic sites that make them conducive for successive metastasis development. Bone marrow is involved and BMDCs are activated, mobilized and undergo a selective homing process resulting in metastatic site tuning that makes it conducive for tumour cells. This process results in a metastatic niche providing support to metastasis-initiating cells, by analogy with the physiological niches that support stem cells in healthy tissues. The local tissue tuning before tumour cell arrival has been labelled *pre-metastatic niche*. The further steps of the metastatic foci, such as dormancy or growth, are depending on several local and systemic factors

transfer genetic information between cells resulting in phenotypic change. Tumours, therefore, seem to lose the exclusivity for most of their typical traits and the notion could not be ruled out that their pathological nature results from unbalanced or untimely activation of otherwise normal physiological processes.

Disclosure The author has declared no conflicts of interest.

References

1. Nowell PC (1986) Mechanisms of tumour progression. Cancer Res 46:2203–2207
2. Hanahan D, Weinberg RA (2000) The hallmarks of cancer. Cell 100:57–70
3. Mintz B, Illmensee K (1975) Normal genetically mosaic mice produced from malignant teratocarcinoma cells. Proc Natl Acad Sci U S A 72:3585–3589

4. Maffini MV, Soto AM, Calabro JM, Ucci AA, Sonnenschein C (2004) The stroma as a crucial target in rat mammary gland carcinogenesis. J Cell Sci 117:1495–1502
5. Bissell MJ, Labarge MA (2005) Context, tissue plasticity, and cancer: are tumour stem cells also regulated by the microenvironment? Cancer Cell 7:17–23
6. Tarin D (2012) Clinical and biological implications of the tumour microenvironment. Cancer Microenviron 5(2):95–112
7. Podsypanina K, Du YC, Jechlinger M, Beverly LJ, Hambardzumyan D, Varmus H (2008) Seeding and propagation of untransformed mouse mammary cells in the lung. Science 321:1841–1844
8. Rubin H (2006) What keeps cells in tissues behaving normally in the face of myriad mutations? Bioassays 28:515–524
9. Demicheli R, Retsky MW, Hrushesky WJ, Baum M (2007) Tumour dormancy and surgery-driven interruption of dormancy in breast cancer: learning from failures. Nat Clin Pract Oncol 4:699–710
10. Demicheli R, Fornili M, Ambrogi F, Higgins K, Boyd JA, Biganzoli E, Kelsey CR (2012) Recurrence dynamics for non-small cell lung cancer: effect of surgery on the development of metastases. J Thorac Oncol 7:723–730
11. Martin P, Parkhurst SM (2004) Parallels between tissue repair and embryo morphogenesis. Development 131:3021–3034
12. Werner S, Grose R (2003) Regulation of wound healing by growth factors and cytokines. Physiol Rev 83:835–870
13. Krause DS, Theise ND, Collector MI, Henegariu O, Hwang S, Gardner R, Neutzel S, Sharkis SJ (2001) Multi-organ, multi lineage engraftment by a single bone marrow-derived stem cell. Cell 105:369–377
14. Badiavas EV, Abedi M, Butmarc J, Falanga V, Quesenberry P (2003) Participation of bone marrow derived cells in cutaneous wound healing. J Cell Physiol 196:245–250
15. Fathke C, Wilson L, Hutter J, Kapoor V, Smith A, Hocking A, Isik F (2004) Contribution of bone marrow-derived cell to skin: collagen deposition and wound repair. Stem Cells 22:812–822
16. Prockop DJ (1997) Marrow stromal cells as stem cells for non-hematopoietic tissues. Science 276:71–74
17. Sasaki M, Abe R, Fujita Y, Ando S, Inokuma D, Shimizu H (2008) Mesenchymal stem cells are recruited into wounded skin and contribute to wound repair by transdifferentiation into multiple skin cell type. J Immunol 180:2581–2587
18. Ji KH, Xiong J, Fan LX, Hu KM, Liu HQ (2009) Rat marrow-derived multipotent adult progenitor cells differentiate into skin epidermal cells in vivo. J Dermatol 36:403–409
19. Rea S, Giles NL, Webb S, Adcroft KF, Evill LM, Strickland DH, Wood FM, Fear MW (2009) Bone marrow-derived cells in the healing burn wound – more than just inflammation. Burns 35:356–364
20. Tamai K, Yamazaki T, Chino T, Ishii M, Otsuru S, Kikuchi Y, Iinuma S, Saga K, Nimura K, Shimbo T, Umegaki N, Katayama I, Miyazaki J, Takeda J, McGrath JA, Uitto J, Kaneda Y (2011) PDGFRα-positive cells in bone marrow are mobilized by high mobility group box 1 (HMGB1) to regenerate injured epithelia. PNAS 108:6609–6614
21. Verstappen J, Katsaros C, Kuijpers-Jagtman AM, Torensma R, Von der Hoff JW (2001) The recruitment of bone marrow-derived cells to skin wounds is independent of wound size. Wound Repair Regen 19:260–267
22. Okuno Y, Nakamura-Ishizu A, Kishi K, Suda T, Kubota Y (2011) Bone marrow-derived cells serve as proangiogenic macrophages but not endothelial cells in wound healing. Blood 117:5264–5272
23. Herzog EL, Van Arnam J, Hu B, Krause DS (2006) Threshold of lung injury required for the appearance of marrow-derived lung epithelia. Stem Cells 24:1986–1992
24. Spees JL, Whitney MJ, Sullivan DE, Lasky JA, Laboy M, Ylostalo J, Prockop DJ (2008) Bone marrow progenitor cells contribute to repair and remodelling of the lung and heart in a rat model of progressive pulmonary hypertension. FASEB J 22:1226–1236

25. Tran SD, Pillemer SR, Dutra A, Barrett AJ, Brownstein MJ, Key S, Pak E, Leakan RA, Kingman A, Yamada KM, Baum BJ, Mezey E (2003) Differentiation of human bone marrow-derived cells into buccal epithelial cells in vivo: a molecular analytical study. Lancet 361:1084–1088
26. Sumita Y, Liu Y, Khalili S, Maria OM, Xia D, Key S, Cotrim AP, Mezey E, Tran SD (2011) Bone marrow-derived cells rescue salivary gland function in mice with head and neck irradiation. Int J Biochem Cell B 43:80–87
27. Theise ND, Nimmakayalu M, Gardner R, Illei PB, Morgan G, Teperman L, Henegariu O, Krause DS (2000) Liver from bone marrow in humans. Hepathology 32:11–16
28. Kleeberger W, Versmold A, Rothämel T, Glöckner S, Bredt M, Haverich A, Lehmann U, Kreipe H (2003) Increased chimerism of bronchial and alveolar epithelium in human lung allografts undergoing chronic injury. Am J Pathol 162:1487–1494
29. Spencer H, Rampling D, Aurora P, Bonnet D, Hart SL, Jaffé A (2005) Transbronchial biopsies provide longitudinal evidence for epithelial chimerism in children following sex mismatched lung transplantation. Thorax 60:60–62
30. Suratt BT, Cool CD, Serls AE, Chen L, Varella-Garcia M, Shpall EJ, Brown KK, Worthen GS (2003) Human pulmonary chimerism after hematopoietic stem cell transplantation. Am J Respir Crit Care Med 168:318–322
31. Tran SD, Redman RS, Barrett AJ, Pavletic SZ, Key S, Liu Y, Carpenter A, Nguyen HM, Sumita Y, Baum BJ, Pillemer SR, Mezey E (2011) Microchimerism in salivary glands after blood- and marrow- derived stem cell transplantation. Biol Blood Marrow Transplant 17:429–433
32. Valcz G, Krenács T, Sipos F, Patai AV, Wichmann B, Leiszter K, Tóth K, Balogh Z, Csizmadia A, Hagymási K, Masszi T, Molnár B, Tulassay Z (2011) Lymphoid aggregates may contribute to the migration and epithelial commitment of bone marrow-derived cells in colonic mucosa. J Clin Pathol 64:771–775
33. Drukala J, Paczkowska E, Kucia M, Młyńska E, Krajewski A, Machaliński B, Madeja Z, Ratajczak MZ (2012) Stem cells, including a population of very small embryonic-like stem cells, are mobilized into peripheral blood in patients after skin burn injury. Stem Cell Rev 8:184–194
34. Tomihara K, Dehari H, Yamaguchi A, Abe M, Miyazaki A, Nakamori K, Hareyama M, Hiratsuka H (2009) Squamous cell carcinoma of the buccal mucosa in a young adult with history of allogenic bone marrow transplantation for childhood acute leukemia. Head Neck 31:565–568
35. Janin A, Murata H, Leboeuf C, Cayuela JM, Gluckman E, Legrès L, Desveaux A, Varna M, Ratajczak P, Soulier J, de Thé H, Bertheau P, Socié G (2009) Donor-derived oral squamous cell carcinoma after allogenic bone marrow transplantation. Blood 113:1834–1840
36. Hu YX, Luo Y, Tan YM, Shi JM, Sheng LX, Fu HR, Liu LZ, Xu YL, Wu KN, Xiao HW, Zhang LF, Yu XH, Cai Z, Huang H (2012) Donor bone marrow-derived stem cells contribute to oral squamous cell carcinoma transformation in a recipient after hematopoietic stem cell transplantation. Stem Cell Dev 21:177–180
37. Avital I, Moreira AL, Klimstra DS, Leversha M, Papadopoulos EB, Brennan M, Downey RJ (2007) Donor-derived human bone marrow cells contribute to solid organ cancers developing after bone marrow transplantation. Stem Cells 25:2903–2909
38. Soldini D, Moreno E, Martin V, Gratwohl A, Marone C, Mazzucchelli L (2008) BM-derived cells randomly contribute to neoplastic and non-neoplastic epithelial tissues at low rates. Bone Marrow Transplant 42:749–755
39. Golfinopouloss V, Pentheroudakis G, Kamakari S, Metaxa-Mariatou V, Pavlidis N (2009) Donor-derived breast cancer in a bone marrow transplantation recipient. Breast Cancer Res Treat 113:211–213
40. Hutchinson L, Stenstrom B, Chen D, Piperdi B, Levey S, Lyle S, Wang TC, Houghton J (2011) Human Barrett's adenocarcinoma of the esophagus, associated myofibroblasts, and endothelium can arise from bone marrow-derived cells after allogenic stem cell transplant. Stem Cells Dev 20:11–17

41. Houghton J, Stoicov C, Nomura S, Rogers AB, Carlson J, Li H, Cai X, Fox JG, Goldenring JR, Wang TC (2004) Gastric cancer originating from bone marrow derived cells. Science 306:1568–1571
42. Cogle CR, Theise ND, Fu D, Ucar D, Lee S, Guthrie SM, Lonergan J, Rybka W, Krause DS, Scott EW (2007) Bone marrow contributes to epithelial cancers in mice and humans as developmental mimicry. Stem Cells 25:1881–1887
43. de Visser KE, Eichten A, Coussens LM (2006) Paradoxical roles of the immune system during cancer development. Nat Rev Cancer 6:24–37
44. Ishii G, Sangai T, Oda T, Aoyagi Y, Hasebe T, Kanomata N, Endoh Y, Okumura C, Okuhara Y, Magae J, Emura M, Ochiya T, Ochiai A (2003) Bone-marrow-derived myofibroblasts contribute to the cancer-induced stromal reaction. Biochem Biophys Res Commun 309:232–240
45. Dudley AC, Udagawa T, Melero-Martin JM, Shih SC, Curatolo A, Moses MA, Klagsbrun M (2010) Bone marrow is a reservoir for proangiogenic myelomonocytic cells but not endothelial cells in spontaneous tumours. Blood 116:3367–3371
46. Madlambayan GJ, Butler JM, Hosaka K, Jorgensen M, Fu D, Guthrie SM, Shenoy AK, Brank A, Russell KJ, Otero J, Siemann DW, Scott EW, Cogle CR (2009) Bone marrow stem and progenitor cell contribution to neovasculogenesis is dependent on model system with SDF-1 as a permissive trigger. Blood 114:4310–4319
47. Quante M, Tu SP, Tomita H, Gonda T, Wang SS, Takashi S, Baik GH, Shibata W, Diprete B, Betz KS, Friedman R, Varro A, Tycko B, Wang TC (2011) Bone marrow-derived myofibroblasts contribute to the mesenchymal stem cell niche and promote tumour growth. Cancer Cell 198:257–272
48. Scarlett CJ, Colvin EK, Pinese M, Chang DK, Morey AL, Musgrove EA, Pajic M, Apte M, Henshall SM, Sutherland RL, Kench JG, Biankin AV (2011) Recruitment and activation of pancreatic stellate cells from the bone marrow in pancreatic cancer: a model of tumour-host interaction. PLoS One 6(10):e26088
49. Jin H, Aiyer A, Su J, Borgstrom P, Stupack D, Friedlander M, Varner J (2006) A homing mechanism for bone marrow-derived progenitor cell recruitment to the neovasculature. J Clin Invest 116:652–662
50. Goldstein RH, Reagan MR, Anderson K, Kaplan DR, Rosenblatt M (2010) Human bone marrow-derived MSCs can home to orthotopic breast cancer tumours and promote bone metastasis. Cancer Res 70:10044–10050
51. McAllister SS, Gifford AM, Greiner AL, Kelleher SP, Saelzler MP, Ince TA, Reinhardt F, Harris LN, Hylander BL, Repasky EA, Weinberg RA (2008) Systemic endocrine instigation of indolent tumour growth requires osteopontin. Cell 133:994–1005
52. Takemoto Y, Li TS, Kubo M, Ohshima M, Ueda K, Harada E, Enoki T, Okamoto M, Mizukami Y, Murata T, Hamano K (2011) Operative injury accelerates tumour growth by inducing mobilization and recruitment of bone marrow-derived stem cells. Surgery 149:792–800
53. Kaplan RN, Riba RD, Zacharoulis S, Bramley AH, Vincent L, Costa C, MacDonald DD, Jin DK, Shido K, Kerns SA, Zhu Z, Hicklin D, Wu Y, Port JL, Altorki N, Port ER, Ruggero D, Shmelkov SV, Jensen KK, Rafii S, Lyden D (2005) VEGFR1-positive haematopoietic bone marrow progenitors initiate the pre-metastatic niche. Nature 438:820–827
54. Quian CN, Berghuis B, Tsarfaty G, Bruch M, Kort EJ, Ditlev J, Tsarfaty I, Hudson E, Jackson DG, Petillo D, Chen J, Resau JH, The BT (2006) Preparing the "soil": the primary tumour induces vasculature reorganization in the sentinel lymph node before the arrival of metastatic cancer cells. Cancer Res 66:10365–10376
55. Shiozawa Y, Pedersen EA, Havens AM, Jung Y, Mishra A, Joseph J, Kim JK, Patel LR, Ying C, Ziegler AM, Pienta MJ, Song J, Wang J, Loberg RD, Krebsbach PH, Pienta KJ, Taichman RS (2011) Human prostate cancer metastases target the hematopoietic stem cell niche to establish footholds in mouse bone marrow. J Clin Invest 121:1298–1312
56. Wong CCL, Gilkes DM, Zhang H, Chen J, Wei H, Chaturvedi P, Fraley SI, Wong CM, Khoo US, Ng IO, Wirtz D, Semenza GL (2011) Hypoxia-inducible factor 1is a master regulator of breast cancer metastatic niche formation. Proc Natl Acad Sci U S A 108:16369–16374

57. Gil-Bernabe´ AM, Ferjancic S, Tlalka M, Zhao L, Allen PD, Im JH, Watson K, Hill SA, Amirkhosravi A, Francis JL, Pollard JW, Ruf W, Muschel RJ (2012) Recruitment of monocytes/ macrophages by tissue factor-mediated coagulation is essential for metastatic cell survival and premetastatic niche establishment in mice. Blood 119:3164–3175
58. Hiratsuka S, Goel S, Kamoun WS, Maru Y, Fukumura D, Duda DG, Jain RK (2011) Endothelial focal adhesion kinase mediates cancer cell homing to discrete regions of the lungs via E-selectin up-regulation. Proc Natl Acad Sci U S A 108:3725–3730
59. Oskarsson T, Acharyya S, Zhang XH, Vanharanta S, Tavazoie SF, Morris PG, Downey RJ, Manova-Todorova K, Brogi E, Massagué J (2011) Breast cancer cells produce tenascin C as a metastatic niche component to colonize the lungs. Nat Med 17:867–875
60. Malanchi I, Santamaria-Martínez A, Susanto E, Peng H, Lehr HA, Delaloye JF, Huelsken J (2011) Interactions between cancer stem cells and their niche govern metastatic colonization. Nature 481:85–91
61. Cheng Q, Zhang XHF, Massaguè J (2011) Macrophage binding to receptor VCAM-1 transmits survival signals in breast cancer cells that invade the lungs. Cancer Cell 20:538–549
62. Wagers AJ, Sherwood RI, Christensen JL, Weissman IL (2002) Little evidence for developmental plasticity of adult hematopoietic stem cells. Science 297:2256–2259
63. Harris RG, Herzog EL, Bruscia EM, Grove JE, Van Arnam JS, Krause DS (2004) Lack of a fusion requirement for development of bone marrow-derived epithelia. Science 305:90–93
64. Zuba-Surma EK, Kucia M, Abdel-Latif A, Dawn B, Hall B, Singh R, Lillard JW Jr, Ratajczak MZ (2008) Morphological characterization of very small embryonic-like stem cells (VSELs) by image stream system analysis. J Cell Mol Med 12:292–303
65. Kucia M, Halasa M, Wysoczynski M, Baskiewicz-Masiuk M, Moldenhawer S, Zuba-Surma E, Czajka R, Wojakowski W, Machalinski B, Ratajczak MZ (2006) Morphological and molecular characterization of novel population of CXCR4+SSEA-4+Oct-4+ very small embryonic-like cells purified from human cord blood—preliminary report. Leukemia 21:297–303
66. Paczkowska E, Kucia M, Koziarska D, Halasa M, Safranow K, Masiuk M, Karbicka A, Nowik M, Nowacki P, Ratajczak MZ, Machalinski B (2009) Clinical evidence that very small embryonic-like stem cells are mobilized into peripheral blood in patients after stroke. Stroke 40:1237–1244
67. Zuba-Surma EK, Guo Y, Taher H, Sanganalmath SK, Hunt G, Vincent RJ, Kucia M, Abdel-Latif A, Tang XL, Ratajczak MZ, Dawn B, Bolli R (2011) Transplantation of expanded bone marrow-derived very small embryonic-like stem cells (VSEL-SCs) improves left ventricular function and remodelling after myocardial infarction. J Cell Mol Med 15:1319–1328
68. Ratajczak J, Wysoczynski M, Hayek F, Janowska-Wieczorek A, Ratajczak MZ (2006) Membrane-derived microvesicles: important and underappreciated mediators of cell-to-cell communication. Leukemia 20:1487–1495
69. Valadi H, Ekström K, Bossios A, Sjöstrand M, Lee JJ, Lötvall JO (2007) Exosome-mediated transfer of mRNAs and microRNAs is a novel mechanism of genetic exchange between cells. Nat Cell Biol 9:654–659
70. Pisetsky DS, Gauley J, Ullal AJ (2011) Microparticles as a source of extracellular DNA. Immunol Res 49:227–234
71. Deregibus MC, Cantaluppi V, Calogero R, Lo Iacono M, Tetta C, Biancone L, Bruno S, Bussolati B, Camussi G (2007) Endothelial progenitor cell derived microvesicles activate an angiogenic program in endothelial cells by a horizontal transfer of mRNA. Blood 110:2440–2448
72. Aliotta JM, Pereira M, Johnson KW, de Paz N, Dooner MS, Puente N, Ayala C, Brilliant K, Berz D, Lee D, Ramratnam B, McMillan PN, Hixson DC, Josic D, Quesenberry PJ (2010) Microvesicle entry into marrow cells mediates tissue specific changes in mRNA by direct delivery of mRNA and induction of transcription. Exp Hematol 38:233–245
73. Collino F, Deregibus MC, Bruno S, Sterpone L, Aghemo G, Viltono L, Tetta C, Camussi G (2010) Microvesicles derived from adult human bone marrow and tissue specific mesenchymal stem cells shuttle selected pattern of miRNAs. PLoS One 5:e11803

74. Antonyak MA, Li B, Boroughs LK, Johnson JL, Druso JE, Bryant KL, Holowka DA, Cerione RA (2011) Cancer cell-derived microvesicles induce transformation by transferring tissue transglutaminase and fibronectin to recipient cells. Proc Natl Acad Sci U S A 108:4852–4857
75. Hood JL, Roman SS, Wickline SA (2011) Exosomes released by melanoma cells prepare sentinel lymph nodes for tumour metastasis. Cancer Res 71:3792–3801
76. Grange C, Tapparo M, Collino F, Vitillo L, Damasco C, Deregibus MC, Tetta C, Bussolati B, Camussi G (2011) Microvesicles released from human renal cancer stem cells stimulate angiogenesis and formation of lung premetastatic niche. Cancer Res 71:5346–5356
77. Del Tatto M, Ng T, Aliotta JM, Colvin GA, Dooner MS, Berz D, Dooner GJ, Papa EF, Hixson DC, Ramratnam B, Aswad BI, Sears EH, Reagan J, Quesenberry PJ (2011) Marrow cell genetic phenotype change induced by human lung cancer cells. Exp Hematol 39:1072–1080
78. Maria OM, Tran SD (2011) Human mesenchymal stem cells cultured with salivary gland biopsies adopt an epithelial phenotype. Stem Cells Dev 20:959–967
79. Boulanger CA, Bruno RD, Rosu-Miles M, Smith GH (2012) The mouse mammary microenvironment redirects mesoderm-derived bone marrow cells to a mammary epithelial progenitor cell fate. Stem Cells Dev 21(6):948–954
80. Theise ND, Krause DS (2001) Suggestions for a new paradigm of cell differentiation potential. Blood Cells Mol Dis 27:625–631

Chapter 11
The Systemic Effects of Local Treatments (Surgery and Radiotherapy) of Breast Cancer

Jayant S. Vaidya

Abstract In general, treatment of solid tumours has been compartmentalized as local treatment and systemic treatment. The only systemic oncological effect of local treatment is supposedly eradication of the primary cancer thereby reducing the probability of further systemic spread. However, as will be described here there are instances where local treatment could impact the outcome in diverse ways. We describe how the modulation of surgery by changing its extent or addition of intra-operative radiation appears greatly impact it systemic effects.

Keywords Breast cancer • Lumpectomy • Targeted intraoperative radiotherapy TARGIT IORT • Relapse • Mastectomy • Reconstruction • Non-breast cancer deaths • Mammoplasty • Surgical trauma

11.1 Clinical Observations

11.1.1 Larger Extent of Local Surgery Appears to Paradoxically Worsen Surgical and Cancer Outcomes

In recent years, the development of new surgical techniques and the availability of newer implant materials has meant that there are increasing numbers of immediate breast reconstruction procedures that allow a woman to wake up after her mastectomy with a newly created 'breast'—a proposition that is attractive to many women facing a diagnosis of breast cancer as well as surgeons performing such a mutilating operation as a mastectomy. A Cochrane review [1, 2] attempted to establish whether there is any demonstrable patient benefit (e.g. psychological) from such procedures

J.S. Vaidya, MBBS, MS, DNB, FRCS, PhD (✉)
Professor of Surgery and Oncology, Division of Surgery and Interventional Science, University College London, London, UK

Consultant Surgeon, Whittington Health, Royal Free Hospital and University College London Hospital, London, UK
e-mail: jayantvaidya@gmail.com

M.W. Retsky, R. Demicheli (eds.), *Perioperative Inflammation as Triggering Origin of Metastasis Development*, DOI 10.1007/978-3-319-57943-6_11

but found no clear evidence to support immediate reconstruction over delayed reconstruction [1]. In another study, the psychological distress at 1 year for immediate or delayed reconstruction was found to be similar to each other and to those who did not have any reconstruction [2]. However, the benefit of performing a breast reconstruction after a mastectomy appears to be considered so obvious that, unlike most other breast cancer treatments, no good randomised evidence has been sought before widespread acceptance and adoption of various reconstructive techniques.

However, such a strategy ignores the fact that many of these take much longer to perform and involve extensive dissection of either local tissues or distant tissues (such as the latissimus dorsi flap or the deep inferior epigastric artery perforator flap—DIEP). New evidence is emerging that suggests these extensive surgical procedures at the time of surgical extirpation of cancer may not be oncologically safe. An interesting non-randomized study comes from the University of Ireland and involved 229 patients. These breast cancer patients underwent immediate breast reconstruction between 2004 and 2009 and the authors found that 23% of patients suffered a wound complication. This complication rate is much higher than seen when only a mastectomy without reconstruction is performed, when it, is usually less than 5%.

Many would suggest that this complication rate is unusually high, but in a more recent study (a rare randomised study published in December 2016) a large Scandinavian collaborative group reported in Lancet Oncology, the first randomised trial of immediate vs. delayed reconstruction with implant + acellular dermal matrix [3], a highly commendable effort. This 142-patient trial had to be stopped early because the Data Monitoring Committee felt it was not safe to continue. When immediate reconstruction was performed, there were many more complications (46% of cases) and re-operations (37%), compared with delayed reconstruction (18% and 15%). So, the high complication rate in the Irish study was not unique.

The most worrisome observation in the Irish study was that those patients who had complications had a significantly lower 5-year relapse-free survival (64%) compared with those without complications (89%), a large difference that could not be explained by any patient or tumour factors. The authors suggest that the increased inflammatory response incited by the wound complications may be detrimental to cancer survival [4]. It will be important to assess breast cancer and non-breast cancer survival in the longer term in the Scandinavian randomised trial to determine if any effect of the complications and timing of reconstruction is evident on oncological outcomes, although the small size of the study may limit the ability to detect all but large differences.

A similar picture appears to arise in the delayed reconstruction setting. A case-controlled study [5] performed in a University Hospital in Norway between 1977 and 2007 which compared 312 patients with delayed reconstruction with 1341 matched controls found a remarkable peak hazard of relapse 18 months after reconstruction, similar to that normally observed at a similar time after the primary surgery. The authors also found that, 'the more extensive reconstruction modalities DIEP/TRAM procedures give rise to a higher early peak in comparison with unilateral implant surgery'. Such a dose-response relationship is usually characteristic of a causal link. They concluded that 'reconstructive breast cancer surgery constitutes an independent stimulating event on the growth of micro-metastases leading to accelerated relapse rates.'

These studies raise the real concern that increasing surgical trauma and peri-operative inflammatory response may be triggering the growth of metastatic disease.

11.1.2 Local and Systemic Effects of TARGIT Intraoperative Radiotherapy Given during Lumpectomy for Breast Cancer

The clinical data in the breast reconstruction studies appears to be supported by laboratory findings looking at wound fluids that collect in the cavity left behind after a lumpectomy. These experiments were performed within the context of clinical trials of targeted intraoperative radiotherapy (TARGIT- IORT) for breast cancer.

In one study [6] that included patients receiving TARGIT IORT, fluid collected in the wounds of patients undergoing TARGIT IORT immediately after a lumpectomy for breast cancer was compared with fluid from those having just lumpectomy. The authors found that wound fluid from normal wounds stimulates cancer cell growth, motility and invasiveness. Remarkably, such stimulation is nearly completely abrogated when targeted intraoperative radiotherapy is given during surgery. There is a sea change in the constitution of the wound fluid in those who receive TARGIT IORT compared with those who do not. These results have been since replicated eight years later, by Zaleska et al. [7] with different experimental conditions.

There also seems to be clinical evidence to suggest that this effect seen in the laboratory may translate into clinical outcomes since the wound fluid is normally absorbed into circulation and it has been postulated that it could have systemic beneficial effects [8]. In the TARGIT-A trial [9–13], 3451 patients undergoing lumpectomy for breast cancer were randomly allocated to receive either TARGIT IORT or whole breast external beam radiotherapy. In the analysis of deaths, there was no difference in breast cancer mortality, which was low in both arms of the trial. However, the trialists found a significantly lower non-breast cancer mortality for the TARGIT IORT patients (HR. 0.47; $p = 0.0086$). The most likely explanation might be due to avoidance of whole breast irradiation. It has long been recognised that inadvertent irradiation of the lung, oesophagus and heart during tangential field radiation of the breast leads to fatal cancers and deaths due to ischaemic heart disease. Therefore, targeted radiation would avoid such deaths. This view has been vindicated by a meta-analysis of randomised trials [14] of targeted vs. whole breast external beam radiotherapy (EBRT) which found that in the breast cancer populations where the breast cancer mortality is low (about 5%), the deleterious effect of whole breast radiation is unmasked and leads to an increased overall mortality—thus using targeted radiation rather than whole breast radiation in such patients leads to an improvement in overall survival albeit by a small absolute amount (Figs. 11.1 and 11.2).

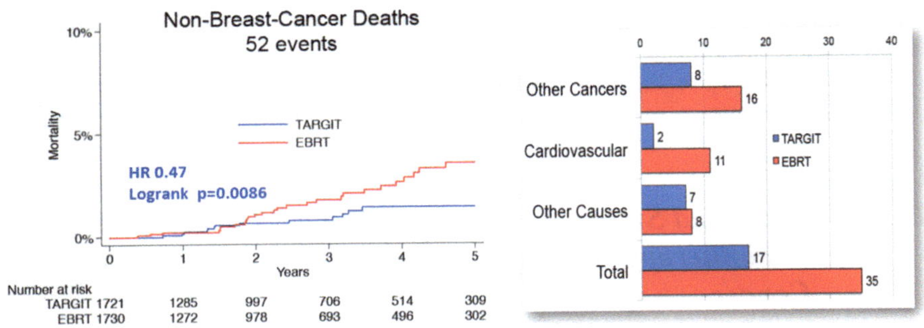

Fig. 11.1 Kaplan-Meier plot for deaths from causes other than breast cancer (17 vs. 35) in the randomised TARGIT-A trial, showing a significantly higher risk of non-breast-cancer mortality with whole breast fractionated radiation given postoperatively over several weeks (EBRT), compared with a risk-adapted single dose radiation delivered to the tumour bed during the lumpectomy operation (TARGIT) [10]

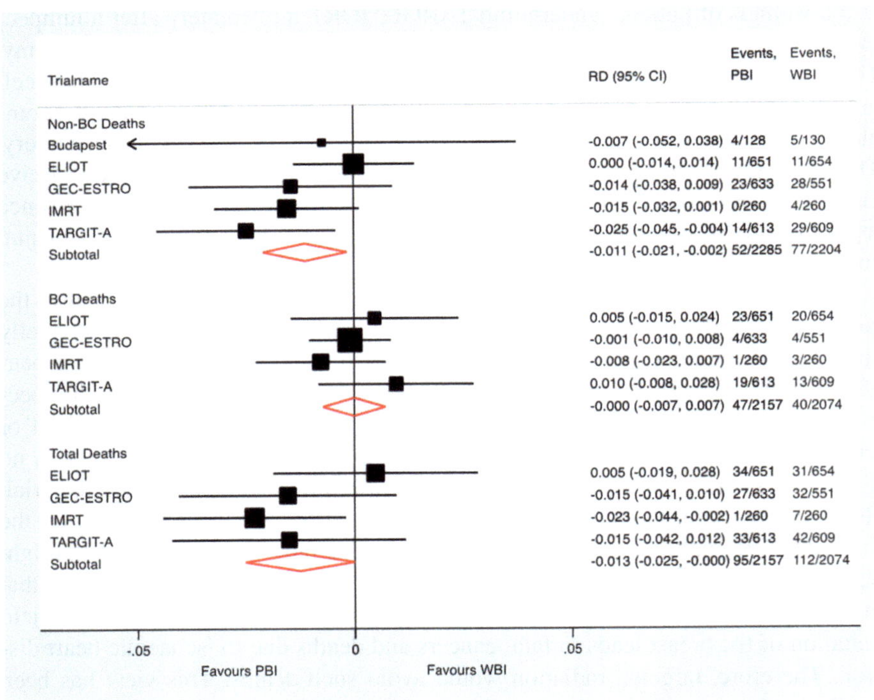

Fig. 11.2 Forest plots representing meta-analysis of difference in mortality between partial-breast irradiation (PBI) and whole-breast irradiation (WBI) with a random-effects model. The trials included for non-breast cancer (Non-BC) mortality were the Budapest trial [5], TARGIT-A [3], ELIOT [6], IMRT [8], and GEC-ESTRO [9]. The median follow-up of all these trials was 5–6 years. Data from only the initial 1222 patients in the TARGIT-A trial, whose median follow-up was 5 years, were included [14]. The Budapest trial was not included in the analysis of breast cancer (BC) deaths or total deaths because these figures were not available

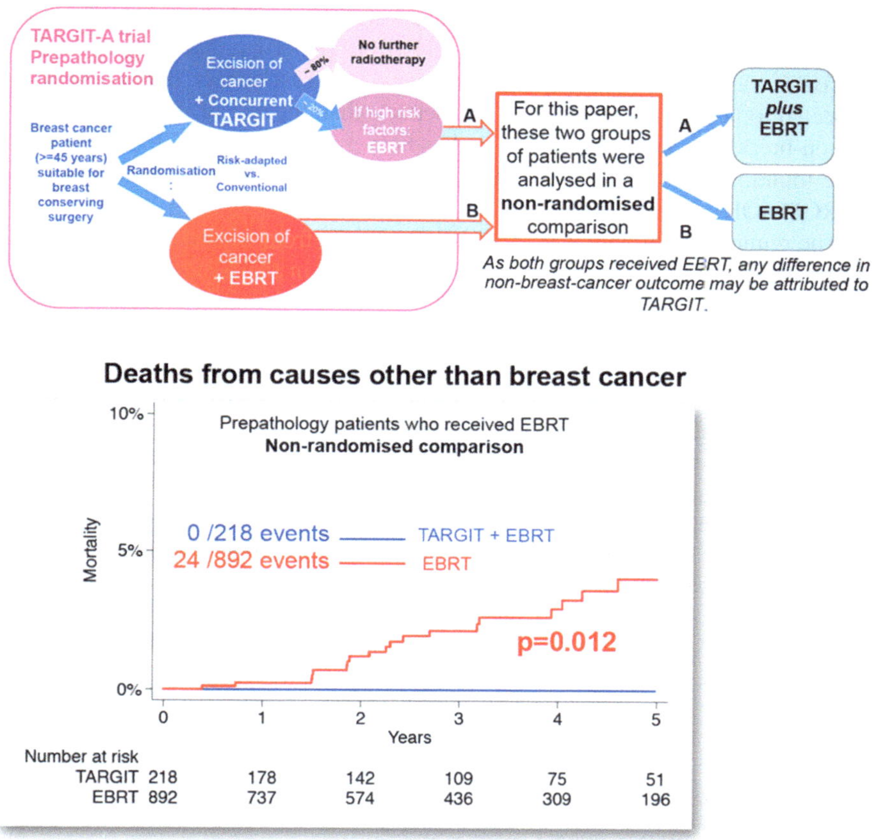

Fig. 11.3 Non-randomised comparison between those who received TARGIT + EBRT and those who received EBRT for deaths from non-breast-cancer causes: (*above*) schema of the analysed cohorts of patients; and (*below*) Kaplan–Meier plot depicting deaths from causes other than breast cancer in prepathology patients who received EBRT—non-randomised comparison [13, 14]

However, there is a twist in the tale. Could the difference in mortality plausibly be due to a *beneficial* effect of TARGIT-IORT, possibly due to its suppression of the cancer-stimulatory effects on the wound fluid? In the TARGIT-A trial, if TARGIT IORT was given concurrently with lumpectomy and if high risk factors were found subsequently, whole breast radiotherapy was added in about 20% of cases—all as specified in the original protocol which followed a risk-adapted design. Therefore, there was a cohort of patients who were randomised to TARGIT IORT and who received both TARGIT IORT and EBRT (Fig. 11.3) as per the protocol.

To try and understand the reason for the difference in non-breast-cancer mortality, a separate analysis [15] was performed: survival from causes other than breast cancer was compared between the two randomized arms but limited to those who had received EBRT. Therefore, the control arm included patients who were allocated EBRT and received EBRT, and the experimental arm included patients who were allocated TARGIT and also received EBRT. The group that received TARGIT + EBRT was characterised by worse prognosis breast cancer but would not be expected to be different—certainly not better—than the rest of the cohort in terms of non-breast cancer co-morbidity, and as both groups received EBRT, any difference found in non-breast-cancer mortality could be attributable to the delivery of TARGIT IORT during lumpectomy.

The remarkable finding was that were no deaths from non-breast cancer causes in the TARGIT + EBRT group compared with 24 in the EBRT group 0/218 vs. 24/892, log-rank $p = 0.012$. Although the numbers are small and the compared groups are not the full randomised cohorts, these data suggest that EBRT toxicity may not be the only reason for the fewer non-breast cancer deaths with TARGIT IORT, and leads to the hypothesis that the local effect of TARGIT on the tumor bed by inhibiting the cancer-stimulating cytokines, may spill over to reduce systemic inflammatory response to trauma and have significant long-term systemic beneficial effects, that might be protective against cardiac and cancer mortality [8].

A more recent case control (non-randomised) study, also found that amongst patients having oncoplastic breast conserving surgery after neo-adjuvant chemotherapy, those who had an intraoperative TARGIT Boost, experienced better survival outcomes than those who received a postoperative EBRT boost (overall survival 96.7% vs. 81.7%, hazard ratio 0.19, log rank $p = 0.016$, and distant-disease free survival 95.1% vs. 69.0, HR 0.23, log rank $p = 0.012$) [16].

11.1.3 Causality

The scientific principle for establishing causality is firstly to show that the factor is present when the effect is seen, secondly to show that increasing amounts of factor increases the effect and finally, removal or abrogation of the activity of the factor reduces the effect. Thus, biologically, it appears that increasing surgical trauma is detrimental to outcome after local treatment of cancer and, if the systemic effects of such trauma are reduced, they may be improved. There have been some data that administration of non-steroidal anti-inflammatory drugs in the peri-operative period reduces mortality from solid tumours [17, 18]. A randomised trial is underway in Belgium to test this hypothesis.

11.1.4 Clinical Implications

The obvious benefit of waking up after a mastectomy with a new breast rather than a flat chest needs to be weighed against the need for a larger operation with the higher risk of complications, longer convalescence, delay in chemo/radiotherapy, with its well known detrimental effects, and the need for several further operations.

From the patient's perspective, a decision about having immediate reconstruction is usually confounded by the significant shock of a new diagnosis of breast cancer and the prospect of removal of the whole breast. A nudge in the direction of "reconstruction is the norm" may be enough to sway someone whose main concern is surviving from the cancer to get convinced that she needs to have it at the time of the mastectomy. The availability of reconstruction can appear to make the prospect of a mastectomy acceptable, even when it is not indicated for oncological purposes. Before all these remarkable data were available and notwithstanding the lack of benefit seen in the Cochrane overview and other studies, it seemed appropriate to offer breast reconstruction as a reasonable option (from both the clinician and patient perspectives) during discussions about mastectomy. Such discussions would centre around patient preferences only, as there was not much evidence either for or against until now.

The same arguments also lead to concerns about the rising trend of using mammoplasty during breast conservation as well as cosmetic operations on the contralateral breast as part of treatment of breast cancer. To us surgeons, the justification for these procedures is 'obvious'—a 'better' cosmetic outcome. Unfortunately, there is a well-recognised lack of good evidence to support the use of major oncoplastic procedures aimed at a better cosmetic result, either for oncological safety or even an improved patient satisfaction about cosmetic outcome [19]. Firstly, potential harms may arise from the additional burden about decisions about a bigger operation, yet another operation, longer recovery, reduced or loss of nipple sensation, psychological distress of decision about the other breast, as well as from the possible oncologic risks of increased surgical trauma and accompanying increased chance of surgical complications. Arguably, if the patient had been keen to have a cosmetic operation, she could have well considered it before the cancer diagnosis. The oncological safety of these more extensive procedures [6] has not been established in randomised clinical trials. One large series from a pioneer in the techniques reports a 5-year recurrence rate of 9.4% [20] which is several times higher than expected, although the authors suggest that the larger size of cancers or extensive DCIS may contribute to the higher recurrence rate. Another study found that use of implants is associated with poorer survival from subsequent breast cancer [21]. A recent study of lipofilling [22] found a high recurrence rate of 1.5% per year (i.e. 7.5% at 5 years). An accompanying editorial from Memorial Sloane Kettering Cancer Centre [23] has warned about the lack of oncological safety and recommended that lipofilling should not be performed outside a clinical trial. Most importantly, patient satisfaction appears to be similar with simple lumpectomy vs. therapeutic mammoplasty [24].

Postoperative radiation may affect the heart in many ways—the coronary arteries causing ischaemia, the muscle causing cardiomyopathy or even the nerves (neuropathy) and the conducting system of the heart, although we cannot find any previous mention of the latter in the literature. One speculation is to consider that post-surgical or post-radiotherapy cardiac neuropathy may be another possible mechanism to explain cardiac mortality as a result of breast cancer therapy. As suggested by Michael Retsky, we are aware that surgery can result in transient systemic inflammation and post surgical peripheral neuropathy has been associated with inflammation [18, 25]. As a possible connection among these effects, immediate irradiation of the surgical wound may contribute to a reduction in inflammation thereby reducing cardiac damage.

Given the new randomised evidence demonstrating a higher risk of complications, as well as evidence suggesting a real possibility of an oncologically detrimental effect of excessive trauma, the most prudent clinical approach is to ensure that patients are fully informed of the evidence that raises a doubt about the oncological safety of therapeutic mammoplasty procedures and breast reconstruction, along with a lack of benefit in terms of patient's satisfaction or psychological parameters.

A material change in relationship between a doctor and a patient has occurred with the publication of the United Kingdom ruling of the Montgomery vs. Lancashire case in early 2015. It is important to recognise that although this is law only in the UK, it could have far reaching implications around the world. The ruling sets a precedent over the process of obtaining informed consent and the need to discuss all options of treatment that the patient may consider reasonable. This is now a legal responsibility rather than just a moral duty and the final decision over the correct application rest with the Courts and not with the medical profession or with patient advocacy groups. Breast surgeons and staff must move away from a single 'recommendation' but offer a list of evidence-based options for patients to consider, along with their risks and benefits. This has wide ranging implications in surgery, particularly in the practice of oncoplastic breast surgery, largely because of near-complete lack of level-I evidence across the field. This is one area where emerging new evidence may require a medical reversal [26].

11.2 Conclusion

Oncoplastic and breast reconstructive surgery takes time to deliver, is expensive to the health system, and lacks empirical proof of benefit to patients. This type of surgery is an anomaly amongst other breast cancer treatments that normally have been tested in randomised clinical trials. Given the recent evidence, in the least, immediate reconstruction, therapeutic mammoplasty, or contralateral 'symmetrisation procedures' can no longer be put forward to patients as a 'standard' treatment but as an option discussed along with the above evidence and concerns about their oncologic safety. The access to and the proportion of patients undergoing immediate (or delayed) breast reconstruction or oncoplastic surgery, should not be used as a measure of quality of a breast service, when there are legitimate doubts about the safety of such procedures. It is now an ethical imperative that these procedures should be subjected to testing in well-designed randomised clinical trials. Such trials may be difficult to set up and perform, but randomisation has always been difficult in surgical trials. In this case, such difficulty could be overcome by an honest appreciation of the current lack of knowledge about oncological impact, or the lack of definite evidence of patient benefit from reconstructive/oncoplastic procedures. Achieving an equipoise is the important first step in that direction.

Most importantly, the popular use of more extensive local surgery appears to have given us an insight into the natural history of cancer—when surgical trauma exceeds its therapeutic value it may be detrimental to outcome—a phenomenon that may open up peri-operative strategies that could be designed to improve outcomes from cancer.

References

1. D'Souza N, Darmanin G, Fedorowicz Z (2011) Immediate versus delayed reconstruction following surgery for breast cancer. Cochrane Database Syst Rev 7:CD008674
2. Metcalfe KA, Semple J, Quan ML et al (2012) Changes in psychosocial functioning 1 year after mastectomy alone, delayed breast reconstruction, or immediate breast reconstruction. Ann Surg Oncol 19(1):233–241
3. Dikmans RE, Negenborn VL, Bouman MB et al (2017) Two-stage implant-based breast reconstruction compared with immediate one-stage implant-based breast reconstruction augmented with an acellular dermal matrix: an open-label, phase 4, multicentre, randomised, controlled trial. Lancet Oncol 18:251–258
4. Beecher SM, O'Leary DP, McLaughlin R, Sweeney KJ, Kerin MJ (2016) Influence of complications following immediate breast reconstruction on breast cancer recurrence rates. Br J Surg 103(4):391–398
5. Dillekas H, Demicheli R, Ardoino I, Jensen SA, Biganzoli E, Straume O (2016) The recurrence pattern following delayed breast reconstruction after mastectomy for breast cancer suggests a systemic effect of surgery on occult dormant micrometastases. Breast Cancer Res Treat 158(1):169–178
6. Belletti B, Vaidya JS, D'Andrea S et al (2008) Targeted intraoperative radiotherapy impairs the stimulation of breast cancer cell proliferation and invasion caused by surgical wounding. Clin Cancer Res 14(5):1325–1332
7. Zaleska K, Suchorska WM, Przybyla A, Murawa D (2016) Effect of surgical wound fluids after intraoperative electron radiotherapy on the cancer stem cell phenotype in a panel of human breast cancer cell lines. Oncol Lett 12(5):3707–3714
8. Vaidya JS, Bulsara M, Wenz F (2013) Ischemic heart disease after breast cancer radiotherapy. N Engl J Med 368(26):2526–2527
9. Vaidya JS, Bulsara M, Wenz F et al (2015) Pride, prejudice, or science – attitudes towards the results of the TARGIT-A trial of targeted intraoperative radiotherapy for breast cancer. Int J Radiat Oncol Biol Phys 92(3):494–500
10. Vaidya JS, Wenz F, Bulsara M et al (2014) Risk-adapted targeted intraoperative radiotherapy versus whole-breast radiotherapy for breast cancer: 5-year results for local control and overall survival from the TARGIT-A randomised trial. Lancet 383(9917):603–613
11. Vaidya JS, Wenz F, Bulsara M, Tobias JS, Joseph D, Baum M (2014) Radiotherapy for breast cancer, the TARGIT-A trial – authors' reply. Lancet 383(9930):1719–1720
12. Vaidya JS, Joseph DJ, Tobias JS et al (2010) Targeted intraoperative radiotherapy versus whole breast radiotherapy for breast cancer (TARGIT-A trial): an international, prospective, randomised, non-inferiority phase 3 trial. Lancet 376(9735):91–102
13. Vaidya JS, Wenz F, Bulsara M et al (2016) An international randomised controlled trial to compare targeted intra-operative radiotherapy (TARGIT) with conventional post-operative radiotherapy after conservative breast surgery for women with early stage breast cancer (the TARGIT-A trial). Health Technol Assess 20(73):1–188
14. Vaidya JS, Bulsara M, Wenz F et al (2016) Reduced mortality with partial-breast irradiation for early breast cancer: a meta-analysis of randomized trials. Int J Radiat Oncol Biol Phys 96(2):259–265

15. Vaidya JS, Bulsara M, Wenz F et al (2013) The lower non-breast cancer mortality with TARGIT in the TARGIT-A trial could be a systemic effect of TARGIT on tumor microenvironment. Int J Radiat Oncol Biol Phys 87(2):S240
16. Kolberg HC, Loevey G, Akpolat-Basci L et al (2017) Targeted intraoperative radiotherapy tumour bed boost during breast-conserving surgery after neoadjuvant chemotherapy. Strahlenther Onkol 193(1):62–69
17. Forget P, Coulie PG, Retsky M, Demicheli R, Machiels JP, De Kock M (2013) Is there a rationale for an anesthesiologist's role against cancer recurrence? Acta Anaesthesiol Belg 64(1):15–24. Review. PubMed PMID: 23767173
18. Retsky MW, Demicheli R, Hrushesky WJM, Forget P, DeKock M, Gukas I, Rogers RA, Baum M, Sukhatme V, Vaidya JS (2013) Reduction of breast cancer relapses with perioperative non-steroidal anti-inflammatory drugs: new findings and a review. Curr Med Chem 20:4163–4176
19. Haloua MH, Krekel NM, Winters HA et al (2013) A systematic review of oncoplastic breast-conserving surgery: current weaknesses and future prospects. Ann Surg 257(4):609–620
20. Clough KB, Lewis JS, Couturaud B, Fitoussi A, Nos C, Falcou M (2003) Oncoplastic techniques allow extensive resections for breast-conserving therapy of breast carcinomas. Ann Surg 237(1):26–34
21. Lavigne E, Holowaty EJ, Pan SY et al (2013) Breast cancer detection and survival among women with cosmetic breast implants: systematic review and meta-analysis of observational studies. BMJ 346:f2399
22. Petit JY, Lohsiriwat V, Clough KB et al (2011) The oncologic outcome and immediate surgical complications of lipofilling in breast cancer patients: a multicenter study—Milan-Paris-Lyon experience of 646 lipofilling procedures. Plast Reconstr Surg 128(2):341–346
23. Cordeiro PG (2011) Discussion: the oncologic outcome and immediate surgical complications of lipofilling in breast cancer patients: a multicenter study—Milan-Paris-Lyon experience of 646 lipofilling procedures. Plast Reconstr Surg 128(2):347–348
24. Eichler C, Kolsch M, Sauerwald A, Bach A, Gluz O, Warm M (2013) Lumpectomy versus mastopexy—a post-surgery patient survey. Anticancer Res 33(2):731–736
25. Staff NP, Engelstad J, Klein CJ, Amrami KK, Spinner RJ, Dyck PJ, Warner MA, Warner ME, Dyck PJ (2010) Post-surgical inflammatory neuropathy. Brain 133(10):2866–2880
26. Cifu AS, Prasad VK (2015) Ending medical reversals. Johns Hopkins University Press, Baltimore

MIX
Papier aus verantwortungsvollen Quellen
Paper from responsible sources
FSC® C105338

If you have any concerns about our products,
you can contact us on
ProductSafety@springernature.com

In case Publisher is established outside the EU,
the EU authorized representative is:
Springer Nature Customer Service Center GmbH
Europaplatz 3, 69115 Heidelberg, Germany

Printed by Libri Plureos GmbH
in Hamburg, Germany